To
Billy

DEVELOPMENTAL POTENTIAL
OF PRESCHOOL CHILDREN

An Evaluation of Intellectual,
Sensory and Emotional Functioning

by

ELSE HAEUSSERMANN

Educational Consultant, Division of Pediatric Psychiatry,
Jewish Hospital, Brooklyn, New York.

With a Foreword by Joseph Wortis, M.D., and an
Introduction by Herbert G. Birch, Ph.D.

GRUNE & STRATTON, INC., 1958

New York   ♦   London

First printing June 1958
Second printing April 1965
Third printing February 1968
Fourth printing January 1971

GRUNE & STRATTON, INC.
757 Third Avenue, New York, New York 10017

Library of Congress Catalog Card Number 57-11741
International Standard Book Number 0-8089-0166-4

Printed in the United States of America (E-B)

Contents

JUL - 7 1976

Foreword

Not so many years ago when I was asked to start a clinical service for retarded children, I had little first hand experience to build upon. Retarded children, I assumed, had varying degrees and kinds of cerebral defects or suffered from some kind of innate stupidity called familial or idiopathic mental deficiency. One of the first puzzles I was called upon to solve was the differential diagnosis between psychosis and retardation, since a number of the children were not only intellectually slow but acted peculiarly too. It took time to learn that the puzzle was often insoluble, because some children had signs of both retardation and disorganization. The children usually came to us with some I.Q. score attached to them after one or another psychometric test (sometimes with an assortment of scores), but if they lacked an I.Q. rating, we quickly supplied one. The widely held assumption was that, given reasonable and ordinary opportunities to pick up information or acquire skills, and then tested with a fair sampling of skills and information, the child's innate capabilities could be measured on a graduated performance scale, in which the average child became the norm.

These assumptions proved to be enormously convenient, because all a pediatrician, psychiatrist or teacher had to do to discover a child's innate capacities was to call the psychologist in to administer a psychometric test. We soon learned that the I.Q. score was being widely regarded as a jargon label for that subtle evanescent thing called intelligence, with the textbooks explaining which I.Q.'s allowed us to call a child an imbecile or idiot. If a child did poorly in school and was discovered to have a low I.Q., it all seemed very simple: the child was being taxed beyond his capacity. If the child couldn't handle the curriculum, the thing to do was to fit the curriculum to the child; and he would be shifted to a low I.Q. or retarded children's class. It would be terribly inconvenient to consider that a low I.Q. might be a *result* of inadequate or improper training, or that many subtle variables, not necessarily the thing called intelligence, might influence a child's performance: sensory intactness, motor coordination, perceptual organization, interest or apathy, energy or fatigue, quickness or slowness, amount of social exposure, familiarity with or ignorance of the test materials or tasks.

Yet the more experience we acquired, the more convinced we became that one could no more understand or encompass a child's mental deficiency with an intelligence quotient than one could evaluate a medical disability by discovering how far the subject could walk. There was no substitute for patient study and observation, sympathetic periods of working together, the posing of ingenious tasks that would inspire the child's reaction and evoke a meaningful performance, and the pooling of information from several different points of view. Yet the clinical frame of reference demanded relatively brief periods of evaluation and the rehabilitation process waited upon some suitable estimate and analysis of the problem.

It was in this setting that the basic value of Else Haeussermann's approach and methods became apparent. For what she did was to ingeniously, sympathetically and persistently explore the child's full equipment and capacities, in a relatively structured series of examinations, formal enough to permit meaningful comparison, but varied enough to tap or plumb each child's open or hidden resources. Avoiding the pressures and temptations to come up with scores, Miss Haeussermann concluded each examination with a *description* and *interpretation* of the child's capacities and performance that provided a solid basis for the rehabilitation process. All of us learned to lean heavily on her perceptive descriptions, and her contributions to staff conferences became indispensable. This description of her methods will certainly provide an invaluable resource for all those engaged in similar work.

A full lifetime of dedicated application to her chosen work, a scholarly interest motivated by her wish to understand and to help—these are not easy to duplicate or emulate; but what shines through this description of her work is a method and style that deserves to be widely imitated. I feel quite confident that this book will represent a solid contribution to the small but growing scientific literature on mental deficiency and cerebral defect.

Joseph Wortis, M.D.
Director, Division of Pediatric Psychiatry,
Jewish Hospital of Brooklyn,
and of the Solomon Clinic
for Retarded Children

Introduction

The use of a method for intellectual evaluation as an instrument that has positive value for the promotion of training and education is an essential feature of rehabilitation. In this area of work one is far less concerned with predicting whether a given child will achieve success in competition with a group of age-mates drawn from the general population, than with the problem of determining the kinds of training and experience that will best promote his own adaptive functional abilities. From this point of view one becomes concerned with the laws of perceptual-motor functioning in a certain seven year old child rather than with the question of whether or not he can copy a geometric figure from a model as well as can other children of the same age. In short, the objective of the examination is to provide information about the positive qualities of a child's functioning; the difficulties he faces in mastering problems when they are presented in the standard manner; and, information about the special circumstances which are needed to create appropriate conditions for learning in the handicapped child. Such an approach, as Miss Haeussermann so aptly puts it, shifts "the burden of proof . . . from the child who is being examined, to the items which test the level of his comprehension."

Obviously this point of view displaces the burden not only from the child to the test item, but from the test item to the examiner. It becomes the responsibility of the examiner to interrelate various forms in which a demand is presented in order to obtain a clearer view of the qualities of functioning of the child as well as of the inadequacies which are revealed in a failure to respond appropriately to a given demand. Such information then becomes a realistic basis upon which special training and educational procedures may be developed.

When a demand of this type is made on the mental examination, it soon becomes clear that although the standard tests of intelligence do provide one with some valuable information, they are inadequate for the purpose. This does not mean that they are poor tests, but rather that they were never designed to answer the questions that arise in a rehabilitation setting. It is of value to explore some of the sources for the differences that exist between the information provided by standard tests of intellectual functioning and the requirements of a rehabilitation attitude.

All standard examinations of intellectual functioning have at least two main objectives. On the one hand they attempt to estimate the degree to which an individual's performances on a set of standardized tasks exhibits the extent to which he has profited from a set of social experiences which are presumed to be generally available. On the other hand a prediction, based upon this test performance, is made as to the probable effectiveness of a subsequent, future set of exposures to environmental influences. Thus their adequacy as assessors of current functioning, and as predicters of future functioning under standard conditions of training are the essential criteria by which the real worth of standard instruments designed for the study of intellectual ability must be judged.

It is clear that the validity of an instrument is dependent upon several factors each of which may exist quite independently of the others. Four of these are especially significant in their influences and deserve some rescrutiny. In the first place the performances which are sampled by a test must be relevant to, i.e., dependent upon, the abilities and capacities which are being estimated. Therefore, tests of reaction time, or of muscular strength and endurance are not items which permit one to obtain a meaning-ful estimate of learning ability. While these tasks may tap other functions, they do not provide the kind of information which is directly relevant to learning ability. Consequently, mental tests are constructed so as to sample performances which are acquired by the individual in the course of his life history and lay especial emphasis upon such phenomena as language acquisition, perceptual and perceptual-motor skills, memory, amount and arithmetic concepts, verbal comprehension, and social judgment. Items measuring these abilities are selected not because they provide a consecutive account of the development of a function, but rather because certain selected levels of demand serve to divide a population into adequate, superior, or inferior performers. Thus in standard tests amount concepts are often measured by means of uniform cubes and the individual is either able or unable to indicate that 4, 5, 7 or 9 cubes have been presented. However, the possibility that the individual who is unable to count 4 cubes correctly is able to count 4 cookies, or 4 bottles is left unexplored. Similar gaps exist for perceptual, verbal, social and all other areas of inquiry.

These gaps are not accidental, but stem from the general philosophy of intelligence test construction. This philosophy can be designated as a theory of invidious comparison. Its object is the determination of the relative performance status of an individual in comparison with a standard popula-tion and not the analysis of any single person's unique organization of functioning. To achieve their objective only episodic data on a wide range of functions are necessary.

A second attitude, basic to the construction of standard intelligence tests, adds still further to the difficulties which attend their use in a rehabili-tation setting. The adequacy of performances as a basis for inferring capacity or ability is necessarily dependent upon the assumption that the experiences necessary to acquire the adequate performances are accessible to the population studied. If such experience is unequally available or if the form in which an environmental event occurs makes it unavailable to the individual, normal development of a function does not occur and the individual's capacities cannot be adequately assessed through a comparison with a standard normal population. In children with sensory deficits, inter-sensory peculiarities, motor deficits, and adventitious motor expressions such alterations of experienced environment occur both as a direct consequence of physiologic peculiarities and as a reactive consequence to limited physical and social environment. Perceptual eccentricities, or bizarreness of social judgment may therefore derive from learned distortions of experience rather than from an inability to learn.

A third feature of standard intelligence tests is their administration. It must be remembered that a standardized test loses its "standard" quality unless it is administered according to an explicitly stated method. If the method of administration is altered the test can no longer be validly used as a normative instrument. It then becomes an inventory of items of performance which can no longer be related to the performances of the standardizing population. Further, if the materials of the test are altered, enlarged, mounted, or presented in non-standard ways the virtues of standardization are lost and reference to general population performance levels become unjustifiable. Both these changes have been introduced in the mental examination of children with modifications of sensory, motor, or neurological organization. Consequently only the episodic limitations of the test items have been retained and the virtues of comparison to a standard population lost.

A final feature of standard tests of intellectual functioning resides in their unity. Items cannot be eliminated without affecting the validity of the total score obtained. Further, a substitution of one scoring standard for another (e.g., using multiple-choice procedures rather than verbal statements in a child lacking speech) changes the level of demand and vitiates the comparative value of the instrument.

At various times workers in the fields of retardation and of rehabilitation have attempted to repair the inadequacies, for their special areas of interest, of the standard tests of intelligence. In the main these efforts have consisted of the piecemeal alteration of existing instruments. Materials have been magnified and made more easily manipulable; scoring standards have been altered to permit of non-verbal responses to verbal items; scores have been pro-rated to include items that could not be administered; and additional materials have been added to modify some aspects of the episodic character of the usual instruments. In a very few instances new instruments have been created to provide us with a fuller picture of the perceptual functioning of the persons studied. However, until the present effort, no full-scale attempt to solve the totality of problems inherent in the positive intellectual evaluation of handicapped children has been forthcoming. Such an attempt had to be based upon a view of the mental examination which assumed a new body of responsibility—a therapeutic educational responsibility—and so involves a fundamental shift in attitude. It is this transformation of attitude from an estimation of relative status to an analysis and inventory of educational and training assets which is embodied in this book.

Else Haeussermann has produced more than a new and highly valuable test in this volume. She has made available to a broad audience a method, a style of work with handicapped children that until now only those of us who have had the privilege of working closely with her have been able to share. It is a style that has evolved slowly in the course of a quarter-century of experience in observing, caring for, teaching, and evaluating children with neurological handicaps. The central feature of her method of work is its pertinence. The child and his problems are her central concern and theories and conceptualizations are used not for themselves, but as instruments for understanding children and helping them to achieve an optimal development. Her test developed over the years as an ever more valuable tool in helping her to accomplish these ends.

As an instrument for the evaluation of intellectual functioning (or more correctly, adaptive capacity) Miss Haeussermann's test is a clinical procedure rather than a psychometric device. In its development her concern was not directed toward the organization of an age-scale of the Binet type, but rather toward defining a procedure which would permit of the longitudinal exploration of psychological functions. Consequently, her method is one which proceeds from above downward, from higher levels of adaptive organization to lower ones, from abstract relations to concrete events. Failure to succeed at a given level does not terminate inquiry, but serves, instead, as a provocation for a deeper probing, for an exploration of the possible causes of the failure in the sensory, motivational, experiential, perceptual or other aspects of the child's psychological organization. The greatest single contribution of the test lies in its presentation of a formulated and standardized procedure which makes such exploration possible. Thus, the results of the evaluation provide one with a profile of the functional abilities and probable developmental potential of the child. These profiles admirably reflect the unevennesses in functioning that are so characteristic of children who are handicapped by central nervous system damage and provide a sound basis for the elaboration of a relevant custom-made educational and training plan.

If this represented the only contribution made by the present volume it would be sufficient to guarantee its worth. However, it also embodies a wealth of clinical experience gained in years of work with neurologically damaged children. The problems of motivating such children, of managing hyperactivity, of controlling distractibility, and even of compiling an accurate developmental history are incorporated into the evaluation procedure. Further, the author directs our gaze toward subtleties of performance which often alone make possible the differentiation of autism and psychosis in children from retardation. What was begun as the report of a new test has emerged as the best available textbook for the clinical evaluation of behavioral functions in the brain-damaged or retarded child.

HERBERT G. BIRCH, PH.D.

Research Associate, Department of Physical Medicine and Rehabilitation, New York University-Bellevue Medical Center; Associate Professor of Clinical Psychology, New York Medical College, Bird S. Coler Hospital

Preface

This manual is written for those psychologists, teachers and therapists, who are concerned with the problem of evaluating the young handicapped child. Some aspects of child behavior which are discussed in the text may be of interest also to pediatricians, orthopedists, neurologists, psychiatrists and speech pathologists in the fields of rehabilitation, child guidance and child study.

The book offers a common sense approach to the educational evaluation of children between two and six years of age, or functioning on that level, who have handicaps in expression and other difficulties.

The experienced psychologist will find here an approach, which makes it possible to demonstrate the individual potential of young children rather than simply to measure their standing within the norm. Such an approach is more desirable in the evaluation of handicapped children when their ability to express themselves by speech or manipulation is interferred with by various factors. Where some areas of functioning may be selectively impaired, individual exploration may be the only means to demonstrate the quality and the extent of preserved and existing potential.

The method presented is the result of experimental exploration rather than of statistical compilation. It does not limit itself to a formula for testing but consists rather of a structured interview, with additional suggestions concerning modification of items methodically, when the clinical evaluation calls for an exploration or for an explanation of deviations or deficits in functioning. Beyond this, approaches are described which may serve to motivate and persuade children, who are inaccessible in a more formal testing situation, to reveal the level and the quality of their comprehension.

The arrangement of the book in four parts should make the use of the educational evaluation a well understood and well learned procedure. The earlier part of the manual is deliberately designed as a training opportunity which will serve to prepare the serious reader to apply the directions given in the later parts.

The first part explains what an educational evaluation is and why it is needed. The second part describes the children for whom the educational evaluation is intended, who should evaluate them, how the structured interview originated and of what it consists.

The third part gives directions concerning the conduct of the interview, describes the items and their presentation and the modifications recommended for given contingencies. The fourth and final part explains how to record the interview, interpret the findings and report the results.

The material for this volume has accumulated over a quarter of a century in the daily work with children handicapped by cerebral palsy. In order to provide effective methods of training and teaching it was found necessary to make an inventory of the level reached by each child in pertinent areas of functioning. Rather than study a given function in the abstract, I tried to find approaches which made it possible to elicit reactions and responses within the physical and intellectual capacity of children presenting a variety of handicaps in expression. The observation and interpretation of the demonstrated level and nature of each elicited response gave clues to the pattern of functioning reached by a child. On the basis of the present functioning demonstrated in this manner the educational and training program could then be planned. In the course of time, the approaches and the materials used to elicit responses from severely involved children with cerebral palsy proved to have value and usefulness beyond the particular set-up in which they were being used.

A three year grant from United Cerebral Palsy Association of New York City made it possible to explore the usefulness of the evaluation method with a widely diversified population of handicapped children at the Division of Pediatric Psychiatry at Jewish Hospital Brooklyn. The findings could be compared and validated in this setting, since each child was examined with standardized tests during a two week period coinciding with, preceding or following the date of his educational evaluation. During the third year of the grant the book was begun. It was completed during a fourth year.

Sincere appreciation is due to Dr. William Cooper, a pioneer in the field of cerebral palsy, who recognized early the value of the educational evaluation and made it possible for me to use and enlarge upon it, not only in the Cerebral Palsy Classes at Public School 135 Manhattan, but also during two summer vacations at the Cerebral Palsy Clinic, Hospital for Special Surgery, New York. Encouragement, stimulation and criticism continued to be given by chiefs and colleagues such as Mrs. Sarah Jane Kinoy, who founded the Cerebral Palsy Class at the Lower East Side Health Center, New York in 1946, Dr. Stanley Zipser, Dr. Joost Meerloo, Mrs. Thea Klein, Principal, Public School 135 Manhattan, Dr. Bernath, Dr. Harnett, Mrs. Rosenson of the Board of Education of the City of New York and Dr. Samuel Wishik, then of the Department of Health, New York City.

Recognition given to my efforts through the long years of experimentation provided constant impetus to proceed, especially since recognition came from such persons and offices as the late Dr. William Featherstone, Teachers College, Columbia University, New York, Dr. Maurice Fouracre, present head of the Department of Special Education of Teachers College, Dr. Joseph L. Stone, Vassar College and the New School for Social Research, New

York, Dr. Heinz Werner, Worcester, Mass., Dr. Kaethe Wolff, Dr. Jay Brightman, then of the State Department of Health, Albany, Dr. Joseph Endress and Dr. Joseph Fenton of the State Department of Education, Albany.

In addition, I owe thanks to Dr. Glidden Brooks and Dr. Arthur Hill, United Cerebral Palsy, to Mr. and Mrs. Arthur Larschan, founders of U.C.P.A. for their loyal and unfailing support, and to Dr. Earl R. Carlson and Dr. Theo Bretcher for their confidence and encouragement during 1942.

Without the grant provided by United Cerebral Palsy Association of New York City the book would not have been possible. The foresight and confidence of that organization is sincerely appreciated. Without the constant prodding, prompting, urging, and the equally constant inspiring, reassuring and confirming by Dr. Joseph Wortis, Director of the Division of Pediatric Psychiatry, Jewish Hospital Brooklyn, and Dr. Herbert Birch, then Chief Psychologist of that division, the writing of the book could not have been executed at this time. I would still be experimenting and collecting material. I am indebted to them also for their helpfulness in reading the manuscript and offering constructive criticism. The team at the division has served as sounding board as well as fellow explorers during the writing of the book and the immediacy of their own experience with the material and their resulting comments frequently have helped to point the way to explanations which were formulated or emphasized. Thanks are due to Dr. Sue Browder, Dr. Arthur Meisel, Dr. Ed. Gordon, Mrs. Lillie Pope and Dr. Jay Rosenblatt of the Morris J. Solomon Clinic, Division of Pediatric Psychiatry, Jewish Hospital, Brooklyn.

I owe the inspiration of this book to hundreds of children, who through the years have helped me to experiment with ways to obtain their responses. Many have taken and maintained a lively interest in my effort and in the meaning it may have for others like them.

Finally I owe thanks to the patience of my family and friends for permitting me the solitude required to write a book.

ELSE HAEUSSERMANN

New York
March, 1958.

Illustrations

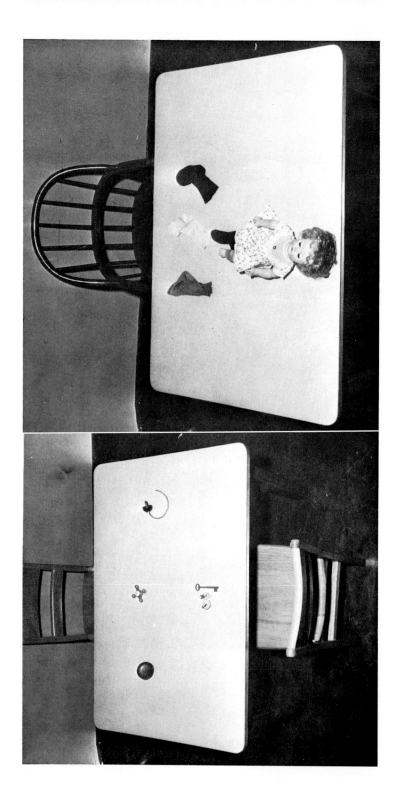

PHYSICAL SET-UP FOR THE INTERVIEW

Fig. 1 (*upper left*). Regular small chair and table. Set-up on child's level for child and examiner. Showing item 32.

Fig. 2 (*upper right*). Arm chair and table. Set-up with slight protection or mild restraint. Showing item 12, in modified form.

Fig. 3 (*lower left*). Relaxation chair with doll representing child. Set-up for physically handicapped child. Showing items 1 and 2.

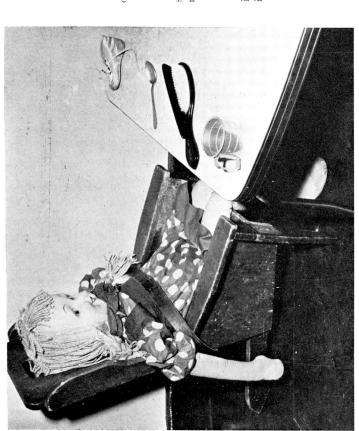

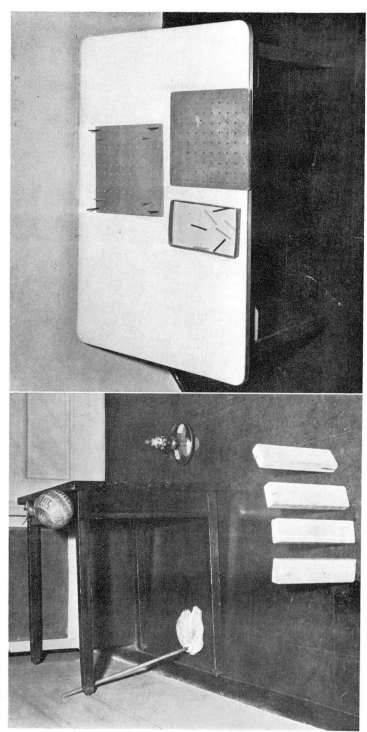

PLATE 1, *Continued*

Fig. 4A. Improvised playpen. Set-up for special needs: playpen arrangement includes some tempting toys.

Fig. 4B. Table facing bare wall. Set-up suitable for distractible child. Showing peg board, one of the materials for modifications.

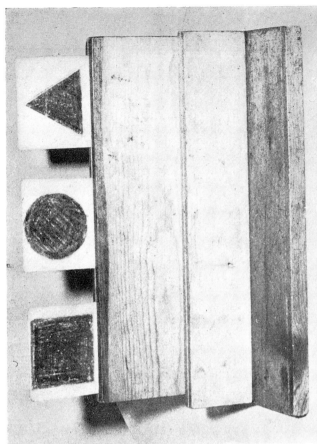

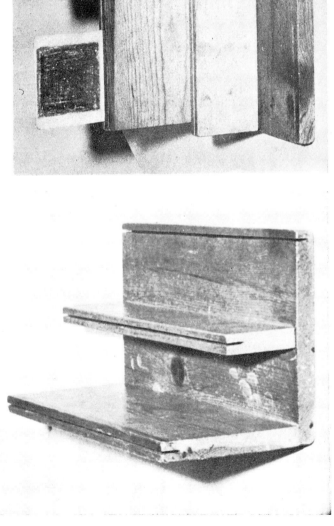

PLATE II. ADAPTATIONS FOR PRESENTATION OF ITEMS

Fig. 5. Wooden stand, side view, to hold materials to facilitate presentation (empty).

Fig. 6. Same, frontview (with cards inserted). Showing items 10 and 11.

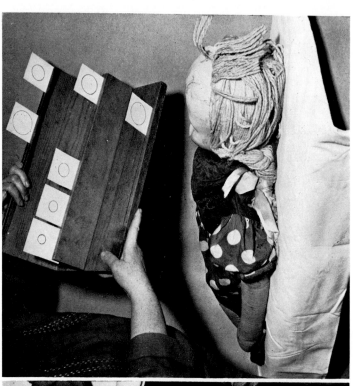

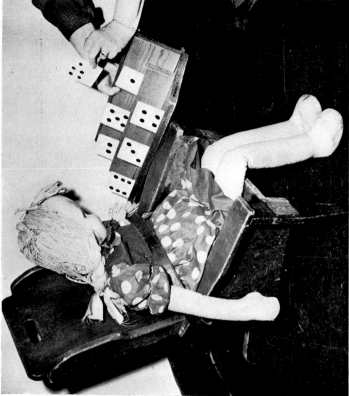

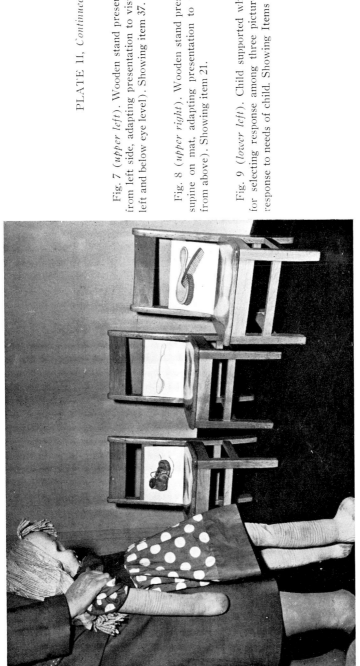

PLATE II, *Continued*

Fig. 7 (*upper left*). Wooden stand presented to child in chair, from left side, adapting presentation to visual needs (here from left and below eye level). Showing item 37.

Fig. 8 (*upper right*). Wooden stand presented to child placed supine on mat, adapting presentation to physical needs (here from above). Showing item 21.

Fig. 9 (*lower left*). Child supported while surveying choices for selecting response among three pictures, adapting mode of response to needs of child. Showing Items 4 and 5.

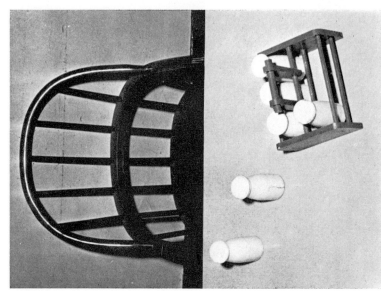

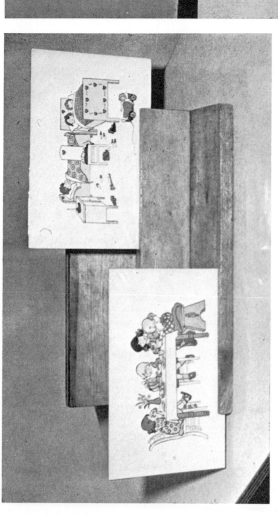

PLATE III. SOME EXAMPLES OF ITEMS USED

Fig. 10 (*left*). Pictures of daily activities of children presented in the wooden stand. Showing items 7 and 8.

Fig. 11 (*right*). Milk bottles with carrying stand for testing of amount concepts. Showing items 24, 25 and 27.

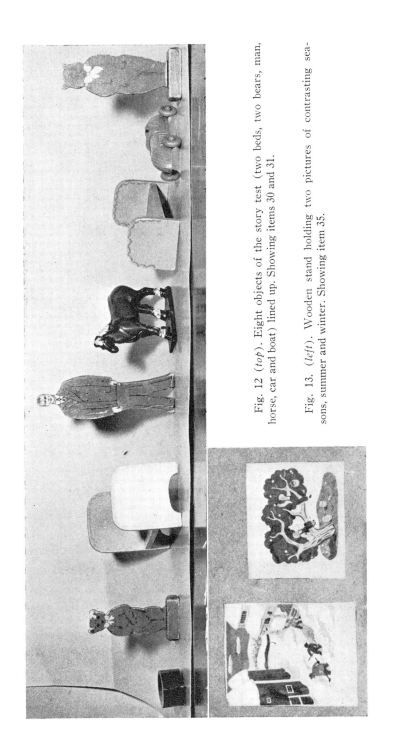

Fig. 12 (*top*). Eight objects of the story test (two beds, two bears, man, horse, car and boat) lined up. Showing items 30 and 31.

Fig. 13. (*left*). Wooden stand holding two pictures of contrasting seasons, summer and winter. Showing item 35.

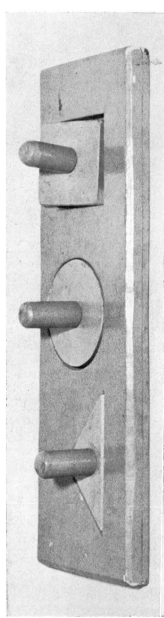

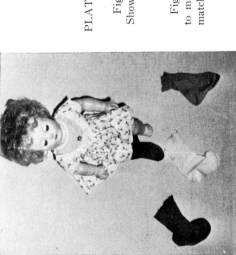

PLATE IV. SOME EXAMPLES OF MODIFICATIONS OF ITEMS

Fig. 14 (*top*). Form board with peg handles to make grasping possible. Showing item 9, downward modification.

Fig. 15 (*left*). Three socks in primary colors (red, yellow and blue) to match sock on doll. Showing item 12, modified downward for color matching in concrete task.

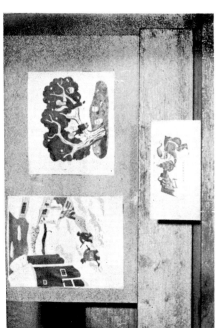

Fig. 17 (*right*). Same as item 35 (pictures of summer and winter landscape) but presentation modified with picture of Santa Claus for use with deaf, aphasic or foreign speaking child; also a downward modification. Showing item 35.

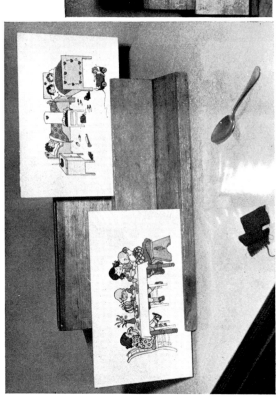

Fig. 16 (*left*). Same as item 7 (pictures of children's activities), but presentation modified for use with deaf, aphasic or foreign speaking child: spoon to "feed," cloth to "cover" children. Showing item 7.

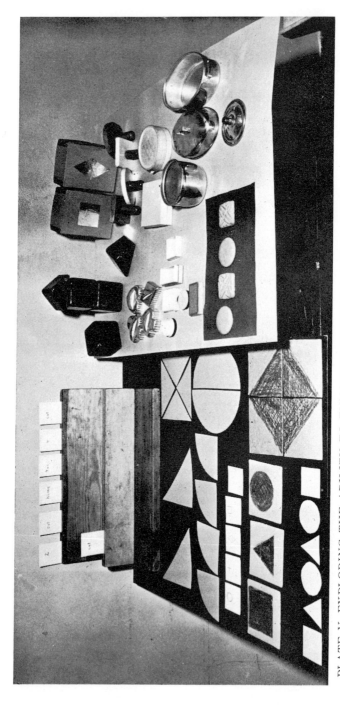

PLATE V. EXPLORING THE ABILITY TO FUNCTION WITHIN A SIGNIFICANT AREA OF FUNCTIONING

Fig. 18. On the left side, display of the complete range of standard items for testing perception and recognition of form and orientation in space: cut-out shapes, cards with basic symbols, wooden stand holding one set of cards, etc.

On right side, various experimental items used to explore the same areas in gradual downward modifications. Showing items 9, 16, 11, 17, 36, 39, 40; also modifications.

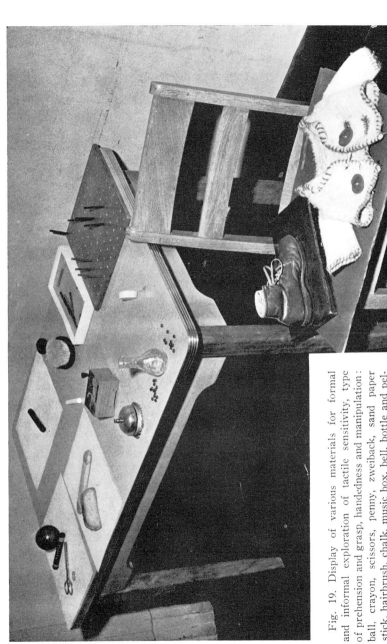

Fig. 19. Display of various materials for formal and informal exploration of tactile sensitivity, type of prehension and grasp, handedness and manipulation: ball, crayon, scissors, penny, zweiback, sand paper stick, hairbrush, chalk, music box, bell, bottle and pellets, peg board and pegs, scotch tape, shoe and doll coat. Showing items 22, 23, 38; also modifications.

1. *Why an Educational Evaluation is needed. How findings are arrived at. What an inventory of developmental levels is.*

Both in Europe and in the United States, methods of teaching children with such obvious handicaps as deafness and blindness have been developed and used over the past two centuries. Methods to train defective children in institutions have been in existence since the beginning of the nineteenth century. The trend in education during the first half of the present century, however, has been to establish an increasing number of facilities and develop programs in public schools to meet the needs of children who are handicapped. The public school class for the mentally retarded child dates back to the earlier part of the twentieth century, while crippled children who cannot be accommodated in regular classes have been taught in special classes since the second decade of this century.

It is interesting to note that it was the physician who preceded the educator in recognizing the problem of handicapped children and in exploring and experimenting with approaches to meet their specialized educational and training requirements. Significantly, the first public school class for physically handicapped children in New York City was started in 1914 at Bellevue Hospital; the first public school class for children with cerebral palsy was started in 1932 at Neurological Institute, Columbia Presbyterian Medical Center, New York City. It is important to keep in mind that the interest in and the responsibility for the training and education of children with handicaps is shared by both physicians and educators.

Educational facilities are being extended to include the more severely handicapped child and the child with multiple handicaps. Recognition of the value of early and systematic training of handicapped children has led to the development of kindergartens and nursery schools for them. With this trend, differential diagnosis and availability of a valid assessment of the educational potential of the individual child have become increasingly important. Especially is this so in the case of children with cerebral defects, since here the consequences of the impairment are not uniform as is true in instances of more clear-cut handicaps, such as blindness or deafness. Even when psychological testing has been successful and the mental age of the

15

child has been determined, subsequent maturation has not always been found to follow a predictable course.

THE EDUCATIONAL EVALUATION offered in this Manual has been developed over a period of twenty-five years. It is the result of a search for practical solutions to practical problems met with in the classroom, and it grew out of the realization that, in planning to meet effectively the educational needs of children handicapped since birth, it is necessary to find out the intrinsic as well as the extrinsic qualities of the handicapping condition as they affect learning. In each child, experiential intake may have been altered in various and differing ways by the existence of the handicap. In each child the present potential for functioning in the areas concerned with learning must be examined for intactness and adequacy.

Use of a standard test determines which of the tasks expected of the majority of children of a given age can be performed and comprehended by a certain child. But it does not reveal how the child has arrived at the solution nor whether he has had to detour impaired areas of functioning in order to respond appropriately to the posed task. Neither does a standard test explore the basis for failure when a task is failed. Yet, in order to plan an effective educational program for an individual child, it is as important to understand the pattern of his learning as it is to know the intelligence level or the mental age he has achieved.

The Educational Evaluation described here determines whether or not a given child can function in all areas related to learning and to developing and what level he has reached in each area. The essential items for this Evaluation have been devised in such a way that neither manipulation nor speech are required of the child who is to react to them, making the test suitable even for children with the most severe physical limitations.

The extent of a suspected difficulty in function in a given area can be determined and explored by the mode of presentation of the items in the Educational Evaluation. Modifications of the items permit a gradual reduction in demand and difficulty so that there can be a gradual retreat to lower levels of functioning within any specific area, until it can be demonstrated conclusively whether or not the child can function at all in that area.

The insight gained into the total functioning of a child through the Evaluation interview provides those responsible for his care with a realistic and reliable basis for planning an effective program of education and training for him. If further investigation of a child's functioning by the pediatrician, neurologist, orthopedist, ophthalmologist or otologist appears indicated, the Educational Evaluation frequently has been found to be of value in pinpointing this. This is especially so in the case of very young or very retarded children. Such children are sometimes found to be unable to cooperate in medical examinations of vision or of hearing, while in the course of an Evaluation interview, limitations of adequate functioning in one or the other of these areas become evident.

The premise upon which the Educational Evaluation offered here has been founded is the clear recognition that only the mutual effort and constant interaction of medical, educational and psychological workers can lead to the solution of some of the problems faced by the child who is handicapped. The need for interdisciplinary communication and cooperation is especially marked in the instance of children with brain defects, since it is sometimes possible for the psychologist and the educator only to pose questions and to describe unusual patterns of failure, while it is the neurologist who will confirm the pattern of functioning and who may be able to explain it on the basis of neurologic impairment.

THE FINDINGS ARE ARRIVED AT BY MEANS OF A STRUCTURED INTERVIEW. Briefly, standard materials are used in a standard mode of presentation. Groups of items are used to sample significant areas of functioning. Within such areas, quantitative age levels are indicated. Other aspects of functioning in addition to those measurable by a quantitative appraisal are explored by means of systematically created situations calling for the maximum functioning of the faculty under observation, for example, hearing or vision. In addition to the intellectual assets, nonintellectual assets such as emotional and social adequacy are evaluated, observed and recorded. Specific deficits, if present, are defined and explored. The physical competence of the child is carefully and systematically observed and described in two ways: the meaning it may have in terms of maturation and the implications it may have for classroom participation and management.

Demands are kept rigid. There can be no compromise in evaluating the response; it is either correct or not. But there is one significant departure from the usual methods. The object of an Educational Evaluation is not to determine if a given child at a given time wants to comply with a request, but to determine if he can, by whatever motivation necessary, perform a certain function, for instance, whether he can discriminate between round and square or between red and blue.

If an item is failed when given in the standard way, modifications are used until it is conclusively demonstrated whether or not the child can function at all in the particular area. The principle of exploring the actual ability to function may necessitate the use of approaches by which a faculty is tapped and an involuntary reaction elicited without comprehending awareness on the part of the child. The object of the Educational Evaluation is to obtain a complete picture of the child's potentials and deficits.

Another reason for the flexibility of the mode of presentation is to permit meeting the demands of a child's physical or sensory equipment. The sequence of presentation may be changed if such a change will enable a child to continue to function at maximum efficiency and without fatigue.

AN INVENTORY OF THE DEVELOPMENTAL LEVELS is the result of this painstaking exploration of the child by means of the structured interview. The findings are utilized to describe the child and his level and pattern of functioning. This represents a departure from the custom of scoring plus and minus and then computing credits or successes in order to arrive at a quotient. The object of an Educational Evaluation is to find the potential for development as well as the obstacles present in the form of specific deficits. The purpose of such an inventory is to provide a realistic basis for the education and training of the individual child.

Experience has shown that there are among handicapped preschool children large numbers who show deficits, limitations and difficulties, both in experiential background and in functional adequacy. The role of the Educational Evaluation is designed to be that of assessing potential so that maximum development may be fostered, rather than to provide a comparison of handicapped children with nonhandicapped ones.

Although it is the role of standard tests to measure a child against the norm, there are many points of contact and similarities in the administration of an Evaluation and of a standard test, and there is general agreement in the results of both procedures. Yet, there are significant differences. The standard test measures a child's performance in comparison to the average, while the Educational Evaluation probes the individual child's specific pattern of functioning. It is considered characteristic of the test performance of children with brain lesions, for instance, to show a spread or scatter of successes and failures over a range of two or more years. Averaging the levels or computing a quotient in such instances only serves to camouflage the true picture and put in its place a number, which does not really tell us anything about the child except how he compares to the norm.

It is possible to compute and to predict on the basis of the findings of an Educational Evaluation. The developmental level of the child in relation to his chronologic age reveals whether he is accelerated, average or below average, and, if the latter, how much he is below average. In the Inventory of Development such a conclusion is usually included. But it is not considered the main objective nor the most important one of the Evaluation. The most valuable contribution is a profile of the child as he is found at the time of the interview.

2. The purpose of the Educational Evaluation as a basis for educational planning

Frequently, a standard test or an Educational Evaluation reveals little that an experienced teacher does not eventually find out for herself in daily contact with a child. The advantage of using a test or an Evaluation interview, however, is that such information, instead of being accumulated over a period of three to six months, can be obtained during one interview session, a session which can be accomplished prior to the placement of the child.

In the case of children with handicaps in expression the systematic exploration of the potential is often the only means of determining the child's readiness for a particular program, be it nursery school, kindergarten or elementary school. The Educational Evaluation is suitable even for children who are so severely involved that they can neither perform manually nor respond verbally on standard tests. Speech and manipulation are not required to react to the items of the Educational Evaluation. This makes it a useful instrument in determining readiness for placement as well as appropriateness of a specific placement.

The utilization of educational facilities is most effective if valuable time does not have to be spent in trial and error before the educational method most suitable for a particular child is discovered. The experience of failure for the child and the experience of frustration and disappointment for the teacher can be avoided or minimized if the child's readiness for a program and his potential for profiting from it are determined prior to admission to a facility.

THE PURPOSE OF THE EDUCATIONAL EVALUATION IS TO PROVIDE A BASIS FOR PLANNING THE EDUCATIONAL PROGRAM by giving the teacher systematic and detailed information about each child. The Inventory of Developmental Levels, which is the result of the Educational Evaluation, describes the pattern of learning as well as the stages reached in various areas, such as comprehension and use of language, recognition of pictorial materials, ability to perceive, differentiate and recall from memory basic symbols, ability to discriminate between colors, concept of amounts, visual-spatial orientation and other fundamental apperceptive assets. Such information about each child gives the teacher a

19

solid foundation on which to base her approach and her expectation concerning his ability to participate and, through participation, to learn and grow. Learning about each child helps her to consider how he fits into the group, with his individual potential and his possible deficits as well.

Detailed inquiry into a child's functioning by means of the Educational Evaluation can reveal weak areas which might otherwise remain hidden until repeated failure has occurred. The object of the Educational Evaluation is not only to detect such areas but to define them once they have been detected. By making available to the teacher this information, the child's specific as well as his general needs can be understood and his participation in group activities can be guided accordingly. Suitable opportunities for growth and development can be planned. Appropriate techniques may be used to accommodate specific learning difficulties in order to increase the child's adequacy in functioning.

The importance of using the Educational Evaluation at an early date is emphasized by the fact that it may be helpful in devising remedial measures for managing difficulties in functioning before wrong habits become ingrained. This may be accomplished by training the child in ways to circumvent specific disabilities, or by attempting to develop poorly functioning areas to greater usefulness when this can be done. If areas of deficit or weakness are pinpointed early, if a thorough exploration of the total functioning can serve to clarify the sometimes existing functional linkage of deficits and poor habits resulting from them, the preschool years can be utilized to start the training or retraining of the child. The benefits to the child can be invaluable if such retraining leads to improved adequacy of his pattern of learning by the time academic instruction is introduced.

The utilization of the preschool years to teach a child how to compensate for defects in function before academic teaching is started is a recognized practice in the fields of blindness and deafness. It might profitably be carried over into educational practice for children with other handicaps.

The usefulness of the Educational Evaluation and the resulting Inventory of Developmental Levels is not restricted to the teacher and the classroom, however. Parents, distressed because the child fails to develop normally, are helped by a reliable evaluation and by an explanation of his difficulties. On the basis of the Educational Evaluation, home training can be planned with the parents, either by the interviewer or by other professional workers interested in the problem. The child's outlook for schooling can be discussed with the parents and implemented when suitable.

The pediatrician in charge of the child is in a better position to advise the parents in their care and training problems when a detailed evaluation gives him a picture of the child's potential and his limitations. If custodial care seems indicated, an evaluation which demonstrates conclusively an inability to function above a minimal level helps in deciding what course is to be taken in consideration of the needs of the child and others involved in the situation.

The neurologist will find the report of the result of an Educational Evaluation useful in rounding out a clinical picture of the child, as will the psychiatrist.

The orthopedic surgeon, the specialist in physical medicine, the speech pathologist and those in other disciplines engaged in the rehabilitation of the handicapped can get valuable information about a given child from the study of the Inventory of Developmental Levels.

In clinics dealing with the diagnosis and treatment of handicapped children, use of the Educational Evaluation can be a valuable addition to existing clinical tools. Clinic teams, including psychologists, social workers, physical, occupational and speech therapists in addition to medical specialists, may utilize with profit the Inventory of Developmental Levels. It will be helpful in the pooling of the team's findings to arrive at a diagnosis, and it will further be useful in planning the treatment, training and education of the child.

3. *Nature of handicaps which present obstacles to testing*

In the previous chapters, the importance of learning as much as possible about a child in order to plan effectively how to train and educate him was discussed, and the necessity of evaluating, in particular, children with handicaps and children who are atypical was described. The suitability and usefulness of an Educational Evaluation for this purpose was stated and the nature of the structured interview was explained briefly.

As will be dealt with more fully in Chapter 4, it is absolutely indispensable to learn about the developmental history of the child and about his habitual behavior within the family, prior to the Evaluation interview. Where such information has been obtained as part of a regular procedure, perhaps by a pediatrician or a social worker, the examiner, after reviewing the available material, may be able to confine himself to asking the parents a few additional questions to round out the background picture as it pertains to the Evaluation interview. To the experienced examiner the parents' report may reveal information of significance. What may appear as a unique, baffling or annoying trait to a parent, who is meeting such behavior for the first time and sees it only in relation to his own child, may be recognized as a specific pattern of deviation by the experienced examiner. Such information will be helpful in defining and differentiating the child's particular problem.

Children who in one way or another are difficult to test with standard tests present a variety of conditions. However, these conditions can be divided into two main groups, each of which has subdivisions. One main group are those children who are able to relate directly to an interview situation and to the examiner but who are hindered in their capacity to react to items for various reasons. They may be handicapped in expression by either speech or manual difficulties, as is true of many children with cerebral palsy. They may be limited in comprehending and in formulating adequate responses due to immaturity, intellectual retardation or foreign-language background. They may have difficulty in vision or in hearing, which interferes with accurate reception of the demand of the task under consideration. Some children with brain lesions who have little or no evidence of motor handicap and who relate well to the examiner may nevertheless experience specific barriers in responding to items.

The other main group are children who have not the capacity to relate appropriately to the interview situation and to the examiner. The reasons for such an incapacity are varied, and differentiation among them is important. Through using various approaches the interviewer may succeed in probing and evaluating the developmental level of a given child and in observing his behavior pattern in spite of the obstacles present. The appropriate approach will depend on the cause of the child's inaccessibility.

In the FIRST MAIN GROUP are children, such as those with *cerebral palsy, who are in direct contact but present physical obstacles to testing.* They can be divided roughly into three subgroupings: children with mild, with moderate and with severe involvement.

Inquiry into the developmental history is essential in all instances because of the interrelatedness of conditions intrinsic and extrinsic to cerebral palsy. The developmental history, which provides information about the age when walking, talking, self-feeding, self-dressing and other natural developmental items have been attained, is important. For example, delay in learning to walk deprives a child of the opportunity to learn about the environment by getting about on his own; it also prolongs his dependence on those who care for his needs. Delay, difficulty or inability in manipulation additionally restrict experiential learning about the nature and properties of everyday things in the environment. Inability to speak, delay in learning to speak, poorly intelligible speech will all contribute in some measure to a delay in learning or to a reduction in the amount of learning; the child cannot satisfy his perhaps normal interest and curiosity by asking questions and obtaining information.

Although some intelligent children who are severely handicapped by cerebral palsy seem to have suffered less from the effects of such limitations than others of equal physical involvement, they are in the minority. Perhaps their capacity to compensate for their restrictions in getting about and manipulating by keener observation of the world about them and by greater alertness to the conversation of those around them may be due to an originally superior endowment, even though on formal testing they may test only in the average range.

Associated handicaps in sensory equipment and in perception, which frequently are present in a child with cerebral palsy regardless of the degree of physical involvement, may be revealed in the developmental history. Or the presence of such handicaps may be suspected by the experienced examiner from the parents' report about the child's domestic behavior. Such information is important because impairment of hearing or vision will have had a serious effect on the child's development, especially since such impairment usually has been present from the time of birth.

Background information, obtained methodically and examined prior to an Evaluation interview, is essential whether the child is mildly, moderately or severely handicapped. This enumeration of the hazards to experiential intake demonstrates how the child coming for the Evaluation interview may have been penalized by his handicapping condition in the sum total of his life experiences.

This applies even to the *child with mild involvement* who has good use of hands and arms and can speak intelligibly, or who is, as some describe him, "normal above the desk" and therefore presents no obvious obstacles to testing. The experienced examiner, aware of the possibility of hidden handicaps and alert to telltale signs, surveys, checks, and probes until he is satisfied that nothing has been overlooked.

The child with moderate involvement may have fair or good use of one or both hands. His speech may be understandable with practice. However, the greater severity of his condition, which still exists and limits him in the present, will have proportionally influenced his previous learning. In the interview situation, he may be able to respond satisfactorily or at least grossly by sounds and partially intelligible words. Manually, he may be able to perform at least to the degree that the meaning or intent of his response becomes conclusively evident. By the nature of his responses to particular items devised for the purpose, the intactness or lack of intactness of his sensory equipment can be grossly estimated.

The child with severe involvement may lack any useful degree of speech and of manipulation. He may lack sitting balance and the ability to hold up his head. He may be unable to bring his hands to the front, singly or together, or if he succeeds in bringing one hand forward, his trunk and face may simultaneously turn away from the table so that he can no longer see what he wants to indicate with his hand. Especially may young children with athetosis be completely incapacitated, although as they grow older there may be some improvement in balance, manipulation and speech.

The items of the Educational Evaluation were originally developed primarily for use with children severely handicapped by cerebral palsy. The mode of presentation is planned so as to elicit the particular kind of response of which a given child with this degree of involvement is capable. The material can be presented even while a child is supine on a bed, table or a floormat (see Fig. 8) if sitting is impossible even in an adjusted chair with a safety strap (see Fig. 3). A method of responding is worked out between the child and the examiner which satisfies both that there is mutual understanding of the signs. These may be as minimal as a smile for affirmation and a frown for negation; or an upward turning of the eyes for yes and a sidewise turning for no; or it may be eye-pointing, which means fixing the regard of the eyes deliberately on a selected answer and holding it there; or it may be a very grossly executed motion of an arm.

When a very young or immature child is examined, it is sometimes necessary to help the child to find a means of expression. A child can be carried or walked toward a small number of widely spaced objects and requested to find the one named by the examiner (see Fig. 9). If he understands, he may be found to strain his whole body toward the spot where he sees the object in question. In this way, he may discover that he can respond even though he cannot speak. Chapter 7 describes examples of motivating such children.

Once a method of responding is agreed upon, the presentation of the items can proceed. The signs can remain the same all through the interview even though the difficulty and abstractness of the items increases. The burden of the proof is placed, from the child who is being examined, to the items which test the level of his comprehension.

Observing the nature of a child's responses to particular items will give the examiner information about the intactness of his sensory equipment, at least to the extent that gross impairment will become evident if it exists. The ability to perceive and to conceptualize is an area of special concern in the examination of children with brain lesions, including the cerebral palsied, and the Evaluation interview is planned so that difficulties in these areas become apparent. Possible interaction of various factors, such as poor sitting balance, visual deficit and a specific visual-spatial difficulty, is investigated. Faulty habit patterns are analyzed. Means of achieving a greater adequacy in functioning may sometimes be suggested to the child by the examiner even during the interview. A description of such findings in the Inventory will then enable continued carry-over in the schoolroom. Early detection of incorrect patterns is one of the most valuable contributions made by the Educational Evaluation.

In later chapters, especially in chapter 7, in which the conduct of the interview is described, more detailed directions for various contingencies are given. It must be remembered that no line of demarcation exists in cerebral palsy and that such terms as mild, moderate and severe are only very gross approximations used for the sake of expediency. Realistically, no two children with cerebral palsy ever exhibit exactly the same impairment. The etiologic factor is a lesion of the brain, but the consequence of such a lesion depends on the cause, time of onset, nature, extent and location of the lesion.

Barriers to testing in spite of good contact may also be found when the following conditions exist: immaturity, retardation, foreign-language background, or auditory or visual impairment. Some children with brain lesions without motor impairment and without severe deviations in behavior may nevertheless present and experience some obstacles in the interview situation in spite of good ability to relate appropriately to the situation. The Educational Evaluation, whose function it is to explore the total child by means of a structured interview, offers enough latitude in the mode of presentation and in the principle of gradual reduction of demands to be adapted to different situations.

Even a child who may refuse to cooperate on formal testing due to *immaturity* or extreme shyness can be put at his ease and, after a warming-up period, persuaded to occupy himself with presented materials in spontaneous play. The potential level of his comprehension can then be evaluated by observing the way in which he uses the carefully selected materials.

Retarded children can usually be assessed with standard tests. Some who are hostile, extremely negative, aggressive or willful, however, may pose a difficult problem on formal psychometric evaluation. With the Educational Evaluation, one does not have to confine oneself to stating that the child refuses to cooperate. Instead, one tries to penetrate the existing barrier. Sometimes, this is possible by using the child's own idiosyncrasy as a means of having him reveal his level of comprehension. A child obsessed with a ball or a toy gun, which he may refuse to relinquish, can be invited to aim it at the material. By using a judicious combination of enthusiasm and casualness, he may be persuaded to shoot at a target which is actually a symbol-card. He may be challenged to shoot all the ones which look exactly like the one the examiner holds up for him to see. If he can aim at the correct choice in a multiple choice until each card the examiner presents has been "killed," he may reveal that he is able to perceive and match symbols. Or he may roll his ball against small towers of color blocks and reveal that he knows the names of colors whispered by the examiner in a conspiratory tone.

Children who neither speak nor comprehend English can be presented with the items by pantomime and demonstration and may give their responses in the same way. Verbal communication is not required of the child in an Educational Evaluation. Some items which test the level of verbal comprehension will have to be postponed or given through an interpreter.

Children with auditory or visual impairment can be evaluated as to the extent of their limitations. An Educational Evaluation is designed to explore patterns of functioning and of resourceful adaptation in the face of handicapping conditions. A child with visual or perceptual impairment may have learned to use tactile clues and auditory clues together with memory and verbal reasoning to compensate to a degree for the unreliability or insufficiency of his perception or vision. A child with significant hearing loss, for example, may have learned to lip-read spontaneously and to pay alert attention to gestures and expressions. By speaking to the child inaudibly, by observing how he handles sound producing materials, hunches as to the nature and extent of sensory impairment can be confirmed or refuted.

Some children with brain lesions who can relate to the situation and to the examiner may yet experience subtle difficulties which penalize them in a testing situation. Most psychologists and teachers are familiar with the child of normal or near-normal intelligence, who shows disproportionate dependence on his mother. Perhaps he walked and talked late, fell frequently, is mildly awkward manually, may have been late in learning to feed and dress himself. In descending stairs he may have to bring both feet to every tread and can not yet alternate, and he may cling to the banister or to an adult's hand. His mild inadequacies in functioning have led to an overprotection on the part of the mother and an over dependence on the part of the child. He may have looked to her to interpret his early speech or the meaning of what he could not adequately formulate or even to speak for him whenever he was pressed to respond to outsiders. He may have expected her to do for him manually what he was slow to learn to do on his own. Although he may be able to relate to the examiner or even be overly trusting and clinging, he may not be ready to leave his mother when he enters the examining room. The basic inadequacies, although mild, profoundly influenced his ability to adjust to new situations and delayed his emancipation from his home.

In the Educational Evaluation subtle difficulties may be revealed, such as delay in recalling appropriate words, concreteness of thought processes, manual clumsiness. While the actual ability to comprehend and reason may be well within the average range, in some areas the level of adaptation may be disproportionally lower. The general pattern of the child may show behavior which resembles the neurotic, but the basis is early or persistent organic inadequacy. The situation is aggravated when instead of receiving parental understanding and protection, the child is under pressure to attain high standards and is punished when he fails to come up to the parents' expectation. Reactive behavior of the mildly inadequate child may take many forms. The Educational Evaluation, exploring underlying bases and existing patterns, can be helpful in clarifying such behavior manifestations.

Another pattern found sometimes in children with brain injury is a peculiar manifestation which can tentatively be termed *two-level functioning*. These children may be found capable of performing under pressure on a level from 6 to 24 months higher than their habitual pattern would lead one to expect. It appears almost as if such children need the proximity of an adult and his constant attention in order to be able to mobilize themselves and to remain mobilized long enough to function at their potential best level. Left to themselves they return to their habitual lower level of adaptation.

THE SECOND MAIN GROUP is composed of children who present obstacles to testing because they lack the capacity to relate appropriately to the interview situation.

The largest subgroup are those children with brain lesions who have one or more aspects of deviation in personality structure or in functioning which render them incapable of reacting normally. Related to this subgroup, but differentiated because their most striking disability is primarily confined to or is most pronounced in the language area, are the children with aphasia. Other subgroups are those children who are autistic and schizophrenic, infantilized or severely retarded. Children who are under an emotional strain also will be unable to relate fully in the interview situation.

The range of children who are more or less inaccessible in an interview situation is not exhausted by this listing. Only the more frequently met problems have been included.

The function of an Educational Evaluation is to assess the developmental level and the behavior pattern of a child, not to make a medical diagnosis. In general, children will be referred for an Educational Evaluation because their condition or their behavior has been noted as unusual and has been causing concern. A medical screening frequently will have preceded the Evaluation interview and a medical report may be available to the examiner.

Conversely, a child may be revealed in the Evaluation interview as presenting unusual behavior patterns or specific problems. In that case, it will be the psychologist who will point out his particular findings to the medical specialist, who in turn will confirm or rule out, explain and illuminate the described findings on the basis of his examination. An experienced examiner may be able to contribute materially to a differential diagnosis.

The examiner concerns himself frequently with appropriate placement in that program of training and education through which a given child can best realize his potential. Consequently, he does not confine himself to evaluation of the child but also periodically evaluates the effectiveness of the educational and training program for the child. Through gradual accumulation of a working knowledge of specific behavior concomitants of various conditions and disabilities, he will learn to recognize indications calling for specific educational management.

Workers in the field of cerebral palsy as well as those familiar with non-motor-handicapped children with brain damage find there is agreement on certain behavior patterns. These patterns are found to be more or less typical of *a number of children with brain damage, whether motor-handicapped or not. It is a pattern which calls for and responds favorably to a specific structuring of the educational environment and of the educational management.* However, this pattern is not found in every child with cerebral palsy or with brain damage, and should not be automatically assumed to exist.

Those children with cerebral defects who do more or less display this pattern present a loosely circumscribed complex of problems. They may be hyperactive or lethargic, distractible or perseverative, destructive or meticulous, verbose or mute, rigid or restless, but whatever quality predominates, it is recognizable as being in excess of the same quality found in any average sampling of retarded children. Disproportional strengths and weaknesses may be present, such as a difficulty in abstract thinking but an extensive vocabulary or an unusually retentive verbal memory but an inability to recall simple geometrical forms. There may be difficulties in visual or in auditory perception and in visual-spatial orientation.

The Evaluation of such a child begins with obtaining and reviewing his developmental history and a report on his behavior at home. It is important to learn to recognize this behavior complex and to differentiate it from manifestations of reactive, neurotic or psychotic behavior. In preparation for the Evaluation interview, the examiner should adapt the physical setting by removing, insofar as is possible, distracting elements from the testing room (see Fig. 4B). During the interview the examiner should seek to explore the child's capacity to receive impressions and to react to them appropriately, making an effort to adapt the mode of presentation of any given item to the specific demands presented by the behavior deviation of the child. The structured interview is used to probe the nature and the consequences of such deviations, with the reactions of the child, both voluntary and involuntary, being observed in an attempt to learn how the child mobilizes himself in response to a stimulus. Lateral probing into suspected areas of sensory or perceptual difficulties may aid in defining their nature and extent.

These problems will be discussed and illustrated throughout the text. In chapters 7 and 9, directions and modifications deal with specific problems and suggestions. The items used in the Educational Evaluation and the method of the structured interview are suitable means to explore the consequences of cerebral defects in the behavior pattern of this category of children who may or may not present physical involvement.

Among the conditions included in the subgroups is *aphasia,* which is believed to be caused by a localized brain lesion. If present in a child, the condition has generally existed from birth although it does not become manifest until the age of language acquisition is reached. The child can hear but is unable to interpret or to use the symbols of language. The inability to understand symbols of language is called receptive or sensory aphasia: the child does not receive appropriately. The inability to produce the symbols of which language is composed and to express ideas by this process is called expressive or motor aphasia: the child does not express appropriately. In central aphasia the child also cannot develop an inner language. A child with receptive aphasia, even if he has no expressive aphasia, will be hindered in acquiring language since he cannot interpret the word symbols spoken by others and cannot therefore, imitate them meaningfully. He cannot, of course, follow verbal directions, and he may not use gestures nor signs nor look for them by watching the expression of a face. In this he differs from the young deaf child, who is usually alert to signs and movements of others. The young child with receptive aphasia often seems completely unaware of the fact that people have a way of communicating by verbal means. He may not only ignore the speaker but show evidence of annoyance or fear of what to him must seem meaningless grimaces and noises. In this he resembles the autistic child. The basis for his behavior and that of the autistic child are the differentiating factors.

The child with expressive aphasia is able to learn to understand language at the usual age. He can follow verbal directions. He has a desire to communicate but is incapable of expressing himself verbally. He may be able to gesture very expressively and point meaningfully, and he may utter sounds and words only to realize their inappropriateness the moment he has said them. He may substitute words, such as calling a telephone a "Hello" while he mimics holding a receiver correctly, or saying "hat" while he draws clearly recognizable hair on a figure and points correctly to his own hair.

The study of childhood aphasia is only beginning. Classes for children with aphasia are almost unknown in the public schools at this time, and educational measures for the various types of aphasic children are in the experimental stage. At present, speech departments and speech clinics are probably the agencies most frequently concerned with diagnosis of the condition as well as with use of rehabilitation techniques.

It is helpful to understand the behavior patterns which may indicate aphasic difficulties of one kind or another. Mild aphasic difficulties, such as marked delay in comprehending communication or marked slowness and difficulty in finding words, should be recognized by the examiner and described in the Inventory of Developmental Levels. Whenever indicated, consultation with a medical specialist with experience in the field should be sought. Mild aphasic difficulties are frequently part of the picture of the mildly inadequate child with a brain lesion, who was described in the first grouping.

Differentiation among the various possible causes of communication difficulty is important but it is not an easy task. The diagnosis of the reason for a lack of language development is arrived at gradually and carefully by a process of elimination of noncontributory elements and confirmation of elements that fit into the picture. Absence of language development and of speech may be on a basis of deafness, aphasia, retardation or autism. Sometimes the cooperation of a team of specialists, such as an otologist, speech pathologist, pediatrician, neurologist, psychiatrist, psychologist, speech therapist, teacher and others may be necessary to arrive at a definite diagnosis. Once deafness, retardation, and autism have been ruled out, the type of aphasia needs to be defined and the extent and severity of the condition explored.

Again, the developmental history is important and frequently it supplies clues about the nature of the involvement.

In the Educational Evaluation, one uses a process of gradually eliminating possible causes for the absence of comprehension of language in a child whom one suspects of having receptive aphasia, and for the absence of speech when one suspects expressive aphasia. Auditory intactness is checked. The level of language behavior is compared to the level of nonverbal behavior in the same child. If there is a disproportionate discrepancy between the general demeanor of a child and his language behavior, with the latter being unusually delayed or poor, one can tentatively rule out retardation as the cause of the lack of language. The ability to relate to persons is observed. While the child with receptive aphasia may be indifferent to his parents, he generally does not lack the capacity to respond to nonverbal management. In this he differs from the autistic child who withdraws from any direct contact, verbal or nonverbal.

Aphasic children may share with the previously described group of brain-injured children certain qualities such as perseveration, distractibility, and forced responsiveness to inessential details. Children with cerebral palsy may have aphasia as well, and it is important to keep this possibility in mind, when examining a child who has adequate hearing and fair organs of speech, yet fails to develop speech or fails to comprehend language. Aphasia may be overlooked in a cerebral palsied child with severe involvement, and educational management will be ineffectual because this associated handicap has not been taken into account in the planning for the child.

Autism and childhood schizophrenia are conditions which render a child inaccessible to a direct approach in an interview situation. Nevertheless, it is sometimes desirable to estimate the developmental potential of the child in order to place him in a suitable educational program. Since the Educational Evaluation requires no verbal responses, reactions to items can sometimes be observed which will give a clue to the level on which the child is functioning. Among young children believed to be schizophrenic or autistic, one meets two distinctly different types of children in the Evaluation interview. There is the child who fiercely resists approach, clings to his mother to the exclusion of everyone else, may resist being taken anywhere even by his mother, may scream ceaselessly but without affect or tears when strangers are present. Yet, within the confines of his own home, such a child may function calmly and with a measure of rationality, adequacy and independence. One also meets the child who wanders around as if living in a world of his own, who barely seems to notice when the parents leave the room, who may hum or talk to himself while using available materials in his own way. He may show affectless clinging even to an unfamiliar examiner and be quite delighted to engage in roughhouse and physical contact, yet be absolutely inaccessible to verbal approach, pantomime or to gestured suggestions or demonstration.

His actions, however, may show a certain coherence and sometimes, while he will not permit himself to follow a suggestion or imitate a demonstration, he will, after a delay, wander near the table where the examiner has placed some item. With an air of secretive nonchalance, he may perform quite competently, although never openly relating himself or his actions to those of the examiner. Children of both types occasionally show a tendency to be excessively orderly and testing in some areas can sometimes be undertaken by using this trait. The examiner can skillfully "spill" a nest of cubes or a formboard or other item to be assembled, and, leaving it there, pretend to be busy in another part of the room. The child, believing himself unobserved, may be found to assemble the toy, often with an aggrieved expression. It may appear that he is annoyed to find order disturbed and is almost compulsively forced to restore it before he once more can return to his withdrawn state. By increasing the difficulty of the demand, such as reversing the formboard, on a subsequent attempt, one may then find a clue to the child's level by observing whether he is able to adapt to the higher demand. The child may inadvertently reveal his ability to hear and comprehend verbal communication by getting his coat or running to the door when the examiner tells the mother that the interview is terminated. This may come after he has acted as if he could neither hear nor understand.

Severe retardation at first glance somewhat resembles autism, since here, too, the child appears inaccessible. The severely retarded child can, however, respond successfully, although only on a very low level. As the difficulty of the demands is increased, he begins to fail or he may stop performing altogether. As it is decreased, he resumes participation, until it becomes fairly clear that it is not autistic withdrawal but inability to comprehend which prevents him from functioning and responding. It is helpful to establish the presence of severe retardation early, if it exists, since severe retardation in the non-cerebral palsied child as well as in the child with cerebral palsy is frequently accompanied by seriously delayed motor development. It is useful to learn to distinguish the child who, whether motor-handicapped or not, does not yet have the intellectual readiness for a certain stage of motor function from the one who can appreciate what is expected of him though he may be physically unable to perform successfully. The latter will profit from rehabilitation through a therapy program, while the former is incapable of cooperating and a therapy program for him may more correctly be delayed until he attains readiness.

Infantilization is qualitatively different from retardation. A child may have been deprived of any incentive to use and develop the potential he may have for functioning. He may be totally unprepared to respond to an interview situation. He may have had all his physical needs attended to by others, been spoken for, been kept in a carriage. This applies even to nonhandicapped children. In the Educational Evaluation interview the potential of such a child may emerge slowly, or it may require several interviews to coax the child out of his pattern of passivity and to awaken some wish in him to be responsible for his own reaction to the examiner. It is important to learn to distinguish between infantilization, autism and retardation.

There will be situations where *emotional* patterns obscure the actual condition. It is always important not only to study the developmental history but also to find out if any recent change in the home situation may have affected the child. An operation or other episode of hospitalization, moving to a new neighborhood, the advent of a new sibling, the loss of a parent, grandparent or even a pet, all can affect temporarily the life of the child. Preoccupation with any of these events will effectively inhibit him in the ability to apply himself during the interview.

An understanding of conditions presenting obstacles to testing is an invaluable asset to the examiner. Only by observing numbers of children and their responses in the structured interview will experience be gradually acquired. Theoretical discussion cannot produce the sensitivity in an examiner which results from observation and experience. It can only provide signposts for those who are ready and willing to explore on their own.

4. Requirements for the evaluation interview: qualities of the interviewer; preliminary background data of the child's individual history; physical set-up

The Educational Evaluation is not a mysterious process. Rather, it is a systematic, commonsense, painstaking investigation of the ability of the child to function in various significant areas. This investigation is made in an objective, standard way. The findings are utilized in a way which relates directly to the child's educational needs.

The first requirements for a successful Evaluation interview are THE QUALITY AND TRAINING OF THE INTERVIEWER. The materials and items offered are, after all, only tools. The skillful use of a tool depends on the training, experience and skill of the person using it.

The interviewer must be trained in clinical psychology, and he must be familiar with psychometric procedures. Ideally, the interviewer should be a person with experience in the teaching of young and of young handicapped children. He must be familiar with teaching programs available for young children with handicaps. He must thoroughly understand child development from infancy to elementary school age. Experience acquired only in clinical contact is not as all-inclusive and practical as that acquired in a living situation and in continued contact. The interviewer needs to have experience and skill in relating to infants and very young children. Preferably, he should also have had experience in the teaching or testing of retarded and defective children. He should not attempt to use the material for the evaluation of children with cerebral palsy without having obtained first-hand experience with them for at least several weeks under the supervision of a psychologist or a teacher experienced in the educational, emotional and physical management of children with cerebral palsy.

The interviewer must also be able to be a cooperative member of a team composed of members of various disciplines and must know how to interpret his findings in a way that makes them most useful to the other members in their understanding of and approach to the child. He should be cautious and suitably modest in his working methods and should not take it upon himself to make medical statements. Findings calling for medical confirmation should be given in such a form that they will contribute to a better under-

34

standing of the child's problem. On the other hand, they should neither be unnecessarily obscure nor should they be permitted to remain ignored by being buried in the report. If confirmation of the findings of suspected impairment in functioning, clarification of the problem and differential diagnosis of the child can be expected to result from further medical work-up, this should be sought.

In addition to his professional qualifications, that interviewer will be most successful who has a genuine liking and sincere respect for young and young handicapped children. He also needs infinite patience and ingenuity. Young children seldom can appreciate and understand the meaning of an Evaluation interview or of any testing procedure. Therefore, adjustments and allowances must all be made on the part of the interviewer and not be required of children below school age. Too, a sympathetic but objective understanding of the problems and attitudes of the parents is indispensable.

The interviewer needs to be willing to venture away from standard testing procedures and to learn about and accept the much more rigorous demands made upon him in the conduct of an Evaluation interview. He should not be a person solely dependent upon a formula but, rather, an investigator intent upon finding out and tracking down elusive clues and subtle difficulties which may interfere with a child's ability to function adequately.

It is necessary that the interviewer spend sufficient time to familiarize himself thoroughly with the materials and the procedure before attempting to use them in the evaluation of a child. After some practice, the simplicity and logic inherent in the Evaluation interview will emerge. It is a systematic investigation of behavior in circumscribed areas. The behavior is elicited by a series of materials which remain essentially the same for all levels. Under the heading of each item in chapter 8, there is a brief reminder of the main area and the related areas being investigated through the use of the particular item. A glance at these will permit the interviewer to know at each instant what he is looking for.

With repeated experience in observing typical reactions at given age levels, the interviewer will soon find himself able to assess the total behavior pattern of the child with some ease. Eventually, it should become second nature for the interviewer to observe the child himself with the same concentrated interest and accuracy with which he observes the child's specific response to items under consideration. Since the Educational Evaluation is an extensive and exhaustive study of the child in a concentrated interview, in the beginning, until an examiner becomes familiar with the material and develops his own deft style of presenting it, it may be advisable and desirable to schedule two sessions for a complete evaluation.

Some of the items are designed exclusively for the purpose of eliciting information on functional ability, which depends on neurological maturation but also on neurologic intactness in the area examined. While children with known and overt brain lesions, such as cerebral palsied children, will obviously not be expected to reveal much additional information on such an item, the interviewer will soon learn to detect subtle awkwardness or almost imperceptible hesitation in children without overt or known brain damage. His knowledge of the performance patterns of the overtly impaired child will have rendered him sensitive to just such observable traits in the child with possible subtle impairment. In chapter 7, detailed directions for the conduct of the interview are given, and the principle of observation of the total behavior pattern is described more fully there.

Although the Educational Evaluation is designed primarily to result in information helpful to the educator, the procedure of the Evaluation interview is one which requires training in psychology. Teachers of young and young handicapped children will not have the background needed to enable them to conduct an Evaluation interview successfully unless they have received additional training in psychological procedures and practices. Recent graduates in clinical psychology similarly will need additional training in child development and practical experience in the educational management of young and young handicapped children before they can expect to have acquired the necessary skill to use the Educational Evaluation appropriately. At the start, they should only attempt to use this material under the supervision of a qualified senior psychologist.

It is foreseen that parents and others in charge of educating and training young handicapped children will use some of the suggestions and procedures described in the text. Utilization of part of the material by such persons, such as ways to elicit responses from a nonspeaking child with cerebral palsy, has occurred frequently during the years the items have been developed, collected and used. Where this has brought about an increased ability of the child to communicate with his parents, it was observed with great satisfaction. But the use of some of the approaches by parents definitely does not imply that a successful Evaluation interview can be conducted by an individual without specific psychological and educational training.

As stated earlier, the Educational Evaluation method is a tool. In the hands of an experienced, skilled psychologist, it will yield the results which are its aims. For such a person this tool can have invaluable usefulness.

The second requirement for a succesful Evaluation interview is the obtaining of and subjecting to critical evaluation THE PRELIMINARY BACKGROUND INFORMATION OF THE CHILD'S INDIVIDUAL DEVELOPMENTAL HISTORY. In clinic settings, this history material is usually available since it will have been obtained by a member of the medical or social service staff. In school settings, it may remain the responsibility of the interviewer to obtain from the parents the pertinent data on the child's early development and present level of achievement in physical functioning and in self-help areas.

Specifically, it has to be determined at what age the child reached the various developmental stages of raising his head, sitting, standing and walking, with as well as without support. It is always enlightening to inquire about the use of a tricycle, with and without adaptations, such as a belt, pedal straps, or back support in the event of a child with cerebral palsy. It is important to learn if a child who is not overtly motor-handicapped has had unusual difficulty in learning to pedal. In the case of a nonwalking, cerebral palsied child the use of a tricycle sometimes has supplied the child with the experience of getting about on his own, and this is important to know. The child's way of managing stairs should always be observed by the examiner himself. Parents sometimes misunderstand expressions like "alternating" or "one per tread" and tend to describe the child's peak performance rather than his habitual pattern; it is the habitual pattern which one wishes to determine.

The development of reach and grasp is important. One has to learn to inquire judiciously since remembered dates are frequently, albeit unwittingly, quite unreliable. It is sometimes helpful to inquire whether the child seemed to favor any certain plaything during infancy since this form of inquiry may aid the parent in recalling more specifically the approximate age when repeated grasping first emerged. Rather than asking when the child began to feed himself, it may yield more pertinent information if the question is formulated in this way: "When he first started to take food by himself, did he rake up some solids with his whole hand, did he pick up a morsel with his fingers or did he perhaps spontaneously reach for the spoon used in feeding him?" This form of inquiry implies that any style of self-feeding is considered an accomplishment and brings more accurate and much more revealing information about the actual levels reached by the child during his early development. Special note should be taken if a parent reports a persistent pattern of throwing of food, spoon, glass or cup when the child was over twenty or twenty-four months old, since this is a pattern not infrequently observed in a number of retarded children. The age when semisolid and solid food was introduced and accepted by the child should be determined. A delay may be an important clue; the basis for the delay will be a different one in cerebral palsy and in retardation.

The age at which the child participated and cooperated in getting dressed, and when he succeeded in undressing partly or completely is important. A physically handicapped child is able to convey his awareness of the dressing process by perhaps offering the correct foot, for sock, shoe or brace, or by anticipating a sleeve in his clothing or a bib at mealtime. With appropriate inquiry the parent may be able to remember such instances. The older pre-school child may at the interview itself demonstrate his level of dressing independence by the way he matter-of-factly unbuttons his coat and slips out of it or else automatically backs up to his mother to be helped.

It is also revealing to find out at what age the child first began to communicate his bathroom needs, regardless of whether he is physically able to care for his needs or must be helped. It is sometimes pertinent to inquire into the training efforts made by the parents if an older child with cerebral palsy is still incontinent.

Washing one's own face is such a controversial issue at certain age levels, especially with boys, that it is an unreliable indicator of the developmental level, but the way in which a child manages to dry his own hands has been found to be most revealing. Many retarded children of five, six and even seven years or older will only dry the palm of the hand and ignore the moisture remaining on the back of the hand. Some autistic children, although remote and inaccessible, will be observed to dry their hands carefully at ages as young as two and one-half or three years. It is not suggested that a differential diagnosis be based on the child's way of attending to his own needs, but it is emphasized that in collecting developmental data, the areas of self-care sometimes yield helpful information.

The development of language deserves most careful inquiry. The time of onset of babbling and of early vocalization, the first meaningful use of sounds for intentional communication, the response to verbal communication and also to nonverbal communication are important factors, especially when, at the time of the interview, language development is found to be delayed. The questions: "How did your child let you know that he was awake in the morning?" or "How did he tell you when he wanted a drink or wanted to come out of the play pen?" sometimes results in valuable information. Whether the child used crying successfully, or was "unusually quiet and undemanding," or seemed indifferent to the parents on waking up in the morning are important clues, especially if the child still presents difficulties in contact or communication. A report of an apparently adequate onset of language with a sudden or gradual cessation of the use of words is revealing and should be noted. A mother's report on a child's response, or the persistent absence of response, to nursery rhymes and stories must be noted down. The child's use of a record player, of radio and television give much information about his hearing and his language comprehension. The length of time he will pay attention, the kind of programs he seems to enjoy, whether he wants the radio turned on louder than the rest of the family needs it, whether he prefers televison viewing exclusively to radio listening or whether perhaps he ignores television and on the radio wants only music programs, all these facts should be elicited from the parents. This information is helpful in the case of the physically handicapped child as well.

As will be seen, information collected in the inquiry about early development often points to one or another basis for the lack of language comprehension and language development. This can then be explored by the use of specific test items.

When investigating the language behavior of children with physical limitation in language production, such as children with cerebral palsy, one should always inquire, tactfully, about the opportunity afforded the child to hear language spoken or to be spoken to. The development of language comprehension and of inner language is not necessarily dependent upon the ability to use vocal language.

Another aspect to be investigated is the age at which the child showed an interest in pictures, either in a picture book, in magazines, or in photographs of familiar persons. If little interest in pictorial material has been observed by the parents, it is always wise to find out if the child watches television, how close he wants to sit to the set and, if he is a walking child, whether he stumbles and falls frequently.

In addition to this information, one also inquires about the present daily routine behavior of the child. One elicits a picture of his play interests, his outdoor play, and his relationship to siblings and to playmates. His attitudes toward the father and others in the home are of significance, as is their attitude toward him. The approximate level of a child frequently becomes quite adequately defined by the parent's description of his domestic behavior.

As already outlined in chapter 3, in the evaluation of a physically handicapped child it is always a must to explore how the handicapping condition may have influenced the amount and kind of experiential opportunities available to him. While the items of the Evaluation interview have been selected with the consideration in mind that the experiences of children with severe handicaps have been restricted, it is necessary to remain consciously aware of the child's limited opportunities in experiencing, learning and communicating.

As previously mentioned in chapter 3, any recent event important to the child's life should also be noted and taken into account. An occasional child may show unreasoning terror when taken to the interview, especially if the interviewer is addressed as "Doctor," or if the interview takes place in a clinic setting. This may be explained by such an event as a recent tonsillectomy, even though the event itself may seem to have passed overtly without making more than a casual impression. If a child does appear unduly apprehensive, it is sometimes wise to omit certain items, for instance, the play with the flashlight which would call for darkening the room.

Children of preschool age are usually neither ambitious nor competitive.

They are still preoccupied with trying to integrate the outside environment into their personal frame of reference. Their attitudes fluctuate and their equilibrium is easily upset. Responses may carry emotional tones which are more important to the child at the moment than would be an objective and uninvolved occupation with the materials presented by the interviewer.

It is wise, as well as considerate of the child's right to dignity and protection, to obtain the preliminary information on his history without his being present.

The third requirement for the Evaluation interview, for which careful preparation is necessary, is the PHYSICAL SET-UP.

The child must be helped to feel safe and comfortable. If available, a small or medium-sized room is preferable for the testing of young children. It should be kept uncluttered and as free from distractions as possible. The floor should be of a uniform and neutral color, preferably dark. Floor-covering of a vivid design, such as checks or contrasting colors, serves only to distract many children. The walls should be painted a light color, and pictures must be kept to a minimum. Outside sounds may be unavoidable, although for the testing of some children with brain lesions, as well as of other young children, a soundproof room would be desirable. A quiet room is time-saving as some children simply are incapable of inhibiting the impulse to rush to the window in response to persistent outdoor noises, an interruption which lengthens interview time accordingly.

The room should contain or have available two adult-size chairs and a regular-size table. There should be some straight-backed children's chairs and a child's table. The table should be at least 36 inches long and 20 to 24 inches wide in order to permit the necessary spreading out of some materials when testing children with involuntary motion. The table surface should be light but not shiny. In addition, there should be available one child-size arm chair and one small relaxation or Adirondack type chair (see Figs. 2 and 3).

Very young or immature children will probably be more at ease if permitted to remain on the mother's lap while mother and examiner are seated opposite each other at the regular-size table.

For many children, a straight child's chair, low enough so the child's heels can rest on the floor, will be sufficient. If the child's feet do not reach to the floor but the size of the chair is in proportion to the table, a box or a stack of magazines can be placed under the child's feet to give him support. The height of the table should be proportionate to the chairs used so that the child's elbows rest on the top of the table. The examiner uses a small chair placed opposite (see Fig. 1). The child should never be placed so that he faces a window directly, unless artificial light is used.

A small armchair is useful when the child has some difficulty with sitting balance. It is also extremely useful when a young child has a habit of toddling away from his seat constantly since the sides of the chair provide a gentle reminder to remain seated. If the table is pushed close to the chair, which in turn is placed so that the back of it rests against the wall, many two and three year olds tend to forget their aimless roamings and let themselves become interested in the presented materials (see Fig. 2). This method of gentle restraint should never be attempted if a child resists or shows signs of frustration.

A relaxation chair of the Adirondack type, which is a reclining armchair (see Fig. 3), will be needed for the child with moderate or severe physical handicap, especially the child with cerebral palsy. The chair prevents the child from falling out. It does not tip due to the construction of the legs, even if the child's involuntary motions are quite wild. If necessary, a belt can be fastened around the child and the chair to give the child an added feeling of safety. The wings on both sides offer a suitable support against which the child can rest his head if physically unable to hold it erect. The wings are shaped so that involuntary shoulder and elbow motion are not interfered with. If the child's feet cannot rest squarely on the floor, a box can be placed under them. Once a child has settled in such a chair, he is able to forget his concern with his balance and can begin to apply himself to the materials presented by the examiner. If a child wants to use gross arm motions to indicate his answers in the interview, the construction of the chair combines enough margin for movement with complete safety. The physical position serves also to prevent undue fatigue.

If the child's physical involvement is so severe that he can be maintained neither in a relaxation chair nor on his mother's lap, a pad or mat can be used to make it possible for him to rest comfortably in a supine position either on a table or on the floor (see Fig. 8).

A useful device when one is attempting to test a child who wanders around with aimless, purposeless disinhibition, refusing or ignoring chairs and sliding off the mother's lap, but who is obviously goodnaturedly aimless rather than purposeful and resistive, is the "playpen" arrangement shown in Figure 4a. The table is placed on its side with the legs touching the wall. The top of the table may need additional bracing by placing a chair against it. It is often possible to lure the child into this play area with a tempting toy. Once inside, the child may be presented with a variety of materials in rapid succession, preferably on the floor or perhaps along the rim of the table. It may in that way be possible to gain and hold his attention, and his use of the materials will enable the examiner to study the level and the pattern of his behavior.

For the truly hyperactive, distractible child who may not permit himself to sit still, who, driven by inner and outer impulses, may flit from corner to corner, it is sometimes advisable to push the table with the presented material flush against the wall so that only blank surfaces surround the child (see Fig. 4B). The child may then focus his attention on the material and begin to use it. He may even absentmindedly seat himself when one pushes a chair into position unobtrusively. Sometimes, he may work on for a while, with the examiner sitting quietly in back of him or to one side and silently exchanging unused materials for those the child has completed, being careful that nothing intrudes within the child's field of vision except the items the examiner hopes to make use of. It is generally advisable to prepare the interview room for such a child before he enters. The test items are kept handy but out of sight until needed. Removable objects, such as a telephone, desk lamp, desk clock, papers and books, inkstand and pen are put away. It is worthwhile to keep on hand a plain dark dress or smock to wear when attempting to test a hyperactive child. By accommodating the child's difficulties, one can sometimes help him to perform at his potentially best level.

Some children will be most comfortable in their carriage or wheelchair, and the examiner may prefer to present the materials on a tray placed across the carriage.

Finally, there will always be some young children who are most at their ease seated on the floor. An experienced examiner of young children is conditioned to this and will never be at a loss under such circumstances. He will simply move his material conveniently and settle down on the floor with the child.

Other modifications of the physical set-up for the Evaluation interview, which are occasionally called for because of a child's emotional needs, will be discussed in chapter 7 as part of the directions for the conduct of the interview.

5. Origin of the structured interview

Before describing the nature and the conduct of the structured interview, a brief review will be given of the way in which this particular form of interview for evaluating children was developed. The principle of the Educational Evaluation will be stated.

Dissatisfaction with the meager scope and limited nature of the information to be gained about handicapped children by means of standard tests led to recognition of the need to supplement such information in a systematic way. One possibility was to utilize the first three to six months of a child's attendance at school or kindergarten for this purpose, making it a period of exploration in trial and error fashion. While this practice, which is employed by many teachers of handicapped children, gives a measure of satisfaction, practical considerations made it a logical aim to find a way in which to accumulate the desired information with an economy of time and an acceptable guarantee of completeness. It seemed wiser and simpler to undertake such an exploration in a concentrated, *systematic sampling interview.*

The Educational Evaluation evolved in a completely pragmatic fashion out of what can best be described as "controlled observation." It arose as an attempt to undertake a concentrated sampling of a child's way of functioning in areas related to developing and learning. On the basis of such a sampling interview, it proved possible to make an *inventory* of the child's levels of development in the areas sampled. The inventory, too, made possible a *more effective educational program,* related to and reliably meeting the specific educational needs of each child.

What was originally intended as an evaluation of sensory functioning and a brief survey of the intellectual level gradually was found to have greater usefulness than had been anticipated. It was learned through repeated experience over more than a decade of observation that the concentrated, systematic sampling of functions related to developing and learning not only served the immediate purpose for which it was undertaken and intended but served as well *to predict the rate of development* and therefore the anticipated time of readiness for educational experiences.

The *selection of materials* used for this concentrated and systematic sampling interview was based on practical considerations. Whenever it became urgent to find a means of sampling another area of functioning or another level within such an area, further items were selected. The selections were based on two criteria: first, the materials and tasks used had to be within the experience, competence and capacity of the children for whom

43

they were to be employed; second, their use had to show reliably what they were intended to show.

The *mode of presentation* was designed in such a way that it could be adapted to children with any degree of physical limitation. Therefore, items were presented as multiple choices, which could be responded to by a glance of the eye or a gross gesture of arm, hand or head. For card and picture material, a stand was designed which could hold a number of cards or pictures at one time, so the child could make his selection by surveying the choices and indicating his response by fixing his eyes on the correct picture or card. This made possible the presentation of the material to a child whether he could sit up, lean back in a special chair, or had to remain on his back and could only look upward. (See Figs. 5, 6, 7 and 8.) Since many of the children tested had speech difficulties, ranging from being unable to produce sounds to having partially intelligible speech production, the items were designed and presented in such a way that *verbal responses were not required.*

Over a period of time, it became evident that here was *a simple and workable procedure to evaluate handicapped children* which appeared to answer a widespread need. Professional workers requested information and instruction about this approach.

In spite of, or possibly because of, the unorthodox and pragmatic way in which the Educational Evaluation emerged out of the realistically encountered needs of an educator of handicapped children, the scope of the information obtainable has been constantly enlarged.

Originally, an evaluation was made of sensory functioning and a brief survey of the intellectual level. In conjunction with the findings available from standard tests, this was thought to yield sufficient information to be used as a basis for educational planning. However, it soon became evident that, while standard tests could reliably demonstrate whether or not a child could perform successfully those tasks which were within the potential competency of his age level, they could not, as a rule, differentiate the reasons for failure to perform. Since it was realized that the fact of failure could have more than the one basis, namely, failure to comprehend, the range of other possible reasons had to be explored. The Educational Evaluation, therefore, came to include an investigation of the various functions necessary to the performance of given tasks. *If a child failed, a sampling of the intactness or impairment of each of these functions* could be made in a systematic way.

Functioning in areas related to developing and learning depends on the adequacy of intellectual maturation, of sensory functioning, of perceptual functioning and spatial orientation and, to a degree, probably also on previous opportunity for exposure to relevant experiences. The more obvious limitations of functions, such as inability to walk, manipulate or speak, are not under discussion here, and their relationship to the more specific area of functions necessary for developing and learning is considered only insofar as they may be interrelated to such areas.

It is possible to measure the adequacy of intellectual maturation quantitatively. The relationship of chronologic age to intellectual maturation forms the basis of the standard tests, of the M.A. or mental age, and the I.Q. or intelligence quotient, as measured by large samplings of the population. But the relationship of sensory functioning to chronologic age cannot be established in a similarly measurable way, if it can be postulated that such a relationship exists at all.

The relationship of perceptual functioning and of spatial orientation to maturation, while perhaps not yet sufficiently explored in young children, is utilized in the usual standard tests by the inclusion of items presumably testing perceptual functioning at a given chronologic level. This assumes that perceptual functioning is intact and that there is a measurable constant relationship to both maturation and chronologic age. It leaves unexplored other possibilities. Such possibilities are: nonintactness of perceptual functioning; delayed maturation of perceptual functioning; intact perceptual functioning in combination with delayed maturation in intellectual areas; intact visual-perceptual functioning in combination with impaired conceptualization, which affects in turn the faculty to deal abstractly with visually perceived symbols; impaired visual-spatial orientation in combination with other factors, such as delayed intellectual maturation, affecting resourceful utilization of means to detour the visual-spatial handicap; physical limitation of trunk motion in combination with limitation of the visual field plus delayed intellectual maturation, resulting in faulty habit patterns and consequent failure to utilize existing potential.

From the few causes cited that can lead to failure on certain items, it is evident that lack of comprehension is only one of several possibilities. But the developmental potential of a child is influenced more significantly by the basis for failure than by the mere fact of failure. This makes it imperative to determine, if at all possible, the reason why an item is failed. The learning pattern is influenced by the particular area of weakness. By detecting the reason why a given child fails, and then *defining the extent and nature of his weak area during an Educational Evaluation,* specific needs for education and training can be determined and suggestions can be made which may help to remedy or minimize his difficulty in the educational process.

The *dual purpose* of the Educational Evaluation became therefore, first, a *sampling* of intactness and second, an *exploration* of the extent and nature of an impairment revealed by the systematic sampling.

The first goal called for uniformity of the sampling process in order to make it a complete and systematic survey applicable to every child no matter how handicapped. The second goal made necessary a provision of flexibility in order to permit an investigation of individual difficulties where they were uncovered. Such an investigation had to be done in a systematic way rather than at random. When a task was failed by a given child, each area of functioning which played a part in the successful performance of the task under consideration had to be explored successively until the weak area could be spotted.

It was found that dual purpose of the Educational Evaluation could best be achieved by the *structured interview*. The two qualities, that of structure and that of interviewing, permitted uniformity in conjunction with controlled flexibility.

An Evaluation is not an end in itself. The principle upon which the Educational Evaluation is based is the belief that the potential of a child with a handicap can only be helped to realization if it is known. It can only become known by means of a *painstaking evaluation of the areas significant for development and learning in the individual child*. The Educational Evaluation aims to provide the means for achieving this.

Both the principle upon which the Evaluation is based and the fact that it came into existence in response to a practical need are responsible for the modifications that still continue to be made so that the information obtainable may be constantly widened in scope. Even at this moment additional items are being subjected to tentative use. An attempt is being made, for example, to develop suitable means to explore the self-concept of the young handicapped child, an area which probably has some significance for evaluation of readiness for therapeutic training. Other experimental items are being used tentatively to extend the Evaluation to older children. Still other materials are being experimented with in an effort to amplify and refine the present items.

It should be noted, however, that the Educational Evaluation in its present form has been used, with satisfying results, with many hundreds of children, some nonhandicapped, most of them handicapped in one way or another, all of whom were tested on standard tests during the same period of evaluation. The procedure of the structured interview has developed gradually over a period of fifteen years of pragmatic use. The structuring guarantees that the procedure will be undertaken with a specific purpose in mind, systematically and consistently. The medium of an interview guarantees flexibility in order to meet every contingency which may be revealed during the procedure.

6.   Nature of the structured interview

In this chapter the nature of the structured interview will be discussed, while the conduct of the structured interview will be outlined in chapter 7. Together, these two chapters constitute the basis for chapter 8, which gives the items of the Educational Evaluation and directions for their presentation. Chapter 9, describing a number of modifications and the indications for their use, complements chapter 8.

The Educational Evaluation is STRUCTURED. There are forty basic items given in a standard mode of presentation. The demand is kept rigid. The sequence in which the items are presented remains fundamentally the same for each interview.

The purpose of the Evaluation is to find out how the child functions and if his functioning is intact in the significant areas under consideration. Therefore, the examiner is required, in addition to noting the validity of a child's response to an item, to observe simultaneously the way in which the child organizes himself to respond and to accumulate gradually during the course of the interview a total picture of the child's behavior pattern as he reveals it in his reactions to the presented situation. The areas which the examiner needs to keep under observation during each item and during the whole interview are:

physical functioning:
    balance and locomotion;
    handedness and manipulation;
    eye-hand coordination;
    self-help functions, namely, feeding, dressing and toileting;

sensory intactness and sensory behavior:
    eye-motion and visual functioning;
    hearing and listening;
    tactile sensitivity;

self-awareness, self-concept, body image;

intellectual functioning:
    language behavior, history of speech development, nonverbal and verbal
        comprehension and communication;
    attention, interest, ability to follow suggestions;
    reactions to impressions;
    perceptual behavior;
    discrimination;
    concept formation;
    association and ability to abstract;

ability to recall;
ability to imitate;
capacity for adaptation, problem solving and insight;
ability to make believe or role playing;
ability to shift and ability to inhibit;
orientation in space, time and sequence;

emotional-social behavior:
attitude to parents;
attitude to examiner;
stability, endurance, resourcefulness, adaptability and perseverance;
sense of humor, frustration tolerance.

Some of these areas can be tested directly by the use of an item and others can be observed indirectly while the interview is conducted, while information on still others will be supplied by the developmental history obtained earlier from the parent. Supplemented by further inquiry during the interview and by actual observation, the evaluation of the child's level of competence in the areas of self-help activities can be completed.

Each item carries a brief listing of the areas which are investigated by means of the item, as well as of other areas which can be observed during the child's performance on the particular item. Since this procedure is an educational evaluation rather than a psychometric test, the active participation and the critical judgment of the examiner is both possible and desirable at every point.

That the areas under scrutiny are listed for each item not only serves to remind the examiner constantly that he is expected to be alert to the total behavior pattern observable while the child responds but also permits him to exercise his own judgment. He will sometimes be able to evaluate which factor may have caused a child to fail on a given item by checking against the listed areas. When presenting the same child with another item, which investigates a related function but where the set of involved areas may be different, he will then be alerted to the specific response of the child and to the meaning of this response. To illustrate: on a given item which tests amount concepts, the examiner may suspect that the child lacks the necessary language comprehension to solve the task rather than that the required ability to deal with specific measured numbers of similar objects is absent. This hunch can then be confirmed or refuted on a later item which tests amount concepts by a nonverbal mode of presentation. If the child actually can comprehend the mathematical operation involved, he will then demonstrate this appropriately on the nonverbal version in which language comprehension does not enter the picture.

The items are presented in a sequence which, step by step, parallels the normal sequence in which various functions develop in children without brain lesions. It is a simple, logical, orderly sequence. Children can recognize familiar objects before they can recognize the same objects in pictures. Therefore, objects are presented before pictures are presented. If the child succeeds in the task presented, these areas of perception and of intellectual functioning are evaluated as being intact. The ability to perceive forms starts with the impression of the mother's face as a vague roundness and the child gradually sees round plates, clock faces, light fixtures. By the end of the first year the quality of roundness has become so familiar that it is on its way to becoming a quality which can be abstracted and recognized when seen under different circumstances. That is why in standard tests presenting form boards, it is found that a percentage of children can place the round block at twelve months, a few more succeed at thirteen months and more than half of them at fifteen months. The ability to perceive squareness gradually develops in a similar way, and even helpless children, such as cerebral palsied ones who cannot sit up in a highchair or hold a toy, develop this ability as they regard windows, frames on the wall, the bathroom mirror, books and the other common square and angular objects in the daily environment. Presented with a round and a square box, they are able to indicate which cover goes on which box. Therefore, matching of forms is presented next in the sequence.

This brief description of the gradual evolving of typical functions, which can be demonstrated by suitable methods of investigation, is given to explain the sequence in which the items are arranged. *The sequence follows the line of development of normal and intact functioning.* The development of such normal and intact functioning depends on the neurologic maturation of the intact organism. The sequence, therefore, closely parallels the sequence of neurologic maturation when it matures at what is considered a normal rate of development.

The sensory equipment is explored as it relates to learning and functioning. It should be emphasized that the Educational Evaluation includes an exploration of sensory areas and of other functions which depend on neurologic intactness and maturation because the adequacy of the capacity to receive impressions and to react to them is directly related to developing and learning. No clinical examination of the functions in question is intended. *The Function of an Educational Evaluation is to evaluate the developmental potential and the learning pattern of the child, not to make a medical diagnosis.*

The Educational Evaluation interview offers a unique opportunity to arrive at a gross evaluation of the sensory equipment. In the case of very young and handicapped children, especially those with handicaps in expression, such as the cerebral palsied and others who are physically, mentally or behaviorally handicapped, a medical examination of vision or hearing is often difficult or unsatisfactory. The evaluation provided for during the structured interview sometimes is the first systematic survey of hearing, vision and tactile sensitivity that proves feasible.

On the basis of this gross evaluation, it is then possible to request examination by medical specialists if it appears indicated. The findings arrived at by direct exploration of functions and by observation of the functional use of faculties in the significant areas by the examiner during the Educational Evaluation interview may contribute materially to the sum of findings of a team of specialists and thus help the medical specialists in their diagnosis of the child.

Sensory functioning can be elicited and observed during a structured interview because the interview situation is designed with the child's emotional and maturational limitations in mind. In a child-centered situation with a child-conditioned examiner, it is possible for the child to relax and to participate in activities which are meaningful to him. By designing and presenting suitable situations and materials, maximum cooperation can be obtained. The child's sensory functioning can then be observed and evaluated. Observation of carefully elicited, involuntary reactions can also provide clues about intactness or impairment of a function even when conscious cooperation is not yet possible in a given area. The ability to receive and to react to tactile sensations, for example, may be explored by attempting to stimulate the child's palm or fingertips by touching them with the bristles of a hairbrush, a piece of ice, chalk, bread crumbs and similar familiar objects. The child's reaction, although involuntary and possibly without conscious awareness, will indicate to the examiner whether the child receives the stimulus or not.

The examiner is required to exercise skill, tact and accuracy. Perfunctory administration of the specific items in question will fail to yield reliable results and information. It is for this reason that the presentation of the specific items is described move by move. Presented with the right mixture of casualness, enthusiasm and a sincere interest in the child's own attitude toward the presentation, the desired results can be obtained because the desired reactions can be elicited. Adults who understand abstractly what they wish a child to do and are intent on getting him to do it tend to give their directions from the point of view of the adult. This is a pitfall to be avoided since such directions fail to elicit the desired reaction. The child cannot participate maximally in a situation which to him is meaningless and incomprehensible.

In the *sequence of items, where to place those testing sensory functions* was carefully considered. It is desirable to evaluate the adequacy of sensory intake early in the interview so that impairment which might interfere with the reception of presented stimuli and thus fail to produce a valid response can be ruled out or detected. Yet, a degree of relaxation and of rapport is desirable before presenting some of these items, in order to obtain maximum cooperation. The investigation of visual functioning, for example, which requires the use of a flashlight and a darkened room, is better placed toward the end of the interview. At an earlier point in the sequence, however, a gross check is provided by letting the child look for a small red pellet on the floor in the frame of a situation which makes this a natural request. It will be explained later how to proceed if either the developmental history or significant failure during the presentation of early items suggests the existence of sensory inadequacy.

A *further consideration involved in the sequence* in which the items were arranged was the fact that *children have a short interest span and become fatigued rapidly*. Many of the items are thus presented in a form which, to the child, looks like an interesting, tempting and often challenging activity which the adult shares with him. Items requiring close visual attention are alternated with others requiring close listening. The gradual progression in difficulty is helpful in *gentling the child along* so that his effort remains at a maximum. At some points, groups of items provide an opportunity for a learning process to take place. As well as holding the child's attention, they make it possible to test whether the child has been able to develop insight into the particular process required for problem-solving in that task.

Deliberately, in specific items, the sequence is constructed in such a way as to provoke a tendency to perseverate. Similar tasks, but with differing materials, are presented in close succession. It can then be observed whether or not the child is able to shift from one set of functions to another without pronounced hesitation or inadvertent perseveration. As a rule, items have been carefully constructed to avoid penalizing children who may have such a tendency by introducing elements which help break a perseverative trend.

In order to arouse the child's interest, the stage is set, when indicated, by use of a stronger stimulus before the more subtle stimulus which actually tests the function under investigation is presented. To illustrate: before introducing the sound blocks which test hearing acuity, noisemakers are used. These alert the child to his own faculty of listening and hearing. A conditioning of this type is more effective in creating readiness for the hearing item, especially with young children, than a verbal request to the same end.

The structured interview is facilitated by the use of the wooden stand described earlier (Figs 5 and 6). Originally developed in order to make possible the presentation of items to physically handicapped children and to facilitate their responses, it has been found that its use with all children, whether handicapped or not, is desirable. It is used for the presentation of most of the cards, which can be inserted into it. By presenting them at eye level, in an upright position, the surveying of the cards is made easier for any child, while an observation of the child's eye-motion and other pertinent aspects of visual functioning is made possible for the examiner, who sits opposite the child. By eliminating the need to manipulate the cards, even for children who have no physical handicaps, since the cards can be indicated simply by pointing, not only is the response speedier but excessive handling of the cards is made unnecessary, which helps to preserve them. It has also been found that placing materials in the stand helps to focus the child's attention on them and aids in lessening distracting elements.

The Evaluation has been designed with particular consideration of the needs of children who are totally handicapped physically. *Manipulation and speech production are not required to indicate responses.* Where some gross motions are desirable in order to make clearer a child's meaning and intent, the examiner is instructed to "lend" his hands if necessary but to let the responsibility remain with the child. To illustrate: when toy milk bottles are to be replaced in their stand so that the child's spatial orientation can be observed, the examiner may assist the child's hand to hold the bottle but will wait for the child's eyes, body motion and signs of affirmation and negation to indicate the spot where the child thinks the bottle should be placed.

But by no means are attempts at manipulation and communication discouraged, even in the case of children who experience great difficulty in these areas. The very purpose of the interview as a medium for the Evaluation is that the natural, usual behavior pattern of the child be given free scope. It is not a stilted, awe-inspiring, rigid session. While the examiner must be able to keep in mind all the facets of the structured interview situation, observe with educated discrimination, store away or note down what he sees and hears, and simultaneously evaluate the quality and the level of the child's performance, to the child the interview must look unhurried and natural.

Any spontaneous attempt on the child's part to participate manually should be anticipated alertly. *The physical competence of the child reveals information* which is important for three main reasons. In the child without physical limitations, it denotes the maturation level. In the child with physical impairment, it gives a clue to adaptations which the child has made, and to the resourcefulness or to the habit of dependency which underlie such adaptations, as well as being indicative of the maturation level. For both, although especially for the handicapped child, it helps the examiner in planning for the child's participation in the classroom and for the assistance the child may require. The attitude of the child toward his handicap becomes observable in his self-sufficiency, persistence, frustration tolerance and, negatively, by his expectation of assistance, his half-hearted efforts followed by quick discouragement, active or passive tantrums. A child's attitude toward being handicapped is an important factor in the rehabilitation program. The degree of self-awareness, self-recognition and self-acceptance can be observed by the examiner who matter-of-factly assumes the child's desire to assist in manipulating or collecting and putting away some of the materials used during the interview.

In a comparable way *the child's spontaneous and elicited manner of communication reveals information* which is significant. It denotes the maturation level in any child, the willingness and ability to adapt and to detour limitations in the speech-handicapped child, and it aids the examiner in determining individual needs in the educational program. The Evaluation has been designed so that the need for verbal responses is eliminated. This was necessary to make it a useful instrument to evaluate even the most severely involved child, who could yet adequately indicate his answers to the whole sequence of items by nonverbal means. But the need for this expedient by no means implies that the faculty of communication is underestimated. Again, as was true in the discussion of physical competence, the combination of the maturation level and of the spontaneous utilization of whatever potential for communication may be present, is studied during the structured interview. The stages of verbal usage must be noted. These stages range from communication by single word to phrase to sentence and from jargon to monologue to the intentional, spontaneous use of language symbols for the purpose of conveying meaning. Only the examiner who is thoroughly trained in normal child development and has had wide experience with nonhandicapped as well as handicapped children can adequately evaluate this area. Experience resulting from clinical practice only, without being re-enforced by actual everyday contact with young and handicapped children in a living situation, tends to remain artificial and academic.

The same stages that are typical for nonhandicapped children are observable also in those children who can communicate only by facial expression, meaningful looks and a resourceful use of clues available in the environment. As an illustration, an immature child handicapped by cerebral palsy, who might be described as being in the monologue stage of language use, may express his wish to terminate the testing interview by looking toward the door and pouting. The more mature child with exactly the same limitations in the production of speech, namely, an inability to produce more than a grunt, would proceed something like this: he would first invite the examiner's attention by looking at him intently and meaningfully. He would then look toward the clock in the room or the watch on the examiner's wrist to indicate the passage of time. Next, he would indicate the door with a determined look or a turn of the body and he would check back to observe whether the examiner had followed his signs. Finally, he would swing his eyes toward the window and check back once more to note the examiner's continued attention and comprehension of his message. The resourceful utilization of clues visible in the room, the ability to assume that people will understand the symbolic meaning "time" when a clock in indicated, his unemotional and rational use of a look toward the door, beyond which he expects his mother to be waiting, and then toward the window to indicate the out-of-doors, which means the way home, all these observable facts reveal to the experienced observer the level of the child's language-usage development.

As was discussed earlier, the child's attitude toward his handicap and the degree of emotional stamina he has can be inferred from his willingness to make the effort to use such means, from his resourcefulness in using them successfully to put his meaning across and from the implied acknowledgment that the unfamiliar adult understands his predicament, which he demonstrates by the intentional effort to impel the examiner's attention to his sign language.

The means of communication employed by children whose language impairment is not based upon physical involvement of the speech apparatus must be studied similarly during the structured interview. Chapter 3 described the more frequent problems encountered in that area.

In this survey of considerations necessary to make the structured interview a suitable medium for the evaluation of handicapped children, *another aspect involved in the sequence of items should be explained.* For the process of painstakingly and systematically sampling the areas related to development and learning, *many of the items serve a dual or multiple function.* Nonintellectual functioning as well as intellectual functioning is evaluated, and sensory intactness is explored.

The arrangement of many of the items is in a sequence of increasing intellectual demand, since it is a sequence which parallels normal development of functions. Yet, performing adequately on each item not only requires and demonstrates the necessary intellectual maturation but also the intactness of total functioning. A systematic sampling of the intactness of functioning, therefore, requires that each child, regardless of his chronologic age, be evaluated on every item of the whole sequence, from the first item up to his present level. This guarantees that subtle disabilities will be detected. The reason for failure on an item even though the intellectual grasp of the child appears sufficient for solving the problem, can be pinpointed, rather than remain undifferentiated, if the particular area of failure has been traced through the whole sequence of items. For example, a given child may experience difficulty of a disproportionate degree in the recall of names of objects or of words in general. This weak area would be pointed up at an early stage when he fails to indicate correctly which one of three pictures of objects was removed. This same child may then be found to fail on a higher level when he is required to find a small outline symbol from memory after brief exposure. By comparing the earlier failure on the lower item with the nature of the later failure on the higher one, it will be possible to demonstrate that it is an inability to commit to memory a name for the symbol rather than an inability to perceive and to recognize a given outline symbol visually which causes the child to fail the item. Since educational methods should be specifically directed at the true weak area of the child rather than be an undifferentiated attempt to teach a child with learning difficulties, this pinpointing of the disability is a valuable part of the Educational Evaluation. The opportunity to spot or rule out such subtle weaknesses is well worth the time and effort required to begin at the first item with every child at his initial Evaluation.

The items exploring sensory intactness were placed at those intervals in the sequence of items which were found most conducive to making them acceptable to young children. For systematic sampling of functioning, all items testing sensory functions must also be presented to each child, regardless of his chronologic age.

In chapter 7, directions are given which explain how to use the sequence of items in the structured interview. In the description of the items in chapter 8, great care has been taken to mark each item unmistakably so that no item will be omitted which is essential in evaluating the total functioning of a child. *The main rules for the use of the items are that the first interview for any child begin with the first item and that the whole sequence of items be scanned for each child.* Only by adherence to these rules can it be certain that nothing is left to chance, that difficulties are either discovered or ruled out, that a child is honestly evaluated and his potentials reliably estimated. The principle of the Educational Evaluation precludes the use of the items for the spurious purpose of a quick check of the present performance level and nothing else.

At later re-evaluations it may not be necessary to repeat the whole sequence. Only the items measuring progress may be needed, unless significant changes have occurred in the physical or neurologic functioning of the child, such as may have resulted from encephalitis or from severe seizures or from progressive conditions of various origin.

There are a few groups of items which test the same area, and, for these, the materials and mode of presentation used is different for younger children, the same area of functioning being tested with slightly changed materials and mode of presentation for older children. Where this occurs, the items are clearly marked. There are also a few items for older children on which a higher demand is made where the item is not given first in the form that makes a lower demand. This is done when presenting the item in its simpler form first would invalidate the response on the next level. These few instances are also clearly marked.

The *recording blank,* which contains the sequence of forty items and the age levels to which they are applicable, serves as a guide to the examiner. Since many of the items have a dual or multiple function, Roman numerals are used to indicate the age range for which an item is to be presented, and Arabic numerals are used to give the age levels at which intellectual maturation is expected to be sufficient for intellectual comprehension of the item. As explained, many items test quantitatively measurable as well as other functioning. Therefore, the age range indicated by the Roman numerals frequently will be broader than that given in the Arabic numerals, since the Arabic numerals apply solely to that range when intellectual readiness can be expected. Chapter 10 contains a description of this blank.

As was discussed in chapter 4, the examiner will find the materials and the sequence simple and logical and he should soon become familiar with the sequence as an organic whole. The practice of starting with the first item in every interview will facilitate familiarity with the materials and with the sequence. The skilled examiner will rapidly learn to arrange the materials in a convenient way prior to the interview. The chronologic age and the developmental history of the child, which are obtained beforehand, will help him to estimate the range of materials which may be required for the particular interview. Items for older age levels for example, need not be prepared when a very young child comes to the interview.

The nature of the materials selected or designed for this Evaluation is such that they are acceptable to any examiner who is at home in nursery schools, kindergartens and classrooms. They are of the stuff with which these environments are equipped. It was in a setting of the natural environment of childhood, not in a laboratory, that the systematic sampling interview was developed. The forty items represent a cross-section of situations any child can be expected to meet in his educational career. The materials and tasks which make up the items were assembled one by one out of real-life situations. Frequently, they recommended themselves because they corresponded so closely to typical and preferred play activities of given age groups. Their concreteness and familiar character enhance their appeal to children.

The age levels denoting the range when intellectual readiness for the item can be expected are typical age ranges. These ranges were arrived at on the basis of clinical judgment, developmental sequences, through comparison with items on standard tests which call for manual or verbal responses, curriculum expectations, and, finally, on the basis of more than fifteen years of use of the materials and thirty years of experience with handicapped children.

It is expected that users of the Evaluation will remember at all times that the procedure offered in this manual resulted from the need to *supplement the information gained by means of standard tests*. It is to be used in conjunction with the results of standard tests. It is not a standardized test in itself, but an educational evaluation.

No doubt, in succeeding years, further opportunity will be available to apply this test procedure to a larger series of normal children. This will allow more effective comparison and will also allow a closer approximation to "standardization." However, no standardized test ever really qualifies as the fully objective measure of intelligence it presumes to be, and I do not believe the value of this procedure would be significantly enhanced by standardization. Its essential character will continue to remain descriptive.

The principle upon which the Educational Evaluation is grounded and the purpose which it serves would not be affected by standardization. The criteria for each item, as it was selected, was that it had to be within the experience, competency and capacity of the children in question and that its use had to show reliably what it was intended to show. The first of these two criteria allows the indicated age levels deliberately to encompass a wide range, so that the somewhat slow and the average child are both within the indicated age range. In order to motivate the child to react to an item, he has to be able to comprehend reliably what he is expected to do. The second of the criteria guarantees the opportunity to observe the child's way of functioning in the area under investigation. Since it is the second criterion which is the object of the Educational Evaluation and the reason for it, the fact that age levels are indicated does not imply that they are used in a way similar to that of standardized tests. There the indicated age levels must have a high correlation with acceptable criteria of intelligence. *Here they must be within a calibrated range.*

It would be a misuse to attempt to use the age levels indicated in this manual as rigid criteria of achieved "mental ages." *They are not designed to be considered so and nothing could be more contrary to the principle of an Educational Evaluation than to subject the material to such misconstruction.*

Chapters 11 and 12 will describe how the performance of the child reveals *his level of functioning as well as his individual pattern of functioning.* It will be remembered that the findings of the Educational Evaluation are described in an inventory and not computed numerically. Nevertheless, a useful description of the estimated level of functioning will result from the procedure, and it will be entirely possible and justifiable to determine whether a child functions on an average level, above average, borderline, mildly subnormal, moderately subnormal or severely subnormal.

With the essential uniformity of the structured interview described and the general rules underlying the conduct of the interview demonstrated, the final part of this chapter will deal with the circumstances and conditions under which a departure from the rigid structure is provided for.

As an INTERVIEW, the Educational Evaluation provides for *controlled flexibility* in order to accommodate individual needs as they become evident during the interview. It is flexibility within the general framework of the structured interview, however. The interview can by no means become a random, unregulated, anarchic, capricious or confused process. The Evaluation is useful only as long as it shows reliably what it is supposed to show. *It must constantly serve the dual purpose of the Educational Evaluation: the sampling of intactness and, if this sampling has revealed impairment of intactness, the exploration of the extent and nature of impairment.* A departure from the rigid structure is indicated and justified when by it the purpose of the Evaluation can better be achieved. This requires that the examiner must know what he is trying to demonstrate and by which one of a series of modified approaches he may be able to obtain the desired information about the child's functioning. Any departure from the structured sequence and from the rigid demand made during an interview must be scrupulously recorded.

Modifications serving most of the needs which may be encountered during an Evaluation interview are described in chapter 9. Frequent references to these modifications are made in chapter 8 at appropriate points in the description of the items.

The examiner must familiarize himself with the modifications before he attempts to conduct the Evaluation interview. Rather than look up suitable modifications after he has run up against a problem or after he has terminated an unsuccessful interview, the examiner should be in a position to recognize and to accommodate many eventualities during the interview and achieve a natural transition to a modified approach. The experienced educator and psychologist may be able to improvise his own modifications in specific situations once he has become at home with the nature of the structured interview and its aims. In an Evaluation interview, an important role is played by the judgment, sensitivity, ingenuity and experience of the examiner, much more so than is true in the administration of a standard test. This manual gives directions to make the task as clear-cut and as graphic as possible, but it cannot take the place of clinical experience nor of individual sensitivity. It will be found in the course of use that the material results in simple and easily recognizable reactions and responses. With some practice the examiner will gain in his ability to evaluate individual responses and reactions, so that typical deviations in responses will indicate recognizable trends in the functioning pattern. The indications for modifications will thus gradually become a familiar pattern, enabling the examiner to retreat smoothly to lower levels in his conduct of the interview.

Since the items are designed and the sequence of presentation is planned so as to correspond closely to the natural stages of usual child behavior and child development, the *need for modifications* admittedly *exists only when development or sensory functioning fall below the range of the test items or behavior is outside the range of the expected.* In chapter 3, a brief survey was made of conditions which present obstacles to testing. Many of the more frequently met conditions, such as motor handicaps and speech handicaps, were considered in the development of the structured interview, and they are accommodated sufficiently by the ways in which the material is presented and can be responded to. There remain, however, a number of instances where adherence to the standard sequence of items or the rigid demand inherent in an item will not yield sufficient information. Such instances are: the chronologic age or the mental age of the child may fall *below the two year level;* the behavior pattern of the child may render him *inaccessible* to direct contact; the sensory equipment may be inadequate and may *prevent reliable reception of the items;* the physical handicap, or a combination of sensory and motor difficulties, may put an *undue strain* on the child in his attempt to respond adequately. There may also be a *combination of any of these four factors.*

The provisions for flexibility in the structured interview makes it possible to use modifications which, in most instances, will help to reveal the information about the child's functioning which is the object of the Educational Evaluation.

The flexibility of the interview must remain controlled. This means that the range of areas listed at the beginning of this chapter is used as a guideline. The task is to elicit and demonstrate the child's pattern of functioning in each area by the use of modified approaches.

This aim will lead to a *downward extension* of the use of the items for the *child who falls below the two year level,* the baseline of the standard sequence. It may lead to a *change in the sequence of items or a departure from rigid demand in the case of the inaccessible child* in an attempt to reach the child and elicit possible reactions or responses. It will call for a *departure from strict sequence in cases of inadequate visual or auditory functioning,* when the need to explore the specific difficulty makes it expedient to use the items testing sensory functions before proceeding with the interview. *A judicious departure from the strict sequence* also is indicated *where the nature or severity of the physical handicap or other valid factors* call for specific opportunities to rest or relax by reducing the stress in one or another area. Finally, the provision of flexibility makes possible an *exten-*

sion laterally into an area or areas if the child's responses point to *a specific isolated difficulty* in one or another area.

This admittedly radical innovation in testing serves the purpose of assessing individual potential for developing and learning. Rather than the instrument of the Educational Evaluation being only for the purpose of measuring a child's level as compared to the level expected at his chronologic age, the usefulness of the instrument is extended to an exploration of the underlying causes when the expected level is not achieved. It becomes possible to probe within any area of functioning and *to determine whether the child can function at all in that area, how he can function and how far he can function.*

It is evident that there must be a *qualitative difference* between the majority of children who can cooperate in the structured interview when it is conducted in the standard mode of presentation and those children for whom modifications have to be used. The advantage is that it becomes possible even in extremely difficult cases, by using modified approaches, to assess the child's true potential quantitatively and *to observe systematically his pattern of functioning as it deviates qualitatively.*

Difficulties in cooperating and in reacting and responding observed during the structured interview will parallel the difficulties the child will meet and present in adjusting to a classroom situation. The examiner, utilizing intensive and systematic observation of the child during the interview and the insight he gains into the motivation for the child's responses, will be able to formulate a descriptive report which will make possible more appropriate and effective management of the child both at home and at school.

Detailed directions for modifications will be outlined in chapter 9. A brief explanation will serve here to familiarize the examiner with this essentially simple idea. The sequence of items aims to sample the gradual stages of the ability to perceive, recognize and discriminate. The sequence leads from objects to pictures, from forms to colors, sizes and sounds and then on to more advanced concepts, associations and relationships. A downward extension in any of the primary areas is possible by gradual steps to ever lower levels of demand. First, the number of choices among which the child is expected to make his selection is reduced. If further retreating to lower levels is necessary, the situation can be made more meaningful by the introduction of a doll to whom the objects, pictures, forms or colors can be related in a natural play situation. If such a concrete situation is still beyond the level of comprehension of the child, the material can be related directly to the child. This can be attempted verbally, and if the verbal request is not comprehended, nonverbally. At that level, the examiner when presenting the first item (see Fig. 3), for example, would approach the child's mouth with the spoon and then with the cup and observe his reaction. He would hold out the shoe in the general direction of the child's foot and gesture as if anticipating the child's compliance with this offer to put a shoe on; in very extreme cases it is even advisable to remove one of the child's shoes and later offer a shoe to the side on which the child is stocking-footed. To check the responses, it is then advisable to offer the shoe and the comb and brush in the general direction of the child's mouth and the cup and later the spoon in the general direction of his foot so that an accidental success or an inconclusive one can be demonstrated.

The area explored remains fundamentally the same one. The material utilized to elicit responses or a reaction remains identical with that used in the standard presentation. The innovation is that by a gradual reduction of demand and difficulty the child's level in the area can be determined.

A different problem on the same item would have to be met by a different modification. For instance, when the child is inaccessible to a direct approach because he is inattentive, withdrawn, driven or negative, more indirect approaches have to be used and the examiner may have to experiment with various modifications until a reaction or response can be elicited. Sometimes a child will watch secretly out of the corner of his eyes while the examiner, apparently ignoring him, uses the materials, perhaps feeding, dressing and grooming a doll. Such a child may be lured into performing if the examiner leaves the material available and appears to become busy somewhere else in the room. Inconspicuous but close observation of the child's use of the objects will then give information about his level of recognizing them. It may not be a reliable clue to his potentially highest level, but it will give a satisfactory demonstration of the minimum level he must have achieved since he obviously must be functioning at least on the level on which he can perform. Thus, the child who uses the spoon and comb appropriately on himself, tries to push his or the doll's foot in the shoe, pretends to drink from the cup or even looks for a faucet from which to fill the cup must be developed further than a child who tries to chew each object indiscriminately, including the doll, or throws all objects to the floor indifferently. Sometimes, a negative child can be motivated to perform by an appeal to this very characteristic of negativism by an examiner who challenges him with pretended unconcern. Such a child may reveal his ability to comprehend verbal communication and to recognize objects if he gleefully throws a ball at each object as the examiner names it or even pushes the object in question off the table when challenged to show how fast he can throw it down.

These examples show how the *same* area is explored and the *same* materials used to elicit a response which gives information about the function which is the object of investigation by the use of the item. Only the *approach differs*.

This explanation should serve to dissuade the reader that the Educational Evaluation and the medium of the structured interview are used subjectively, constitute hit and miss guesswork, or that hints are provided to help a child "succeed." A useful evaluation is only guaranteed if the examiner remains an objective observer of the levels on which he can motivate the child to respond. Any need for departure from the standard mode of presentation obviously shows that the exact level of the child cannot be correctly evaluated as equivalent to the assigned age levels. Since the aim is to explore the true potential of the individual child, it is only commonsense to modify the presentation or the demand if a standard mode of presentation fails to reach the child's level. The examiner who can accept this innovation and can learn to go below or outside the range of the standard sequence is here given the opportunity to achieve this objective.

It is important to remember that rapport with the child and the spontaneity of the interview must not be allowed to suffer by a need for a departure from the usual method. Since the materials frequently remain the same, no abrupt departure from the previous standard presentation need become apparent to the child.

7.   Directions for conducting the interview

The most effective use of the material offered in this manual will be made by the interviewer who has familiarized himself thoroughly with the text, the items and the recording form, who has accepted the principles of the Educational Evaluation and the validity of using a structured interview, and who has learned to become less psychometrically minded. Such an examiner will use his skill to establish rapport with the child and will make the items of the sequence serve the purpose of the interview in a systematic, sensitive and flexible way. With practice, he should be able to commit his observations during the interview to memory and only record the interview after the child has been dismissed.

Since every examiner will develop his individual pattern of conducting the Educational Evaluation, only fundamental guidelines will be stressed. Suggestions to facilitate the interview will be explicit and practical. They are intended to take the place of a course of demonstration in training the examiner in this method, which resembles testing but also differs from testing. The externals of the interview situation will be covered by a description of the way the room and the materials are prepared. General suggestions dealing with simple, but carefully worked out, techniques of introducing children to the interview situation may prove helpful, especially since it is foreseen that many of the children interviewed will be handicapped in one way or another. The technique of observing the total behavior pattern of the child will be discussed as well as approaches to meet specific difficulties presented by some of the more frequently found atypical conditions. With such directions as a background, his professional training, skill and judgment will enable the examiner to develop his own ways of using the test material.

A brief summary of the role of the examiner and of his equipment at this point may serve as a survey of the tools, the field of action and the objective. The equipment is composed of the materials used for the sequence of items. The frame of reference is the educational setting appropriate to the child's age, be it nursery school, kindergarten or elementary school. The recording form closely reflects this frame of reference, just as the materials represent it. The explicitness of the clear-cut and immediate purpose of the Evaluation circumscribes and channels the task of the examiner. That task is to determine the child's readiness to profit from an educational program; the Evaluation is never an end in itself.

The recording form (chapter 10) contains headings under which is entered a description of the child's physical and sensory functioning as it relates to learning and developing. Space is provided for the recording of specific responses to the sequence of forty items, as well as for a description of any modification in approach used. Other headings provide space for a description of language behavior and for notes on the over-all behavior pattern. Finally, there is space for a summary: a statement of the levels of functioning, of the causes for poor performance, of abilities, assets and probable potentials, as well as for a formulation of conclusions and recommendations. The report (chapter 12) of the findings about the child is condensed and abstracted from these notes entered on the recording form.

The sequence of items is designed to parallel natural situations and demands made on children in school settings. If functioning is found to be intact and adequate in the responses to test items, it will probably also be intact and adequate in the respective school setting. If it is found to be inadequate and not intact during an Evaluation, the same deficiencies and obstacles will also hinder the child in an appropriate adaptation to school situations. The very nature of the items, incidentally, should help to enable the examiner to learn about and to recognize the adaptive qualities demanded of children at the various levels of school settings. Here, the examiner who has familiarized himself with teaching and education, either through vicarious experience or by actual practice, will be at an advantage, as will the "educational psychologist," a professional worker more prevalent in some European countries than the "clinical psychologist," who predominates in the United States. The functioning pattern of a child, as it is revealed during the interview, must be constantly related to and checked against the background of the school setting, which is the frame of reference for this whole procedure.

Each examiner will work out his own way of dealing with the necessary array of technical equipment. The experienced examiner of young children knows that it sometimes creates difficulties if a book of instructions is placed prominently on the worktable, within view and reach of the child. He also knows that some children will become intrigued with his writing utensils and activity if he is seen taking notes. If time has to be taken out for elaborate entries and consultation of a manual, the child may be found to discard assigned tasks, demand to scribble on his own part, or wander off. It is thus preferable to use the manual and the recording form as unobtrusively as possible. Thoughtful preparation of the room and the materials will facilitate smooth and rapid conduct of the interview. An examiner who uses the Evaluation material frequently may find that as he learns to make the interview sequence and technique his own, he needs to depend less and less on the technical tools. Repeated experience in observing typical and atypical responses to the same items enables many an examiner to learn to recall the particular responses obtained during a specific interview accurately and vividly. It is then possible to postpone the recording of the interview until after the child has left. It is true that perhaps one or another colorful incident may be lost in this way, but the loss will be compensated for by the greater compactness and continuity of the total interview, which will actually result in a more pertinent picture of the child.

One of the main characteristics of the Evaluation, as has been emphasized in previous chapters, is the transfer of the burden of proof from the child who is to be tested to the items which test his level of comprehension. This is necessary because children with handicaps in expression and manipulation may be prevented from performing any but the most minimal signs or signals to indicate a response. Because in each instance such signals will depend entirely on the particular physical limitations, there cannot be a convenient uniformity of signals. The response may be as slight as a purposeful motion of the head, hand, finger or foot, or it may even be as minimal as a perceptible, voluntary shifting of the eyes. The Evaluation, therefore, has to consist of a scale of progressively more difficult or more abstract situations to which a child can continue to respond with his sign of affirmation or negation. When it is considered that the Evaluation includes an investigation of all pertinent areas of functioning, the scope of the interview is seen to be a substantial one. The examiner must learn to look for a multitude of possible responses to a wide range of concrete and abstract situations. He must learn about the various ways in which children with severe handicaps may be able to indicate their responses and he also must learn how to elicit such responses. The criterion, which remains constant and by which responses are judged, is the adequacy or inadequacy of the child's comprehension of the item responded to.

This review of the role of the examiner serves to highlight the relative importance of the various factors in the Educational Evaluation interview. Although the tools and the technique are essential, the keystone is the examiner who uses the tools. Upon him is placed the crucial part of the burden of proof. His willingness to dedicate himself to the task of exploring the potential of a child beyond the formula-use of tool and technique will determine the quality and quantity of information which will be available about the child. This may appear to be a severe burden and it is certainly more demanding than the administration of a psychometric instrument. The user of this material will soon discover, however, that with practice the habit of observation of the total child will become second nature and that it is a worthwhile and satisfying habit. He will gain increased insight into children and will be able to describe and explain them and their educational needs more completely when reporting his findings. The more children he sees and studies, the more he will find to see and to study in each child. He will discover that his changed way of studying children will carry over in his use of other test instruments, to the benefit of the children and the usefulness of his contributions.

The basic guidelines for planning the conduct of the interview are:

1. The first interview with each child begins with the first item.

2. The whole sequence of items in the recording form must be scanned for each child.

3. The emphasis is shifted from sole attention to the correctness or incorrectness of responses to a simultaneous, systematic observation of the total behavior while responding.

4. The items represent the means to elicit typical responses in significant areas; they are tools and as such are subordinated to the purpose which they serve, namely, the evaluation of intactness of functioning.

The interview technique will profit from judicious attention to the following considerations:

a. The age-group in question is traditionally one for which reasoned and ready compliance with a formal situation cannot be taken for granted. Therefore, the successful conduct of an interview with a preschool child will depend largely on the skill with which the examiner learns to temper his approach to the individual child; adaptations will have to be made on the part of the examiner since the child cannot be expected to appreciate the reason for and the meaning of such an interview.

b. The items of this sequence had to be purposely planned to be of such a nature that minimal responses, of which even the most severely physically involved child is capable, will serve to indicate reliable responses; therefore, the reduced need and scope for active manipulation tends to lead to restlessness with some very active children, unless high motivation and interest can be maintained by presenting the items in rapid succession.

c. Familiarity with the items and with the sequence will contribute materially to the habit of making mental notes of pertinent responses and patterns; this is desirable because the spontaneity and the smooth progress of the interview will be interfered with if there are frequent pauses for note-taking. The examiner will be wise to plan in such a way that time will be available immediately after an interview to record his findings and impressions while all pertinent details are still fresh in his mind.

d. Until an examiner gains enough experience with this method to develop his own efficient pattern of using the material, it is advisable to plan two sessions in order to complete an evaluation.

The time required ranges from forty-five minutes to two hours or more. The briefest session the author has ever conducted took only thirty minutes and, paradoxically, was conducted with a bright, severely handicapped, six year old girl with cerebral palsy who could neither sit, stand nor speak. She was interviewed while resting on her back on a floormat, with the examiner kneeling beside her. She responded reliably, speedily and correctly to every item presented to her, using nothing but her eyes to point out her answers. (For illustration, see Fig. 8.)

The prospective examiner may have gathered from the description of the origin and nature of the structured interview and of the difficulties presented by handicapped children in the testing situation that his previous training in administering tests may not have adequately prepared him for conducting an Evaluation interview. Not only must he learn to recognize and elicit responses which may be performed in unusual and minimal forms but he also must learn to enlarge the focus of his inquiry from sole attention to an isolated response to a simultaneous observation of total behavior. Not only is he to present a sequence of items but he also must be prepared to modify an item or the sequence.

While it is expected that the user of this manual will be well trained and qualified, it is recognized that the best academic preparation cannot initiate an examiner into the innumerable and unforeseeable eventualities of actual interviews with children who are handicapped. Since the examiner is asked to acquire some novel habits of conducting an interview, it is felt that it is not a presumption but an obligation to provide some form of guidance.

What will be offered, then, will be comparable to an invitation to enter an interview room and sit in for the beginning of an Evaluation. An opportunity to observe the by-plays and innuendos representative of some or many situations and of one or several children can be provided in this manner. The beginning of an interview will be described. Since problems in functioning tend to be magnified in children handicapped by cerebral palsy and since some of the same problems, although perhaps more subtly manifested, may also be found in the functioning pattern of children with other handicaps, the discussion will deal with the problems encountered in testing children with cerebral palsy. Not every one of the eventualities listed and discussed here will be met with in a single interview with a given cerebral palsied child. Also, some of the problems found in testing children with cerebral palsy may never be encountered in the testing of children without cerebral palsy. But the technique of constant and alert observation and the knack of resourceful, immediate adaptation to observed deviations in functioning can best be illustrated by a slow-motion demonstration of the conduct of an interview with a child with cerebral palsy.

More and more evidence points to the possibility of neurologic concomitants of conditions of reduced intellectual functioning. Malformation of the brain, subtle and minimal brain damage may be present in a child even though he may show no or little motor handicap. The examiner of handicapped children needs a thorough grounding in the observation of the child with cerebral palsy to sharpen his powers of observation. Slight hints of malfunctioning resembling typical difficulties seen in the pattern of a cerebral palsied child will prompt him to explore more specifically the performance of a child in whom no gross neurologic signs are present.

DIRECTIONS FOR THE CONDUCT OF THE INTERVIEW properly begin with the concrete preparations necessary to make the interview simple, smooth and effective. Chapter 4 described the requirements for the interview in a general way. In the concrete situation, here and now, it is the task *to prepare the environment and the child himself*. Therefore, the preparation of the room and the material will be described and the introduction of the child to the examiner and to the interview room will be discussed.

Before the interview the examiner should read or obtain the data on the developmental history of the child. This is described in detail in chapter 4. Since it is impracticable and unwise to make the child wait, it is preferable that this part of the preparation be accomplished in advance of the interview. An experienced examiner will be able to conclude from the developmental data and from a description of the child's domestic behavior much about the way the child appears to function. The anticipated level of functioning, as well as possible deviations in functioning, may be revealed by comparison with the typical patterns with which an examiner learns to become familiar.

It is necessary to meet with the child and the parent briefly before attempting to start the interview. This is probably best done in an office or waiting room. This brief inspection of the child, together with the recorded material available about the child, will inform the examiner as to the physical set-up which will be required and the range of items which may be needed. If the child is old enough to comprehend, the examiner should introduce himself not only to the parent but also to the child. When feasible, the examiner may then say: "As soon as I have all the toys and things ready, you can come in and then you and I will look at them and play." The reaction of the child to this invitation should be observed carefully for an indication of the child's readiness to accompany the examiner alone or whether he will need his mother with him. The location of the bathroom should be pointed out to the parent so that the child can be taken before the interview; this will save time later on.

The examiner then prepares the seating arrangements and the materials which will be needed. The physical set-up is discussed at length in chapter 4. (See also Figs. 1, 2, 3, 4A, 4B and 8) The examiner selects a suitable chair for the child and places a corresponding chair for the examiner, removes the other chairs from the work area, arranges the lighting, being especially careful that the child will not face a window and have bright light shining in his eyes. If it appears likely that the mother will have to be invited in because the child needs her presence, a regular-size chair is placed for her. This chair should be somewhat in back of the child and to the side. This arrangement will suffice to reassure most children that the mother is near but will allow them to become involved in the interview without feeling a constant obligation to work for her approval. Some young children will have to start the interview on the mother's lap, either due to their young age or to shyness, but it may later be possible to place them in a chair if they become engrossed in activities. Except for the very distractible child, who is placed with the table pushed up to the wall and with his back to the room to cut out all possible distractions (Fig. 4B), the child and examiner sit opposite each other, with the table between them (Figs. 1 and 2). The table should be approximately 36 inches long and 20 to 24 inches wide and low enough so that the child can rest his elbows on the table surface. Comfort and safety in the seating arrangement is especially important, when the child is physically handicapped. With young and shy children, it is important to remember to avoid carefully any need for the examiner to move physically between the child and his mother. At least during the early part of the interview, some children become panicky when this occurs. Knowing his mother is at his side, while the examiner sits opposite safely separated by the table, often gives the child a feeling of safety, which is helpful to start off the interview in a favorable atmosphere.

Before the child is taken to the room a suitable toy is placed on the table, or perhaps on the floor if the child is still in the creeping stage. This toy might be a musical spinning top, a large ball, a doll, a picture book or the hundred-hole peg board if the child has fair to good hands. (This peg board is one of the modification toys in the set.) The purpose of this is to deflect the child's attention from the door which will be closed behind him, and perhaps from the examiner, who at that moment is still a stranger to the child, to a familiar and neutral object. The more familiar or tempting this "warm-up" toy is, the quicker will be the child's initial occupation with it. Some children seem almost to shut out the examiner by their intensive or pretended interest in the toy during the first few minutes. If they are given such a breathing spell, during which some will quickly take in the room or look at the door calculatingly, they frequently will then welcome an approach from the examiner.

The materials of the sequence are lined up in the order in which they will be needed. This order is available in the recording form (chapter 10). The recording form states the age ranges, both the range within which items can be presented and the one by which intellectual readiness normally can be expected. On the basis of the preliminary review of the record and the brief inspection of the child prior to preparing the room, the examiner can have made an approximate estimate of the upper limit the child will reach and have chosen his materials accordingly. If it appears likely that modifications will be needed, these are also placed ready. Lining up the materials in the order in which they will be presented makes it possible to find each item as it is needed; this cuts down or eliminates a constant dependence on the recording form or the manual during the interview.

A convenient way to arrange materials is on an inexpensive six by one foot shelf, fastened to the wall with brackets and high enough so that children cannot reach it from the floor. It can serve to hold the whole series of items in the order in which they will be used. Such an arrangement is especially helpful when hyperactive children or very retarded and uninhibited children are to be tested. The child will not be distracted because he cannot see what is on the shelf. He will not be tempted to finger every item or to sweep the material to the floor, as he might do if the material were more accessible. He will be better able to concentrate and to confine himself to the tasks presented by the examiner, which permits his true potential to be determined more reliably.

If the materials are to be lined up on a table, the table holding them should be in back of the examiner's chair, out of reach of the child and partly hidden from view by the examiner. This will make it possible to keep up a steady flow of materials to the child and to return each to the supply table in exchange for the next item.

Materials that are especially attractive, such as the bells, music box, milk bottle set and the flashlight, are placed either so that they are hidden by bulkier materials, such as the box containing the story objects, or are covered with a towel to screen them from view. The sound blocks are placed so that the softest sounding one can be identified quickly by the examiner at the appropriate moment. The flashlight is checked so that no time need be wasted in last minute adjustments once the interview is underway.

Pencils, crayons and plain sheets of paper should be kept on hand. Large hexagon-shaped crayons are more suitable for small hands and for children with manual difficulties than thin round ones, and crayons are preferred to pencils by most children of preschool age. A supply of tissues must be kept within reach; these may be needed when a child sneezes or drools; tissues are also used for certain modifications that involve hiding or wrapping up objects for testing purposes.

General outlines for the physical set-up were given in chapter 4. Suggestions about various ways to adapt the physical set-up to the personality and the needs of given children will be found there.

Only after all or most of the expected eventualities have been provided for is *the examiner ready to call for the child.*

The following description is of general measures that will serve to introduce most children smoothly and successfully into the interview situation.

These measures have been found workable with many children over many years. There are, of course, children who enjoy the challenge and attention which testing involves; there are others who have been prepared appropriately by their parents for the experience; and there are friendly, outgoing children who have been in nursery school or kindergarten and who look forward to the session as a form of playing school. With all these robust little people the examiner will use his own approach. But, in general, the situation is not one of the child's own choosing and the examiner needs to win the child's confidence and cooperation. The examiner should be in control of the situation, and this can be accomplished best by anticipating the child's possible reactions before they get out of hand. It is for this reason that thoughtful preparation for the first few minutes of the interview pays off in the long run.

The Evaluation begins with the first contact with the child. As the examiner returns to call for the child, it will be possible to *observe the child's readiness to accompany the examiner alone, his necessity for having his mother come along, or unusual difficulties he presents.* Unless the child is in obvious distress, crying, angry or fearful, the examiner, child and mother start casually for the interview room, with the examiner talking about "the nice time we are going to have." If the child holds back, clings to the mother or looks worried, the examiner invites the mother into the room matter-of-factly and may precede mother and child into the room, immediately indicating to the mother where she is to sit. On the other hand, depending on the child's observed readiness, the examiner may let the child precede him into the room and tactfully dismiss the mother quietly, informing her of the approximate length of time the interview will take or just saying cheerfully: "We will see you when we are finished."

A nonverbal but friendly management of the child for the first few minutes of the interview seems to be more reassuring for many children than verbal communication. It absolves the child from an obligation to speak, which is especially important if he is shy, immature or has poor speech. This kind of nonverbal management is very different from a "silent treatment," which would only serve to bewilder the child. Rather, it is a smiling, friendly, surehanded concern with the child's comfort and should give a feeling of mutual preparation for a pleasant visit. It should help to make the child feel that he and the examiner will be able to get along with each other. If a child is quite verbal and if he is responsive to conversation, the examiner will of course respond in kind.

Once the child has been gentled into the room, the examiner must be willing to lead a double life. Overtly, he must be relaxed, seem leisurely and show deep interest in and response to the child's own reactions to everything he suggests. Inwardly, he must be alert, concentrate on the essentials, keep his goal in mind, which is the evaluation of intactness of functioning, commit to memory all observed aspects of the interview for later recording, evaluate responses and behavior constantly and adapt readily to deviations in functioning and in behavior with suitable modifications. He must slow down or speed up the tempo of the interview to meet the child's needs. He must remove materials skillfully after they have been used.

If, after a few moments, a child who apparently was ready to remain without his mother changes his mind and decides that he wants her after all, the examiner casually complies without giving the impression that this is unusual or a big concession. If, however, a child expresses a wish to see his mother halfway through the interview, it is best either to let him go to "tell his mother how well he is doing," or perhaps go with him to give this reassuring information and then lead him casually but firmly back to the room.

The seating of the child will differ with his physical and emotional status. The nonwalking child will have to be helped to his chair and may need aid in unlocking his braces, if he wears them. The child who is heedless or awkward is helped in order to forestall the chance of a fall at this critical first moment. The child who silently refuses to sit down is left standing tacitly, with his chair in back of him. If the mother tends to become insistent or impatient, it may be helpful to say quietly: "It's all right. He can stand until he is ready."

The examiner, sitting down at some distance from the child, can divert the child's attention from any misgivings he might have by casually starting to use the "warm-up" toy, unless the child by now has begun to do this on his own. If the child needs a little time to look around, familiarize himself with the room, or perhaps express himself to his mother, the wise examiner waits pleasantly but expectantly and continues casually to play with the toy with a general air that suggests anyone can join in the fun. If a shy or inhibited child then shows signs of approaching the toy, it can be pushed closer with a cheerful smile or a comment: "That's right. You play too." When the child begins to enjoy himself, the examiner must judge whether the child is ready to have him join in or still needs a little period of grace in which to play alone. If the latter is the case, the examiner can become strategically occupied with a more distant article. In most instances, this interlude only takes a few minutes, but these few minutes frequently decide the course which the rest of the interview will take.

The observations which can be made about handedness, motor development, visual functioning and other areas during the child's initial occupation with the toy will be described later when observation techniques are discussed. At this point, comments will be limited to management of the interview prior to the presentation of the standard test items. The examiner now begins to gather the objects of the first item (chapter 8, see also Fig. 3), and when the child begins to look a little bored with his solitary play, starts to line up these objects slowly before the child. If the child does not or cannot spontaneously push or lift his first toy toward the examiner when he sees something new coming up, the examiner may say: "Are you ready?" or "Are you finished with this?" and simultaneously hold out his hand to receive the toy. There is seldom any objection to a change of scenery at this point, especially if the examiner calls attention to the new objects with a pleasant: "Look what I have." Any verbal comment of the child, such as naming the objects as they are lined up, is received in a friendly manner; it is also stored away as part of the observations made on the child's language behavior which the examiner will continue to make all during the interview.

By the time the first objects are lined up before the child, he is usually quite ready to be directly and verbally addressed by the examiner. If he did not sit down immediately, he probably has settled down in his chair almost automatically by now if resistance has been avoided by avoiding any sort of admonition or pressure.

As a rule the interview can then begin as directed in chapter 8. It is wise to have the material for the next item ready as one removes the previous one. It will help keep the child interested if he does not have to sit before an empty table and wait idly. It will also induce him to release his hold on some interesting material after it has served its purpose rather than deciding to play with it a while in his own way.

The child who finds it unusually difficult to come into the interview room needs to be approached with great caution. It sometimes is worthwhile to take one or two toys, such as a spinning top, a music box, a ball, a doll or a small toy car to the room where the child is waiting. If the child is crying, the examiner ignores him at first and instead sits down near the mother and casually begins to speak with her. This can go on for a few minutes, during which time the examiner may continue to ignore the crying in a friendly and unworried manner, perhaps patting the child's shoulder or offering him a tissue to wipe his eyes. If this can be done with the right combination of unconcern and comradely friendliness and with a complete absence of impatience or remonstration, the child will frequently begin to get a little curious or even bored. Still respecting the child's reserve, the examiner can then try to begin using one of the toys without directly addressing the child but with a general air of inviting him to join in. With some children, it is even a helpful trick to drop the toy accidentally or in some other way to pretend to put oneself in a mildly ridiculous position and to persuade the mother to join in a spontaneous and hearty laugh about it.

Care must be taken lest the child mistakenly suspect that the laughter is at his expense. Sometimes a child will try to have the examiner repeat the mistake in order to have his mother laugh again. As the child gradually ceases to cry, he may be given one of the toys to hold, if he is so inclined. It is then advisable to suggest to the mother that she carry him in the interview room, even if he can walk alone, adding the comment: "There are some more nice toys in there." On the way in, a remark should be made, ostensibly to the mother and in an undertone but in such a way that the child will surely overhear it, that is some praise of the child's looks, or his nice suit or dress, necktie or hair ribbon, new shoes or nail polish. Frequently, such a device disarms and wins over the child because he senses that the examiner is on his side and blames neither him nor his mother for the preceding fuss. The calm and unhurried manner of the examiner makes him feel that his crying was accepted and understood. In consequence, such a child frequently becomes quite responsive and trusting in a very short time. Frequent praise at the beginning of the interview and perhaps even a few spurious successes, if necessary, will then pave the way to a successful session.

More severe conditions of real emotional disturbance and how to manage them in order to gentle the child into the interview situation will be discussed toward the end of this chapter.

One commonsense consideration, which is frequently overlooked, is the need to select that hour for the interview which is one of the child's natural waking hours. This is especially important when testing young children who still nap once or twice daily. It is also wise to select a suitable hour when one plans to test an older child who reportedly has a disturbed sleeping cycle, possibly being wakeful part of each night and habitually sleeping late into the forenoon.

As the interview gets under way, it will sometimes become necessary to *help the mother to understand and accept her role*. As a rule, it will be sufficient to ask her to let the examiner take over, so that the child will not become confused by conflicting instructions. There are some instances, especially with very young or immature children, where the mother will need to be drawn into the situation. The materials will have to be related to her, or they may even have to be presented by her under the direction of the examiner, until the child gradually becomes able to respond directly to the examiner.

The simple and familiar character of the first objects helps most children to forget their reservations, if any, and to become intrigued in a favorable way. Rapport is then quickly established. The older child rapidly loses any apprehension he may have had about his capacity to cooperate, since he, too, begins with the first item, which is simple for him. It may be necessary to explain to the more sophisticated four or five year old: "We have to do these baby games first." Or: "If you were little and I said, 'Give me the shoe,' what would you have to give me?" Such an approach makes the simpler tasks acceptable if a child has any qualms about being asked to do something that appears too easy. The confidence gained by initial successes frequently generates a momentum which carries the child happily through the early part of the interview.

Similarly, the child who has difficulty in verbal or manual performance frequently is helped in his initial adjustment to the examiner and the testing situation by the concreteness, simplicity and size of the first objects. They and the elementary demand of the first item provide him with an opportunity to experiment with, practice, or be taught some form of responding and to arrive at some sort of understanding with the examiner about signals or signs within his physical capacity. The examiner has occasion to study the child's answering technique or to help him develop a means of responding.

A brief enumeration of the observations which the examiner can make during the initial play period follows. In addition to serving as a natural and informal medium of establishing rapport, this period teaches the careful observer much about the child's way of functioning. The technique of observing behavior minutely and of continuously and immediately interpreting it during the interview starts with the first contact and ceases only with the termination of the interview. As the sequence of items brings into focus one significant area of functioning after another, each area is subjected to investigation by the systematic use of this technique of educated observation.

The extent and kind of findings will differ with the "warm-up" toy which has been used. Simpler toys, which may be indicated for use with young and shy children, will yield less information than will the more elaborate toys, but to the trained observer any activity of the child tells something pertinent, and even the absence of activity has its meaning. The toys described here are by no means the only ones that may be useful, but they do have special appeal. One, of course, never uses the actual test items for this purpose, except in desperate situations. Toward the end of this chapter, some instances will be discussed.

The following are samples of some of the observations that can be made:

If a *ball* is used, it can be observed how the child manipulates the ball, whether two-handedly, whether by pushing it or by kicking it with his foot; whether he throws, rolls or bounces it; whether he shows resourcefulness in retrieving the ball if it has rolled under the table; whether he engages in reciprocal games with the mother or even the examiner or prefers to play by himself and how long he remains interested in the activity.

If the *spinning top* has been used, it can be observed what length of time the child watches without interruption; whether he attempts to make the top go by himself and which hand he uses; whether he succeeds and what his reaction is to success or failure. Any verbal or nonverbal communication during the initial play period is observed alertly and responded to readily. The spinning top is an especially suitable toy for breaking the ice with very young, very inhibted and also with very severely handicapped children. Since it moves, it is sufficient just to watch it from a safe distance; it is possible to remain completely passive and yet evince an interest in this toy. Where interest and attention are brief, the continued motion of the toy recalls them again and again. Since the motion eventually stops, there is occasion for the child to demonstrate a termination of interest or else give a show of demand for a repetition of the experience; either of these reactions reveals something about the child.

If the "warm-up" toy has been a *picture book,* observation will reveal the way in which the child manipulates and uses books: whether he turns single pages or several at one time; whether he holds the book right side up or not; whether he looks at the picture with comprehension or only enjoys the tactile experience of handling a book; whether he names some picture spontaneously or perhaps looks at those his mother has named; whether he wants to share his enjoyment of the book or refuses to share it; how long he remains interested in the activity; or, finally, whether, having been overestimated, he wants to tear, chew or throw the book. If this should be his only response, it is best to substitute for the book, quickly and in a friendly way, the ball or the spinning top. If this arouses a storm of protest, a sheet of paper to tear up and throw on the floor might be substituted. The examiner will, in the meantime, have revised his initial estimate of the child's probable level.

The use of the *doll* will show which hand the child uses to approach it; whether he can hold it appropriately or not; whether he spontaneously begins to undress or explore the doll, or perhaps hugs and kisses it; if a doll nursing bottle is offered, whether he brings it to the doll's mouth (or perhaps to his own) appropriately or not; whether he mimics in the handling of the bottle some realistic activities, such as shaking the bottle, fixing the nipple, or holding it against his face as if testing the temperature of it; or perhaps whether his very concrete way of thinking prevents him from wishing to use it until some actual liquid has been poured into it for him. It can be noted whether he addresses the doll, verbally or nonverbally; whether he mimics a sucking sound when "feeding" the doll; whether he wants to share his play or not, and how long he remains interested.

As can be seen, information becomes available, in this informal and preliminary way, concerning the child's level in self-help activities such as dressing and feeding. Comprehension and awareness of the feeding and dressing process precede the semidependent or independent use of such functions and the child therefore tells by his behavior something about his potential. Where there is delayed language development, an observation of a mimicked sound made during this play, be it a sucking noise, a pretended crying of the doll, or perhaps a tune hummed while playing, is an important finding. The nature and cause of the delay in language development are difficult areas to explore and every positive finding will contribute to an accumulation of observed data useful for arriving at an eventual diagnosis by the specialists studying such a child's problem.

The toy of preference when the child has fair to good hands is *the hundred-hole peg board and pegs.* It is a self-explanatory toy, acceptable to most children and appealing to a wide variety of age levels. It can be used by a very young or very retarded child, who may be persuaded to imitate inserting a peg or two if the examiner places the peg in his hand and guides it conveniently over the board. It may be used by a creative and imaginative child to make complex designs or to plot a landscape with streets and fences, lawns and flowers, by ingenious use of the color pegs. Within these two extremes, most preschool children will be able to find their own level of using this material. The observations which can be made by an alert examiner while the child occupies himself in this way will be enhanced if pegs are placed on both sides of the board, for instance, in a flat box and its cover. The type of grasp, the preferred hand if any, whether both hands have an equally good pincer grasp, transfer of pegs from the nonleading hand to the leading one, accuracy and firmness of insertion, all these and other telltale ways of using the match-sized pegs give informtion about manual functioning. Selection of colors; attention to the placement of the pegs; resourceful ways of gathering the pegs, such as filling the nonleading hand and holding the supply ready for rapid use by the leading hand; the use and the degree of complexity of designs; the use and the level of imagination when projecting ideas on the board, all these factors reveal something about the child's intellectual maturity. Accuracy in finding the appropriate holes; filling rows without skipping holes; placing pegs in rows from left to right systematically; meaningful use of one or another color and other observable facts give clues about the adequacy and the level of development of visual functioning. The tendency to bunch pegs in one spot, consistently ignoring one side of the board; strained peering at a distant part of the board; fumbling for holes or skipping holes without apparent notice of the empty spaces between filled stretches; dropping of pegs and upsetting placed pegs while retrieving fallen ones; a tendency to slide pegs slowly over the board until they are caught by a hole, these and similar observations may reveal limitations in visual functioning or in eye-motion. If such performances are observed in a child with strabismus, or in one who must hold his head at a peculiar angle while inserting pegs, the examiner is particularly alerted to the possibility of difficulty in visual functioning. This can then be probed further during the presentation of the first few items of the interview and will have to be taken into account in the form of presentation and in the sequence of presentation; the items testing visual functioning may have to be used before going on with the rest of the interview. If the difficulty is mild, the manner of presentation may be adapted to the difficulty, the material being placed within the space that the child is reliably able to spot and to scan. If it is severe, postponement of the interview until after there has been a medical examination of the visual functioning may be necessary, or if the child is resourceful and cooperative, perhaps those items which do not depend on great visual effort may be presented and the others postponed until an eye check-up has been possible.

The level of social maturation also is often revealed during this play with the "warm-up" toy. A child may offer pegs to the examiner, invite him to use the side of the peg board nearest him, comment sociably about the mutual activity. Language behavior frequently can be observed when a child spontaneously describes what he is making with the material.

These then are the preparations leading up to the actual presentation of the sequence of items in the structured interview. To summarize: The room has been prepared. The materials have been lined up conveniently in the order in which they will be needed; the manual and the recording form are within reach but not prominently displayed. The child and the examiner are seated opposite each other and the preliminary play period has helped to establish rapport between them. The objects of the first item are on the table and the child and the examiner are ready.

The examiner has stored away in his memory the pertinent data about the child's developmental history and has a preliminary idea of the items which will be needed for this particular child. He has referred to the recording form and checked the Roman numerals for the age range when items are to be presented and the Arabic numerals for the age levels when children are expected to succeed on the item; he thus knows quickly what each succeeding item will be. He will begin the sequence of forty items with the first item, no matter what the age of the child is, and he will scan the whole sequence for those items placed later in the scale which are marked clearly: "Not to be omitted." These are the items testing sensory functioning.

If the child is not able to speak, he will have obtained from the parent a description of the child's signs or mode of communication, if any. Perhaps the child, under the guidance of the parent, has already demonstrated his signs for the examiner.

Proceeding to the fictional representative interview, which was proposed as the most graphic means of training the examiner in this technique of Educational Evaluation, a description can now be given of how the examiner has to function when he presents the items to the children with cerebral palsy and at the same time learns to understand their answering technique and observes systematically their total way of functioning.

The first consideration has to be with the safety and comfort of the seating arrangement. Even when sitting *balance* on a straight chair has been achieved by the child, it is frequently advisable to use the arm chair or the relaxation chair for the interview. This is so because long habituation to precarious balance may have resulted in a persistence of poor habits: the child may have learned to be content with sitting rather tensely and moving very cautiously, keeping his head forward and avoiding sudden motions of the arms or of the trunk if past experience has taught him that such exertion may lead to falls off the chair. He may be more concerned with maintaining his balance than with performing for the examiner. Confining himself to looking cautiously only forward and through a very narrow arc to left and right, he may fail to see materials lined up to the extreme left or right. Failure to perform correctly on the first item can be the result of poor sitting balance or poor habits retained from earlier poor balance rather than a true reflection of his intellectual level. But since the examiner also wants to study his potential for functioning in a school setting, when a suitable item is reached the examiner can suggest that the child use a straight chair, helping him to it at a point during the interview when this can be done naturally, perhaps after a search for a pellet dropped on the floor (item 22b). Since the next item calls for some manipulation, involving as it does a pushbutton bell and a music box (item 23), the examiner will then have an excellent opportunity to observe in what way the child is limited in adequate use of his physical equipment by poor balance, poor habit or fear of falling. Children sometimes are not cognizant of their self-imposed restrictions, and teachers, occasionally encouraged by therapists, may wish to give the child as much practice as possible in maintaining sitting balance on a straight chair in the classroom, once he has achieved this coveted stage. Thus resulting restrictions in functioning may be discounted. The Evaluation aims to detect such pernicious interrelationships of the handicapping condition, as they affect the ability to function in the classroom.

A limitation in scanning a wide arc, once the examiner has recognized it and its implications, will prompt him to spot the same manifestation if present in a physically normal child. Such a child may fail to look left or right due to mental retardation with consequent lack of initiative or curiosity. The examiner will also be alerted when a child misses materials at one or the other side of the table to possible limitations in the visual field. Each cause will require a specific accommodation in the presentation of materials to the child, depending on the specific difficulty. Thus, the child with poor balance is placed in an appropriate chair and is then encouraged to look systematically all the way from the left end of the table to the right end as he scans the possible choices of responses. The child who fails to look anywhere except directly in front of himself because the degree of his retardation is such that he is not able to appreciate the significance of the situation or the need to make an effort is trained during the interview. The examiner can lift up each object in turn, causing the child to look, or he may rap on the table next to each object to attract the child's attention, or he may guide the child's hand from object to object to help him perceive them manually and visually at the same time. The child whose difficulty appears to be a limitation of the visual field is made aware of the fact that objects are visible at each extreme end of the table as well as in the center. If he then can learn to discover each object by turning his head, he is encouraged to use this means of circumventing his handicap, or else the materials are moved until they are all within his field of vision.

The child may have poor head balance. His head may drop forward or to the side. It may be thrust backward by strong muscle pull. Another child may have seizures or petit mal and drop his head forward suddenly and unexpectedly. It sometimes is necessary to pad the edge of the table nearest the child with a layer of folded towels, which can be fastened with strips of adhesive tape or scotch tape. The construction of the relaxation chair is such (Fig. 3) that the child can rest his head against the wings of the chair and perhaps maintain it stabilized in that manner for brief periods of application to the tasks. Frequent rest periods are indicated for such children. Some children with a hyperextended back or a backward thrust of the head, although they are perhaps able to sit in the relaxation chair, may be more comfortable on their backs or even on their stomachs on a table mat or a floor mat (Fig. 8). Materials can then be presented placed on a tray with a rim and in the stand, depending on the item.

Use of the *upper extremities* may be interfered with in various ways. The child may be unable to use one or both arms. He may be able to use two, one or no hands. He may have a fair-functioning hand on the side of his poorer arm or shoulder, while he may have no control over the other hand even though that arm may have a fair range of motion. He may be able to grasp with his fingers but have no ability to release or to maintain the hold. In the functional use of arm, hand and trunk, he may be forced to turn his body as one piece, so that his trunk turns away from the table as his hand tries to approach it; by the time his hand can reach forward, his eyes may face away from the front and he may no longer be able to see what he is trying to reach or point to. Initial handedness may be confused by the fact that the dominant side may also be the more affected one, so that his manipulation will appear to be a series of hesitating attempts when, in reality, he may try instinctively to start an activity with the leading hand, only to substitute the nonleading but less involved hand for a second attempt, in his drive to succeed. Involuntary motion of shoulder, arm or hand may interfere with any useful function. While the items can be responded to with only eye-pointing or signs of assent and negation, the spontaneous use of the upper extremities is observed carefully since they affect the functioning of the child in the classroom and his potential for future manual activities.

Younger children with cerebral palsy sometimes cannot be made to understand that they need not exert themselves but can indicate their responses by looking at the right answer. They may have the same drive to touch and manipulate as young nonhandicapped children and some retarded older ones. Young children also may not yet be aware of the fact that they are handicapped; they may not yet have observed that not everybody has the constant difficulties which they experience every time they try to use their hands. While the examiner then has to wait and watch them struggle laboriously, it will at least be possible to observe what resourcefulness they can muster and how persistent they can remain. Some children, when failing to reach the desired spot with the hand, will triumphantly bring the face close to the object or card selected in a multiple choice item and touch it with the nose or the tip of the tongue.

Whatever the child's pattern, it will need careful observation. One child may be able to use only one arm. As he attempts to lift this arm and guide it to the selection he wants to point out, he may appear to indicate indiscriminately always the object or card on that particular side of the table. Only when one observes his eyes and facial expression to judge whether he strains to reach the correct spot but is physically slow in doing so or whether he actually fails to appreciate the difference between the items, does his intent become known. Another child may still have a pattern of bilateral approach, or else his one arm may ape the motions executed by the other arm, or the only way he can reach for objects may be by a sudden scissor-like clasping with both hands. The involuntary motion and the vagueness in approaching the correct choice may appear to the inexperienced observer or to the unobservant examiner to be an inability to decide between choices or an intentional ambiguity, offered on purpose in the hope that one of the two answers might be correct. With his eyes, however, the child may have picked out the correct answer immediately. An expression of purposeful effort until he has reached the correct spot, and perhaps an expression of relief when he has succeeded in getting his hand there finally, would be further proof of the child's initial plan.

Appearing to fumble for the correct answer can also be observed in the functioning of those children who have to turn the trunk away from the table in order to bring one hand to the front and of those who may be handicapped visually by an alternating strabismus. The former may no longer be able to look at the material by the time the hand is brought forward and they may appear to grope undecidedly or may even pick up the wrong object. The examiner must be willing to wait until the child indicates that he is satisfied with his choice lest this fumbling manner be mistaken for indecision. If the response appears inconclusive, the examiner should bring the selected object into the child's field of vision after the child has reached a decision. The child can then be observed for an expression of satisfaction with a terminated performance (correct or incorrect) or for recognition of the fact that, due to being unable to see while reaching and having misjudged the distance or direction, he has pointed out the wrong answer.

The child who has an alternating strabismus of one or both eyes may experience a similar difficulty to the above. His eyes may have turned inward or outward by the time he reaches for what he has just seen, so that he, too, has to depend on his touch and his remembered estimate of the position of the material or make an attempt to focus one of his eyes anew, in order to respond by a correct grasping or pointing.

Responses like these, which, to the uninitiated or inexperienced, look like random attempts to guess at the right answer or even like meaningless involuntary motions, are actually the outcome of hard work on the part of the child. Not only must he decide upon the correct answer but he must also try to make his unruly body obey his bidding. Another pitfall which may trap the unwary examiner of the young or immature child with cerebral palsy is that a child may have received training in reaching, grasping and placing of objects by an occupational therapist, and having been told that he is brought to the interview to "play some games" and being unable to appreciate the significance of an Evaluation interview, he may neglect to listen to instructions carefully when first starting to work and may try his best to demonstrate his achieved proficiency by industriously picking up the test objects one after another. He will have to be instructed, on his level of understanding, that, "Today we are playing a different kind of game," until it is evident that he is ready and able to get the idea. Sometimes, with a child who comes to the interview with this kind of previous conditioning, it helps to challenge him by simply changing the emphasis one places on the words in the request. Instead of asking him to "look at" or "give me" or "show me," one might say: "Can YOU give me the cup? or: "I wonder if you can find the SHOE." In this way, he may eventually be able to switch from the previous set of mind which he has learned so obediently.

Some of the patterns and deviations which an examiner will observe in children without cerebral palsy will be reminiscent of those described in the discussion of problems that may be encountered in testing children with cerebral palsy. They will assume more meaningful importance because they can now be related more directly to causes and effects of such deviations. They also will probably be spotted more alertly by an examiner who has learned to watch the total functioning of a child during an interview. Some of the deviations more frequently found when testing large numbers of retarded, physically normal children are: awkwardness of grasp; delay in the emergence of pincer grasp; unevenness of emergence of pincer grasp on both hands; delay in establishing a dominant hand, with a tendency to transfer objects from hand to hand as if experimenting to establish the greater usefulness of one or the other hand; delay in unilateral approach to objects; and apparent lack of sensitivity in fingertips. Some of these characteristics show up on the specific items probing these areas, such as the pellet and bottle item, the winding of the music box, the tapping of the pushbutton table bell. A child may be able to pick up pellets with ease with one of his hands, opposing thumb and index finger normally, while with the other hand he may use a raking motion or grasp pellets with the thumb opposed to three or four fingers. When winding the music box, some children cannot execute a complete circular motion with the crank. These findings are important for two reasons. If such subtle delays and difficulties are detected in the functioning of a child who has no gross neurologic defect, they point to the possibility of subtle impairment or pathology; the examiner can then contribute this data as an aid to the neurologist in establishing his diagnosis. Since such manifestations of delayed neurologic maturation or impaired neurologic intactness are not present in every retarded child, many of whom have excellent manual abilities, these findings can not be considered incidental; they may eventually lead to a better insight into the cause of the retardation. The other aspect of the importance of these observable findings is their direct implication for the potential for functioning of the child. Obstacles which the child meets and demonstrates during the interview will correspond to obstacles he will meet and present in a training and educational program. He will be slow in learning to unbutton and button his clothing if his type of grasp is palmar rather than pincer. Shoelaces will baffle him. His hold on a crayon or pencil will be awkward. He will be unable to complete a circle with pencil on paper if he is unable to complete the circular motion required to wind a music box crank. This in turn will influence the performance of which he is capable when he is asked to "draw a man;" while the intent may be appropriate, the result will look like the product of a younger or more retarded child. The same difficulty will be present when he tries to turn a doorknob or a key. He may be clumsy in self-feeding activities. He will find it difficult to manipulate scissors.

The functional linkage of handicap and performance needs to be explored in every case during the Evaluation interview. In that way the technique of educated observation serves the frame of reference, which is its justification: the educational setting and program for the child.

Returning now to the fictional interview, it can be appreciated how the first few minutes, by means of the technique of systematic observation presented here in slow motion, have already resulted in a considerable sum of information about the functioning pattern of the child. The headings on the first page of the recording form will have become more pertinent, as the reader can begin to project this information upon the blank spaces. Before going ahead with a description of modes of responding other than the ones just demonstrated, it is necessary to sound a warning.

The examiner has to guard against two extremes, that of misreading a correct but fumbling performance as a demonstration of failure and that of interpreting wishfully the incorrect performance of a handicapped youngster as correct but inaccurately executed due to the motor difficulty. Not all fumbling is meaningful. One has to observe the intent of the visual regard, the facial expression, whether the attitude is that of blind persistence or of trial and error. Persistence in the face of a handicap, for instance, is an impressive and admirable asset and augurs favorably for the child's future adaptation to his handicap. But prolonged persistence and mechanical repetition of an act, without accompanying employment of judgment, sometimes indicates an inability to learn from experience or a tendency to perseverate. The examiner thus must learn to use his judgment in assessing the meaning and quality of the child's reactions.

Two other cautionary notes should be included here for the novice in the field of cerebral palsy. Even after an examiner has undergone a training period under the guidance of a teacher or psychologist specializing in this field, he should examine himself frankly for his own attitudes. One tendency is to become uncritically enthused in the natural reaction of respect and admiration which the resilience and the uncomplaining effort of young children with difficulties in physical performance arouse in the able-bodied adult. The other, no less important but fortunately less common, is the feeling of repugnance which assails some nonhandicapped persons when in the presence of someone with a handicap. An examiner must learn to recognize and analyze his reactions and work through his subjective emotions. Unless he can develop an objective yet sympathetic professional attitude to handicapped children, he will not be successful in his work with them. Humanizing the testing interview leads to making it a mutual endeavor, with the child being motivated to demonstrate cooperatively what he can do and the examiner evaluating sincerely the performance level, difficulties and potential for further development. A child who senses that an examiner is either uncritically overindulgent or else embarrassed, perfunctory or impatient will not be able to enter into a mutual relationship of effort simply because no such relationship will exist. Even a young child will respond when his reserve is respected, his person accepted and his cooperation solicited in an appreciative, surehanded, kind and leisurely manner. The little hurdles, such as problems with the production or intelligibility of his speech, drooling, accidental spilling of materials, can be surmounted by an attitude of comradely acceptance of his predicament. Such an attitude assigns to the condition its proper status; it leaves inviolate the child himself and his relationship with the examiner.

Observation of the *language behavior* proceeds informally during the whole interview and specifically during the presentation of many of the items, starting with the first one. The reaction of the child to verbal communication, during the introduction, the "warm-up" play period and during any incidental conversation between parent and examiner is observed obliquely. A discussion of special difficulties and their management in the interview situation will be found in the final part of this chapter; the associated problems which may be found in the language area, both in children with cerebral palsy and those with other handicaps, will be considered there. The present discussion, therefore, will be focused upon the more general aspects of comprehension of language, modes of communication and the production of speech by the child with involvement of the speech apparatus.

The development of comprehension of the spoken word presupposes exposure to the usual opportunities to hear language spoken and to be addressed individually, repeatedly and directly. If a child has been deprived of any or all such opportunities, the development of comprehension of language will be interfered with in proportion to the deprivation. If all has gone well, it can be expected that the child with cerebral palsy will have developed an understanding of simple verbal communication commensurate with his age level. A failure to do so would indicate impairment of one kind or another in this area.

The inability to speak due to physical involvement of the speech apparatus does not have any direct relationship to the development and growth of language comprehension, although it certainly will have consequences because of the passive role which a nonpracticing, nonverbal mode of communication imposes. The development of inner language will not be interfered with if there is no impairment other than that of the physical speech apparatus.

The challenging task facing the examiner of the child without speech production or with severe limitations in speech production is to find the level which the child has achieved in comprehension of language and the level which he is using in communicating, as well as his mode of communication.

An evaluation technique which depends largely on the observation of manifestations of comprehension, rather than on performance, requires a knowledge of the levels of communication. When this is present, it is possible for the examiner to appraise readiness for developing a mode of communicating on any level in a child who uses neither appropriate reactions nor signs at the beginning of an interview, as well as to elicit responses from a nonspeaking child who has not yet developed a mode of communication by signs but may use appropriate reactions. This statement, however, is not offered without caution and some misgivings. Work in this field is still in the empirical stage, and each examiner must learn to experiment, gauge, coax and try. He also must be able to concede defeat if his most resourceful approaches yield no success. The statement has been made only because in over twenty years of actual work, there have been large numbers of children who could be brought during one interview from a stage of action-response to the stage of using a sign, and another group who could learn to indicate a response by action even though they could not learn to understand the use of signs.

While the problem of eliciting and developing modes of communication presents the greatest difficulties at the lower age levels, a discrepancy between a child's level of comprehension and communication is sometimes found in older children also. Such a child may apparently understand and enjoy a story on a four to five year level but lack understanding of how to demonstrate his comprehension. There is also the possibility that the desire to communicate may be weakened through continuous frustration.

The items of the Evaluation, which was developed for use with non-speaking children, provide a scale which samples comprehension of language on successive levels. The problem, which is inherent in the functioning of the children in question, is that there cannot be uniformity in their modes of response. Where younger children are concerned, the problem is also complicated by the fact that the level of communication which makes responding possible is at first achieved only fluctuatingly and tentatively. The examiner needs to be familiar with this aspect of language development in the young child. Therefore, a brief outline will be given, tracing the growth of the function of communication in children.

Observation shows the following stages:

1. Unaware communication by whole bodily motion, such as the raising of both arms to be picked up.

2. Action-response to gestured request, such as lifting a foot when a shoe is offered.

3. Mute action-response to a verbal request, such as opening the mouth when asked, "Open your mouth."

4. Inquiry (forerunner of verbal question), as when the child looks inquiringly at his mother when something goes wrong, for instance, when a balloon breaks.

5. Imitating a familiar word-sound on request, such as "Bye-bye."

6. Naming a familiar person or an object upon seeing it again, almost in the manner of greeting or recognition, such as saying "Baba" or "Bottle."

7. Action-response to verbal request with simultaneous parroting of the request, e.g., when told, "Bring me baby's shoe," does so, saying, "Baby shoe," with a rising inflection.

8. Action-response to verbal request with repetition of the request in the manner of an announcement, e.g., when told, "Shut the door," does so, then announces, "Shut door," and waits for a comment or says, "Good boy," himself.

9. Action-response to verbal request, followed by a verbal utterance which shows the beginning of appropriate adjustment to the person speaking and which is made with an air of accomplishment, e.g., when told, "Get your coat," does so and as he hands it to his mother, may say, "Steven bring coat."

10. Simple questions around own concerns, such as: "Where ball?" or "Where Daddy go?"

11. Naming (and often simultaneously pointing to) an increasingly larger number of objects and perhaps some pictures; may name articles of clothing, animals, cars, man, book, etc.; and in pictures, perhaps baby, mama, or lady.

12. Simple word combinations to express an emotion, declare an intention, or voice a fear, such as, "Mommy home," "Steven walk," or "Go bye-bye," "No bed," "No needle."

13. Answers to simple questions: when asked, "Where is your sister?" he may say, "School (kool)," "Here Susie," "Susie go school."

Just as the first steps in walking are not used to reach a goal but are attempts to practice a new skill, that of upright locomotion, so also are first words not employed for the purpose of intentional communication. But just as goals could be attained before the walking stage and during the time when first steps are still being practiced by simply creeping directly to the goal, so also nonspecific, egocentric communication can be accomplished by actions and bodily motions before words are produced and at a time when they are first formed and experimentally produced.

At first the child saying "Bye-bye" is not aware that he is using a word and that this word (or symbol) is used in connection with parting. In a few months, however, he will be able to use it with intent and in suitable situations. Similarly, at first, although he may be able to say "bottle," the word is recalled by him only upon seeing his bottle. He cannot yet utilize this incipient skill to inform his mother that he is hungry. Without the stimulus, visual or tactile, of the familiar object, he cannot yet summon the word-symbol. Neither is he ready to formulate an idea nor to use names of absent things.

As he progresses from one stage to the next, the child gradually begins to use an increasingly greater number of word-symbols, and almost imperceptibly he begins to discard the nonspecific action-response and replace it with the use of word-symbols. In the beginning, words are used in combination with gestures and inflections which serve to supplement the intended meaning; one and two word sentences must serve to carry the idea. Words and word combinations still center around the child's own emotions, comfort and wishes. Appropriate use of verbal communication to respond to questions or requests requires the ability to become a little more detached from this self-centered world of childhood. Communication is at first rarely spontaneous; in response to requests, communication is initially fragmentary, then partial, then adequate in a simple way. The rate of this development will show individual differences; there are late and early talkers just as there are late and early walkers. But the sequence will be grossly the one governing the development of communication in any child.

Reduced to essentials, the levels progress from a nonspecific language of behavior by appropriate action to the use of word-symbols in an experimental and egocentric manner to the beginning of an intentional and conscious use of word-symbols for communication in response to one who elicits it. At this level the use of words or language with the conscious intent of expressing or conveying an idea spontaneously is found only infrequently.

The levels of communicating in children with physical involvement of the speech apparatus run parallel to the described stages. The child with cerebral palsy may not be able to get around and may not be able to use his hands, in addition to his inability to produce speech, but when intelligence is not impaired, the growth of inner language will follow the same stages, as long as environmental conditions are reasonably favorable.

The mode a child uses to manifest that he has comprehended a verbal request will reveal on which level of communication he performs. At an early level there will be an action-response. A correct action directed toward the test materials will conclusively demonstrate that the child has comprehended the verbal request. At the level on which word-symbols can be used by the nonhandicapped child for the conscious and intentional purpose of communicating his response, a sign can be used by the nonspeaking handicapped child. The ability to understand that signs can serve to convey meaning requires the same degree of comprehension necessary to an understanding that words can convey meaning.

Some children with cerebral palsy fail to employ signs for communicating a response to questions or requests although, theoretically, they may be on the level where this form of communication could be expected of them. In the nonretarded child with cerebral palsy, this may be due to an unenlightened environment, which, by overlooking or ignoring possible earlier attempts of the child to make signs, has discouraged and prevented the development of this form of communication. It may be due to an absence of resourcefulness in the child or to the fact that action-responses have served him well and neither he nor his family have experienced a need to change the response method. It may be due to infantilization of the child, who, due to physical helplessness, may still require the care given an infant and of whom nothing is expected in return.

The task of establishing a means of communication with the child who cannot produce speech due to physical involvement of the vocal apparatus will be simplified if the examiner keeps in the back of his mind the stages of the growth of communication in nonhandicapped children. In the manifestations of communication of the nonspeaking child, equivalents of such stages will then become more easily recognized. Such recognition will aid the examiner in judging whether the child may be ready and able to progress to the next level, and whether an attempt during the interview to prod and coax the child ahead a little might be desirable.

Assuming that there is no hearing or other handicap which interferes with the reception of language and that it is possible to concentrate on the pattern of responding and communicating, the first step is to check the limitations which the physical handicap imposes upon the ability to indicate by signs. Thus, while the examiner is occupied in an initial period of eliciting those modes of communication which the parents have described as the ones used habitually in the home, his mind will simultaneously be busy going over pertinent aspects of the child's body which can play a role in nonverbal modes of communication. It will be the pooling of these factors: the physical equipment, the level of communication achieved and the reported means of communicating at home, which will give information about the potential in this area. Anything that limits the mobility and balancing of the head, whether poor head balance or hyperextension of the back and neck which forces the head backwards and prevents free movement, will probably mean that the child cannot make, and will not be able to learn how to make, the signs of nodding the head for assent and shaking the head for negation. The same difficulty will interfere with eye-pointing, since it may be impossible to maintain a steady regard on a given spot. Severe strabismus will also interfere with the use of eye-pointing for the purpose of responding. Facial grimacing makes it difficult for the observer to interpret the child's expression reliably, and it will depend on the presence or absence of head balance in such a child as to whether he may be able to learn to use signs made by moving the head or not. If head motion is not under his voluntary control, it will have to be observed whether trunk motions are possible, or whether voluntary intentional motion of arm, hand or finger is possible, or, perhaps, whether he can use his foot to indicate responses. The kind of signal he can learn to make will depend on which part of his body can be utilized for the purpose.

Physical limitations must also be taken into account in the presentation of the materials so that failure will not occur on the basis of inability or poor ability to inspect the materials. Whether accommodation is accomplished by stabilizing the child's head against the wings of the relaxation chair or against the shoulder of the examiner, or whether materials are brought into the field of vision by holding them up singly or by placing them lower for a child whose head is habitually lowered or by placing them higher for the child whose eyes are staring upward because his head is pulled backward by strong muscle-pull will have to be decided in cooperation with the child. In one extreme case the author had to place the materials on a regular size table to the left of the low chair in which the child was strapped, with her back curving and her head twisted back and toward the left. In this distorted position, which was her habitual one due to the severity of the impairment, she was able to indicate her comprehension of the materials by smiling for assent and pushing out her lower lip in a pugnacious manner for negation.

Fortunately, such extreme and severe involvement is not the rule. The nonretarded child with cerebral palsy frequently develops an amazing resourcefulness in finding means to contact a person who is willing to be contacted. In instances in which this is the case, one is then not limited to the one or two ways in which responses are indicated but can supplement them and can sometimes confirm an inconclusively demonstrated response by the child's way of communicating incidentally with smiles, chuckles, grunts, meaningful looks and revealing facial expressions.

During the initial period of eliciting those modes of communication which the parents have reported, it will depend on the severity of the handicap, on the maturity of the child and on the reliability or, conversely, the inconclusiveness with which he habitually communicates whether the examiner will decide to begin with the first item or instead postpone it in favor of a brief practice period in order to learn to know the child's response pattern better. If the child is quite young and immature and his answering technique is still changeable and vague, it is probably best to use a practice period. If the parents have reported the signs used for assent and negation, the examiner can use questions of simple content to elicit them. He might point to the child's mother and ask, "Is this your mommy?" and await the child's sign for assent. Next, he might hold up the mother's handbag or umbrella and ask, "Is this your hat?" or, "Is this Steven's hat?" (using the child's own name) and expect the sign for negation. If more practice seems advisable, the examiner can use familiar elements in the room in his questions, such as touching the door and asking, "Is that a door?", then touching the mother's hand and asking, "Is this your shoe?" (or, "Steven's shoe?"), until the child's responses become conclusively recognizable to the examiner and the child feels assured that the examiner can understand his answers. Confirming comments must be kept on the child's level, such as, "Good for you," or, "Steven is showing me, aren't you?" (using the child's own name). This will convey to him that his signs are received and accepted. After three and one-half or four years of age, the nonretarded child usually can understand the request, "How will you show me 'Yes'?" and, "Now, show me how you can say 'No'." The child will then demonstrate his signs. If necessary, some practice can be provided by pointing to a chair and saying: "Is that a chair?", then pointing to the child's mother and saying, "Is this Santa Claus?" and waiting for the child's signs. Similar right and wrong questions can be used alternatingly.

Signs which have been reported by parents and which have been observed in children as young as two years old range from the conventional nodding and shaking of the head for "Yes" and "No," to a slight motion of the eyes toward the forehead for "Yes," sidewards to whichever direction the child can manage for "No." Other children use a smile for assent, a frown for negation; protruding lower lip for negation; sticking out the tongue for negation; fixed forward position of the trunk for assent, violent turning away of trunk and face to one side for negation; raising one or all fingers or whole hand for assent, pulling hand and arm toward the body for negation; tapping the floor with the foot for assent, pointedly stiffening the foot and holding it still for negation; one forward drop of the head for assent, a deeper forward drop of the head and keeping it down for a longer time for negation, with a glance following the signs to judge whether the "hearer" has understood the answer. Some children can and do use sounds even if they cannot produce words. Some of these sounds have been observed: "mmm" said with rising inflections for assent, an almost similar "mmm" but with a drawn-out and disappointed-sounding tone for negation; "ah" for assent, "ooh" for negation; throwing a kiss with a distinct lip sound for assent, saying "aaah" in a rejecting way for negation. Some children, while they use a recognizable sign for assent, use nothing for negation, so that the conclusiveness of their decision cannot be checked; one child had developed a screwing up of the left cheek and closing of the left eye for assent, using this sign reliably and appropriately, but he assumed a blank or bored expression when a sign for assent did not answer the situation. This behavior seems to mark a half-way point between the intentional use of signs for the conscious purpose of communication and the level just below.

It seems to correspond to that level of communication in the normal child on which the child is able to fetch in response to a verbal command and simultaneously repeats the command in an echoing fashion. At that level the normal child probably expresses his refusal by ignoring the command or perhaps by teasingly running away. In the physically involved child who cannot run away, an assumed indifference or withdrawal behind a blank expression might be the equivalent.

The nature of some of these signs suggests that they grew out of responses made spontaneously by the child at one time or another that were then taken up and used by the family until, with steady encouragement and acceptance of their use, they gradually became habitual and well established. In a few of the cruder ones, one can almost divine the flavor of "baby-talk," or whatever must take the place of baby-talk in a nontalking child.

Those children who do not, or physically cannot, use action-responses, or who have not yet developed any signs, or who do not use signs consistently and reliably will require more and a different kind of practice to establish communication. It is permissable to use the first item for the purpose of practicing responding. This may mean that the item has to be discounted when evaluating the child's responses since prolonged exposure to the materials makes them learning materials rather than testing materials. The experienced examiner, however, will realize that inability to comprehend does not suddenly evaporate; if comprehension eventually can be manifested by the child, the potential to comprehend on this level must have been present and only a means of manifesting such comprehension was absent.

When the examiner has surveyed the child's physical potentials and limitations for any means of physically executing some mode of response, he must then speculate about the probable level of comprehension and potential communication. This level will become evident in the series of attempts to solicit the child's cooperation. As the level gradually emerges more clearly, the examiner can use that form of request which most closely corresponds to the child's potential for physically reacting as well as to his intellectual level of indicating to the examiner that he has comprehended. As cooperation becomes possible and established and the child gains in the willingness or ability "to play with the examiner" and in the confident awareness that the examiner understands his way of responding, an attempt may then be made to develop in the child a greater awareness of the fact and the possibilities of communicating. Sometimes, a latent ability can be helped to fruition in the short space of an interview.

Action-responses are possible below the level of conscious and intentional communication; they correspond to the earlier levels in the growth of communication, and they can be observed in children from ten or eleven months of age up. But an action-response that indicates the child has selected from among four objects the one which the examiner has requested presupposes comprehension of language and the ability to remember a heard commission long enough to allow time for consideration, rejection and selection among the various choices. The task may be further complicated for the child by interruptive physical events which interfere with both the selection and the appropriate communicating of the choice to the examiner. The examiner will learn to weigh nuances in a child's correct response. These may range from a fragmentary, fleeting focus, in an echoing manner, on the named object, the child reaching for it almost automatically if his eye happens to spot it before the trend of the task is lost and performing the task without being fully cognizant of what originated the performance, to conscientious, intelligent cooperation. The latter would consist of an acknowledged reception of the verbal request, a distinct reflection about its meaning and a deliberate selection of the correct object, indicating it with an air of terminating the task.

How fragile the young child's ability to enter into intentional, spontaneous communication really is can be deduced from the minute steps in the response pattern: from unawareness with fragmentary ability to attend in an echoing fashion, to noncommunicating but reliable participation of the character of conditioning- or training-reflexes, to a conscious, cooperative following of verbal requests just short of spontaneous, nonverbal communition. One has the feel of coaxing the child along, cautiously and gently pulling him by a slender thread. If he is physically too involved to demonstrate his level by performance-tests, this sensitive establishing of communication is our only way of reaching the child and of finding out what goes on in his mind.

The level of response to which the examiner attempts to guide the child during the practice period depends on the readiness of the child. The desirable goal is to attain the level where the child understands that he can communicate by giving a sign. If he can be brought to that level, the signs can then be used to check whether an inconclusive response, given by means of eye-pointing, was conclusively intended. Some of the more advanced items can only be responded to by signs for "Yes" and "No" unless a child can perform manually. However, the intellectual level for understanding that one can communicate by the use of signs would be reached normally before the mental age at which ability to solve these items could be assumed.

The use of eye-pointing is possible on a lower level than that necessary for the intentional, conscious use of signs. Here, too, nuances can be discerned. At first the child can respond without really appreciating the nature of the interview nor the systematic structure of the contact, which to him looks like play and should indeed be made to look like play. His response is fragmentary and inconsistent, and he attends briefly and inter-mittently. If his glance falls on the correct choice while he still remembers the verbal instruction, he may indicate by his facial expression, a smile or a grunt that he has spotted what the examiner has asked for, but he is not choosing among a series of answers. A higher level of eye-pointing is achieved by the child who is conscious of the fact that he is following a request and who begins to scan the material systematically, being aware of the presence of several choices and the need to decide upon the requested answer. The technique of eye-pointing can be used on any level and is not limited to the use of responding; it can also be used to initiate communica-tion. The child described in the previous chapter who utilized the objects visible in the room to communicate spontaneously by eye-pointing and by inviting the examiner's attention (or "listening") to the voluntary direction of his glances illustrates this point. Eye-pointing is often used spontaneously in conjunction with other signs by children with cerebral palsy. Since eye-pointing and nonverbal communication is unconsciously or consciously used by all of us under certain circumstances, from the fond parent who mutely indicates to another adult some exploit of his child, to the librarian who "eye-points" to the "Silence" sign above her desk to hush a talkative customer, this form of communication should not present great difficulties to an examiner.

For a large part of the sequence of items, eye-pointing is the response of preference because it is a rapid and relatively effortless, nonfatiguing means of indicating choices. The number of children who are physically too involved to use it is fortunately very small and these can be presented with the items in a form which calls for affirmative and negative answers. A growing awareness on the part of the child of the function and the possi-bilities of eye-pointing, which may result from practice during the interview, can sometimes be coaxed along to an awareness of signs and to a subsequent insight into the possibility of using other signs to indicate and to communi-cate. Other earmarks of intentional communication revealed incidentally during the session as the child warms up in this vis-a-vis situation with an understanding and appreciative adult may be a cue that the child matura-tionally has reached that level of communication where it is possible to use signs. It is then worthwhile to attempt to develop signs during the inter-view. This can be done by the interviewer setting an example. The exam-iner might greet any successful response of the child with an emphatic nod for "Yes"; he might use an emphatic shake of the head and a loud "No" as he picks up the rejected choices one by one to remove them. Before long the child may imitate such signs and the examiner would then use a suit-ably enthusiastic expression of pleasure to compliment the child on the clever way he is using "to show what he means." In this way the child may be helped to incorporate the signs into his "vocabulary." Training can also be attempted by gently holding the child's head and helping him to nod it, perhaps saying, "Steven (using appropriate name) is a good boy," while the examiner also nods his head. Then the head can be gently moved in a negative answer, with the examiner saying, "Steven is not a puppy dog." If the child is timid or shy, the examiner might demonstrate first with a doll and then ask the child if he wants to play this game too. The child may even surprise himself and the examiner by nodding for an answer, even before being shown by passive motion.

Over the years, parents have frequently reported that their child "seemed to have much more to say" and that they could understand him much better after he had been tested. The interview, of necessity, sometimes turns into a learning session as well as being an Evaluation. It is perhaps this aspect of the Evaluation which, by unlocking a previously uncommunicating child, reminds the examiner that his technique is an art as well as a skill.

Attempts to discover the child's potential level and mode of responding, if he appears unable to apply himself spontaneously and voluntarily, start with the use of the standard situation. The first four objects are lined up and the examiner observes the child for incipient or adequate reactions as he offers a series of approaches. The formulation of the request can be experimented with, starting with: "Give me . . ." "Look at . . ." and "Show me . . ." If there is no reaction or response, the request can be changed, perhaps to: "I can see a shoe. Can Steven (using the child's name) see a shoe?" Or: "Can Steven (can you) find the cup?" Or: "Where is the spoon?" If this does not result in the child's reaching for the object (or any of the objects) in an action-response, or looking at it, in an eye-pointing mode of response, an object can then be pointed to or held up and the examiner may say, "Look what I have. Is that a shoe?" and observe the child for a sign of recognition or agreement, even a glance at his own shoe. Other attempts may be made by asking the child to "give" or "show" his mother the object in question, since perhaps he may be more willing to relate to her. If there is still no reaction or response, the number of choices can be reduced to two and the approaches repeated. If a smaller number of choices proves successful in eliciting a response, it may indicate that the child is intellectually unable to handle the task of making a selection from among four choices, not that he has no mode of indicating his response, be it action-response or eye-pointing. However, it may also mean that he is just getting the idea and that he might now be able to continue with the standard number of choices and can be given the next items in the standard presentation. This can only be evaluated and decided empirically.

A child who fails to show any recognizable sign of an attempt to react or respond may fail because he is mentally retarded and does not comprehend what is expected of him. This eventually calls for the use of the item in a modified form, which is given in chapter 9. But before assuming that failure to respond is based on mental retardation, a different approach can be used to help the child find a way of responding. Some severely involved children who have never had to respond to requests simply have not had an opportunity to develop a mode of response. They may be bewildered by demands made upon them since they cannot think of a way to act. They may be accustomed to sitting by passively when visiting and cannot adapt at once to a structured situation which tries to involve them. They may be resigned, discouraged and reduced to immobility. It is then advisable to place the four objects at various, easily accessible places around the room. (Fig. 9 shows this approach with the picture material.) The examiner then helps the child to walk by supporting him around the hips or under the arms (children with braces and kneelocks will probably need to have the locks attended to) and leads the child to each object, calling his attention to it, so that he learns their positions. Then he is asked to "Find . . ." each item in turn, as directed in chapter 8. The child who comprehends will pull and strain to reach his choice, guiding the supporting adult toward it and perhaps regarding it triumphantly or touching it. Some children will insist on picking up the object since they have been told to "find" it and do not yet understand the figurative sense of the word, or of words. The examiner, having only the usual number of hands, is sometimes hard put to help such a literal-minded little performer grasp the object while simultaneously supporting him under the arms, but by sliding one hand from the back under the child's arm and supporting him with the forearm, the hand can be used to assist the child in reaching for the object. Ignoring his attempt to manipulate the object would serve to confuse the child and to retard his learning to respond.

He can only learn if one starts on the level of which he is capable. After the child has found the four objects, item 2 can be presented in the same manner, as directed in chapter 8. Some children learn relatively quickly once they have found a way of indicating their response, and it then becomes possible to return them to their chair and present the next items on the table. If the practice period has convinced the child that his actions have served to show the examiner that he can follow a command, he may be willing to continue "showing." He then finds that the attentive and appreciative examiner is able to understand his meaning when he touches or looks at the selected choices, even though they have now been brought close and are lined up on the table before him. Each response should be confirmed with a suitable word so that the child's confidence in his own ability to make himself understood becomes stronger. For some children, it seems to be a revelation to suddenly find that they can express themselves in these ways and they glory in the new discovery; some who start the interview most unpromisingly will be found to work untiringly, as if to reward the examiner for having shown them a way to let the observing mother find out how much they know and how hard they can work. Timid children can perhaps be persuaded to try this technique of "walking around to find" after the examiner has demonstrated it with a doll. Children who do not seem able to respond appropriately and who perhaps enjoy the exercise of being walked around but show no goal-directed action under this maximum stimulation, or those who push the objects to the floor gleefully, are most likely not ready intellectually for this level of presenting the item and a suitable modification (see chapter 9) will have to be used.

The suggestions offered here can be helpful also in work with other children who do not use verbal communication. Knowledge of the gradations in the growth of language behavior makes it possible to recognize subtle suggestions and cues in the behavior patterns of deaf, aphasic, autistic and retarded children, who may be equally mute in the interview situation. The nonverbal communication of each child and of children displaying a particular disability can differ widely. One must remember, too, that these disabilities are not mutually exclusive; the autistic child may also be retarded, for example.

Children with cerebral palsy will be more readily understood and their attempts to communicate more alertly observed and accepted by an examiner to whom it has become evident that while a child may be nonspeaking, he may be far from noncommunicating.

To round out the discussion of language behavior, it should be repeated that many children with cerebral palsy can speak and that where speech production is possible and has been developed, it is of course utilized in the testing situation, both to supplement responses and to study the language pattern.

The examiner who has learned to read the "language" of behavior will be able to learn much about even very severely handicapped children with cerebral palsy. Some children reveal problems of eating or sleeping when items 7 and 8 are presented. They may react emotionally to the pictures, perhaps turning away violently from the picture showing the children in beds, thereby giving a clue to their own nightly battle with the mother about going to sleep or being left alone in the bedroom. Inquiry can then confirms such findings. The experienced examiner may be afforded insight into a child's attitude toward a sibling or one of the parents by an unsolicited, spontaneously displayed emotional reaction to the figures in the story in item 31. A valuable by-product of the Evaluation interview can thus be information about the inner life of a child who can do nothing about informing the persons around him of his difficulties because he cannot speak. The examiner, reporting such findings, can contribute to the understanding of the child by the teacher, therapist and social worker. In turn, they will be able to utilize the findings in their guidance of the parents. The constructive use of such by-products of the Evaluation interview may aid in bringing about a more appropriate and happier environmental management of the child by his family.

A description of the language pattern of those children whose functioning renders them incapable of responding on a two-year age level, which is the baseline of the Evaluation, will be found as an implicit aspect of the modifications of the items described in chapter 9.

To adapt successfully to the demands inherent in an Evaluation interview, the sensory intake has to be adequate. Our next concern in this fictional interview, therefore, will be with *the sensory functioning* of the child with cerebral palsy.

If earlier medical examinations of hearing and vision have been equivocal or have not been attempted because of the child's physical handicap, speech impairment, or both, the findings in the sensory areas uncovered during the interview will contribute to a gross check of sensory intactness. Also, the description of the presence and nature of impaired sensory functioning given by the examiner can be used to point up the need for examination by a physician if this has not previously been undertaken.

Information contained in the child's developmental history and verbal reports by the parents of their estimate of the child's vision and hearing should be carefully reviewed. With the prevalence of television in the American home, the inquiry can conveniently bring out telltale hints of difficulties in vision or hearing by eliciting a description of the child's behavior in relation to the television set. It can be inquired how close he wants to sit to the screen; whether he wants to face it always from the same side rather than from the front; whether he wants the sound on louder than the rest of the family needs it, whether he is able to watch through a whole program or begins to get restless or bored quickly; whether he is disinterested in television and only responds to music; whether he has any favorite programs and the nature of such programs. Answers to questions like these can give clues to specific visual and auditory limitations and will prompt the examiner to be on the alert for them.

The behavior pattern of the child during the first few items gives the examiner an opportunity to survey *the visual functioning* and to spot difficulties, if they are present. Adequate performance on the items using pictures, simple cut-out forms and color blocks indicates that vision is grossly intact. Inadequate performance on these items, however, does not necessarily indicate the presence of impaired vision since failure can also occur on the basis of lack of comprehension. If there is a poor performance and the reason is not clearly apparent, the examiner must begin to check. If an experimental presentation of the item or items in a form permitting lowered intellectual demand results in an improved performance, the reason for failure in the standard presentation would not have been visual inadequacy but insufficient comprehension. If a lowered intellectual demand does not bring about an improvement in the performance, the possibility must then be considered that impairment of visual functioning may be responsible for the poor performance. Poor visual acuity and even blindness is sometimes not suspected in the very young child with cerebral palsy, especially if the child cannot walk (and so does not stumble or bump into furniture) and if he cannot reach for objects because his hands are physically too involved (and so it is not suspected that he may not attempt to reach because he does not see familiar faces, toys and the bottle, spoon or cup used for feeding him). He may turn his head toward familiar voices because he hears them and not because he sees the speaker.

Some difficulties in visual functioning are obvious at first glance. The examiner will recognize, or will soon learn to recognize, strabismus, nystagmus, or a peculiar position of the head while trying to focus. The effect of the particular condtion must be observed closely as the child mobilizes himself to function in response to presented items. Other difficulties are less conspicuous, but the conduct of the interview, with the examiner sitting across from the child, makes possible a careful survey. In observing eye movements, the examiner will be able to recognize such deviations as difficulty in focusing, intermittent or constant difficulty in raising or lowering one or both eyes, poorly visualized fields or complete visual field cut-off. Ataxic vision may interfere with a child's capacity to respond to some items. The interrelationship of physical posture and visual functioning must also be kept in mind, especially in the event of poor head balance or of hyperextension of the body forcing the head into an unnatural position where it is held more or less immobile, the direction of the gaze of the eyes being severely restricted by the position of the head. Poor sitting balance may also reduce the ability to look in all directions, because the child may deliberately avoid movements which might jeopardize his safety.

The habit of total observation is formed only gradually. Initially, the detection of visual impairment may not be as quick, sensitive or complete as it will become with practice. The items of the sequence are planned so that impairment which affects functioning will be revealed as the interview proceeds, even if it has been overlooked at the outset.

With experience and with increasing skill in using the Evaluation items flexibly, the examiner will learn to employ specific items for the purpose of a cross-check in order to confirm or rule out hunches about suspected difficulties in functioning. He will learn how to pinpoint subtle impairment and how to probe its severity and permanence.

Should the performance of the child during the first four items suggest a definite possibility of visual impairment, it may be worthwhile to use item 22 a and b to cross-check, if the child is young, and the same item plus items 14 to 16 if the child is four years old or over. The elementary nature of the pellet and bottle item (item 22) makes it useful for children from two and one-half years of age up. If difficulty in manipulation is not too extreme, it can be observed whether the child can see all the pellets piled up next to the bottle and reach for them without having to feel around manually. Sometimes, a consistently inaccurate approach, such as over-reaching or under-reaching in the approach to the bottle neck when inserting pellets, points to nearsightedness or farsightedness, respectively. The task of letting the child find a pellet on the floor has been found very valuable for a quick screening of gross visual defect. Even a severely involved child with cerebral palsy can look for the pellet if the examiner holds him around the middle, with the child's hands and knees on the floor (if he wears long leg braces, the kneelocks have to be unlocked for kneeling). The child is asked to indicate the position of the pellet for the examiner to pick up if the child himself cannot grasp it. If a child searches with his hands, with or without making a simultaneous attempt to look, it is a very strong indication of real visual difficulty. If the performance appears to have been successful accidentally, it can be repeated a few times, with two or three pellets placed a few inches apart.

With children who function on a four-year level or over and for whom the large pictures of objects have posed a definite difficulty (item 4, see also Fig. 9), it is possible to identify visual difficulty as the basis for the poor performance by a quick cross-check with the sound blocks, items 14 to 16. Especially valuable for this purpose is the task of grading the blocks by degree of loudness (item 16), which requires comprehension of the concept of serial grading, while visual acuity is unimportant. The weak area will emerge quickly. If a test on a two-year level, which for a successful performance depends on vision, has been failed, and a test on a four-year level, which for a successful performance does not depend on vision, is not failed, visual impairment is clearly responsible for the earlier failure and the area of difficulty has been isolated.

The performance of children with strabismus deserves close scrutiny. A constant or even an intermittent strabismus of one eye may cause a child to use only the other eye habitually in order to avoid blurred vision or double vision or other discomfort. A resourceful child may be able to adapt himself to this one-eyed sighting by remembering to look around and by using appropriate scanning motions. Depth perception may, however, be affected. A less resourceful child may not compensate and may restrict himself to viewing to the front and on his one good side. An alternating strabismus can be a very serious handicap since it makes fused vision practically impossible. It cancels out sighting now with the one, now with the other eye, unpredictably and irregularly, and the child must attempt to adapt with compensatory head movements. His attempts to focus on an object or line of print resemble the attempts of the athetoid hand to reach and grasp an offered object. If this handicap exists in a child who also has poor head balance, the difficulties are almost insurmountable; some function can be obtained by using enlarged materials and placing them at the farthest possible distance at which they can still be seen accurately; the field to be regarded will then be at least intermittently in full view of the child. Eye-hand coordination may be affected in a child with strabismus. He may turn his head away deliberately from an object, after he has marked its position, before reaching for it lest his unpredictable vision may cause him to misdirect his hand.

Difficulties in lowering or raising the eyes above or below a certain level are sometimes found in spastic children. Both eyes may move together, but just so far; or one eye may remain fixed for a while as the other one is lowered or raised, making it impossible for the child to perform the systematic progression of the regard of the eyes needed for reading. As he comes to the end of a line and tries to return his gaze to the beginning and drop it down to the next line, one eye will conform while the other one will remain fixed, until, eventually, it also will join the other eye and the child can then focus both eyes until the next time he comes to the end of a line.

Another difficulty exists when a given area is only poorly visualized or not visualized at all, causing the child to miss materials in a particular location. Some children are aware of their difficulty and try to adapt to it. Attempts at adapting, such as the peculiar position in which the head is held, turned to the side or lowered sideways to the shoulder, while the child tries to see out of the corner of one or both eyes, may be a clue to the difficulty. A suspected deviation in functioning occasionally needs to be demonstrated conclusively. The color blocks (items 12 and 13) are a suitable vehicle for this. The examiner can experiment with various placements of them for the purpose of determining, first, where the child can reliably spot materials and, second, where he seems to visualize them poorly or not at all. The blocks may be spread out or moved close together, or placed all on one side of the table and then on the other. Blocks can be placed within the suspected area of poor vision and the child told about such placement. It can then be observed whether subsequently he may remind himself to look on purpose, perhaps by turning his head searchingly, or whether he lacks such resourcefulness.

The presentation of the small cards in the wooden stand is a further aid in narrowing down this and other types of deviations in visual functioning. Frequently, the child himself will voluntarily indicate where he can see the cards best (or, if he is younger, where he "wants" them), and thereby, consciously or not, assist in circumscribing possible areas of limitation.

During the presentation of the flashlight and the sparkler toy (item 33), a demonstration of limitations in eye motion and the existence of poorly visualized fields or fields not visualized at all is provoked. Children will be observed who stop following the sparkler toy with their eyes, as it is moved slowly up and down. Some will follow it up to eye level and then simply wait until it comes into sight again. The child with precarious head balance has to be observed shrewdly, since it maybe that he does not dare to raise his head for fear of bringing it back too far. Children who do not yet walk or have just recently learned to walk may fail to follow in a downward direction; in them, visual functioning may improve spontaneously as balance improves or as the child becomes habituated to an awareness of space and spatial directions. The child who spends his days in a wheelchair or carriage has no need to look other than forward, sidewards and upwards, which may delay an awareness of, or a suitable reaction to, things below his accustomed horizon. Repeated rechecks will help establish whether there may be improvement or whether the apparent restriction is a permanent one and unrelated to the delay in upright locomotion. Occasionally, a child will turn completely around his own axis in order to spot the reflection of the flashlight on the wall after he has lost it temporarily, only discovering it again when one of his eyes falls upon it; if this performance is observed frequently, it may indicate that the child is not able to spot the reflection with the other eye, for instance, at eye level or shoulder level, eight or ten inches from center to the suspected side. This hints at a limitation or even disuse of the one eye.

The presentation of the items has to be adapted to limitations in eye motion, once the limitation has been defined. Objects such as the color blocks, the story toys (items 30 and 31, see Fig. 12), and the hardware items (item 32, see Fig. 1) which cannot be seen when on the table surface by a child who is unable to lower his gaze can be placed on a tray or perhaps on the base of the wooden stand and held at a height at which they are visible to the child. Use of the stand facilitates accommodation of various limitations. The inserted cards can be presented at any angle, below eye level, above eye level, from one side or another, closer or farther away, wherever they can best be seen by the child. (For some examples, see Figs. 7 and 8.)

Accommodation of the possible difficulties found in children with ataxia calls for other expediencies. Some of these children experience discomfort or dizziness when called upon to look at material closely for any length of time. The more resourceful child has learned by experience that the dizzy feeling goes away when he looks into the distance, and this gives a clue to the way to present the material to an ataxic child. The facial expression, unwillingness to fix the gaze for a prolonged time, or a verbal comment on his discomfort by the child himself should tip off the examiner when there is ataxic vision. In milder cases, it may be sufficient to provide brief periods of inactivity. If the child does not look into the distance of his own accord, the examiner can shield the stand from view and so suggest a pause in the effort. It is better not to begin to converse, so that the child senses that the task is still unfinished. Many children will indicate spontaneously when they are ready to take another look at the material. If the difficulty seems more severe, it is best to give the child the benefit of the doubt and present the material in a form which will allow the child to demonstrate what he knows without being penalized by the mode in which the presentation is made. The cards can be placed at various spots around the room at the child's eye level, such as on window sills, desk, and table. The color blocks and the sound blocks make suitable props against which to lean them. The child is then asked to walk around, or is helped to walk around by being supported under the arms, until he has become familiar with the available choices of cards and their location. The testing then proceeds as usual, except that the child, instead of eye-pointing or reaching for the card he chooses, has to guide the supporting examiner to it. The activity and the necessary distances between the cards provide enough pauses for the child's eyes to remain free from discomfort.

Observations made of the area of vision are not confined to deviations but extend also to habits of visual functioning and their levels of development, such as the systematic left-to-right scanning motion of the eyes. As a child surveys his choices in the stand, such as the cards with configurations (item 37), the small black outline symbols (item 39) and the word pictures (item 40), the examiner watches the movement of his eyes. If systematic eye-sweep is not present, the sample card, which the examiner holds in his hand, can be moved slowly from the child's left (the right side from the examiner's point of view) to his right, over the cards in the stand, to suggest this systematic direction; or each card can be indicated individually, with the motion again leading in the same direction, and the child invited verbally to start looking from this side (pointing to the child's left) to the other side. It is then observed whether on succeeding items the child will spontaneously begin to use a left-to-right progression of the eyes.

Left-handed children sometimes tend to look consistently from right to left. Unless retrained, such a tendency will pose difficulties in the beginning reading program at school. Some right-handed children appear to have left-eye dominance. This may be observed when item 34 is presented, when the child is required to look, or sight something, through a tube. Some of these children will also be found to tend to survey rows from right to left.

Apart from the importance which a description of such incipient difficulties will have for the child's teacher, who is concerned with establishing effective habits of visual functioning in her pupils, the tendency for right-to-left progression has implications for the presentation of certain test items. The examiner must be on the look-out for a reversal of direction when the child tries to line up, as requested, such materials as the color shadings (item 20) and the circles in ascending serial grading (items 19 and 21; see also Fig. 8). An apparently confused performance, such as a frequent attempt to place the correct next choice to the left or "incorrect" side of the preceding card, may in fact represent a deep-seated habit. If this is the case, it is wiser to let the child arrange the cards in his own way, or perhaps even to change to a right-to-left line-up in a deliberate second demonstration. The issue at stake for the moment is insight into the concept of serial grading rather than the child's ability to conform to the direction in which materials are conventionally lined up.

Through the use of educated observation, being constantly watchful not only of the result of the performance but the nature of it, probable causes of poor performance often become gradually more apparent. The lists of areas at the heading of each item in the chapter giving the directions for presentation (chapter 8) will provide a ready means of checking areas of functioning and eliminating as a cause for poor performance those found intact. The principle of modifying an item if it is failed in the standard form leads to an identification of weak areas. An illustration is the provision for cut-out forms (item 9) for a child who has failed to match the forms printed on the square cards (item 10). If the child demonstrates the ability to match the forms in cut-outs, his inability to succeed on the symbol cards would not mean that he cannot perceive forms. It might mean that he cannot perceive figures against a background or it might mean that he fails to appreciate the significance of the fact that there are various forms visible on the cards, but, in that case, his failure would be caused by conceptual immaturity or conceptual difficulty, not by an inability to perceive the various forms.

Whenever further inquiry appears desirable in order to learn more about suspected limitations, this is undertaken either by going to lower levels of functioning or by probing laterally within the same level. Such inquiry often serves to clarify why a certain child cannot learn under given conditions, whether he may be able to learn under different conditions and what these conditions are. Suggestions for his training program can then sometimes be offered.

For the teacher who is responsible for the educational planning for the individual, it is frustrating to have the child's difficulty labeled simply "perceptual disturbance." An accurate description of the child's performance in the weak area and a statement of the probable cause of poor performance should be entered in the report. If teaching techniques can be suggested, they should be definite and detailed. Personal contact between teacher and examiner should be cultivated.

In view of the present incomplete understanding of difficulties in perception and in spatial orientation, a team approach seems to offer the best prospect for eventual clarification of the causes of disability and the retraining methods that will be most effective for the individual child. The examiner's most valuable contribution is his descriptive report of the nature of deviations in functioning. Other contributions must come from the medical specialists and from the experienced teacher, who has a responsibility to share her observations and to help devise approaches for meeting difficulties.

We know that neurologic and intellectual maturation play a role in the attainment of competence in the area of visual perception. We know something of the interrelationship of one area of learning and another; for example, it is known that an amount concept disproportionly low in relation to over-all functioning may in turn affect the ability to deal with simple form and space percepts or may actually be a manifestation of a general disturbance in that area. Too, delayed or confused laterality appears to influence adversely the capacity to deal competently with simple tasks in spatial orientation and the reconstruction of simple patterns from memory. A lack of, delay in or denial of eye-hand coordination sometimes is present in a child who performs poorly in this area. Some children will be unable to copy a drawing of a cross or square when they are looking at the strokes they are making, only to succeed when doing the same task with averted eyes, and showing by their proud visual examination of the finished product their correct appreciation of the adequacy of the performance. One such child volunteered an apologetic, "My hand knows, but when I look, my eyes get me all mixed up." Some children are observed to turn pictures upside down in order to perceive them correctly. This has been tentatively ascribed to an incomplete reversing of the image on the retina by medical specialists, but medical substantiation is difficult to obtain in young children. The child can only demonstrate his deviating way of functioning; having always perceived in this way, he is unable to describe how it differs from the conventional.

Involuntary eye-motions as well as limitations in eye-motion, as described as part of the observations during the fictional interview with the child with cerebral palsy, certainly points to an organic basis for some difficulties in perceiving reliably, consistently and adequately. Observation of the actual visual behavior must parallel observation of the end-product of a performance in this area if a contribution is to be made to an understanding of the problem. In the instance of children with cerebral palsy and of those who may have brain defects but are without motor handicaps, individual observation is the only means of discovering the potential and the difficulties; neither the examiner nor the teacher can afford to take unimpaired functioning for granted nor expect automatic progress to occur simply by exposing the child to an educational program.

The learning of self-help skills and the adjustment to a classroom will be influenced by existing visual limitations. While the effects of some difficulties are almost self-explanatory, others may be less obvious unless the interaction of handicap and functioning has been pointed out. The examiner needs to relate his findings and observations constantly to the frame of reference of the Evaluation, the school setting of the child. In his report the most useful comments will be those which a teacher can immediately translate into her classroom experiences. Examples of the interaction of limitation and functioning in the daily routine include: the child who cannot adequately lower his eyes and thus may not be able to button or unbutton his coat; he may not be able to write and read if the material is placed flat on the table and will need to have it placed on a slant, the degree of which will have to be worked out with and for him. Or again, the child who cannot raise his eyes may not be able to see the blackboard or see experience charts placed above his eye level.

While these are conspicious difficulties, the effect of severe strabismus or of a visual field cut-off, for example, may not be so clearly evident in the classroom. The teacher will be aware of its influence on academic learning, but she may not discover that the same limitation may seriously impede or discourage a child who is just learning to walk with inanimate support. As the child tries to reach for support, he may fail to grasp correctly because he miscalculates a distance or height. He will take many falls and may avoid independent walking altogether.

Lack of adequate depth perception may be responsible for fearful clinging to the banister or a refusal to descend stairs alone, since such a child, although he may be able to walk safely on level ground, cannot judge the actual height of a tread and consequently feels unsafe.

Both child and teacher can be spared frustration and anxiety if these and other effects of impaired visual functioning are described simply and clearly in the examiner's report.

Every opportunity for maximum functioning must be provided during the early years, which means that observed deviations in visual functioning should be brought to the attention of the medical specialist so that they can be confirmed or ruled out, corrected if possible and retraining instituted when indicated.

While these observations have been centered around the child with cerebral palsy, the method of painstaking observation is the same for any interview with any child. The examiner will be in a position to detect subtle difficulties in visual functioning and to appreciate their implications for the performance of the child. In the evaluation of children with diagnosed or suspected brain defects, explanations of the nature of perceptual disturbances found may be helpful. The illustrations of how findings are submitted to cross-checking with suitable items may have demonstrated the usefulness of flexibility in the structured interview. Perhaps, too, the description has helped to convey an impression of the immediacy and intensity of the evaluation procedure.

There is a great need for research in this area of deviate sensory functioning in young children, and no examiner should consider himself limited to recognition and observation of the visual difficulties described here, but should make his own observations and add his own contributions.

Evaluation of *auditory functioning* in the fictional interview with the child with cerebral palsy calls for a review of those aspects of the developmental history which are concerned with the production of sounds, emergence of first words, and development of speech, and the parents' estimate of comprehension and of hearing. The child who, because of physical involvement of the speech apparatus, has no or very little intelligible speech must be observed for behavior reactions which would indicate that he can comprehend simple verbal communication. These were described earlier in reference to language behavior.

The report of the parents may be very helpful or it may be noncontributory. It will be helpful if the observations they give to substantiate their estimate of the child's comprehension and hearing are conclusive evidence of the child's ability or inability to hear and to comprehend. It may be noncontributory if the parents either underestimate or overestimate the child, assuming that he is retarded and cannot be expected to understand or else assuming that the child understands everything they tell him without being in a position to substantiate their claim.

Evaluating the auditory intactness of a child with multiple handicaps requires a careful study of his behavior and of all factors which may have had a bearing on his previous opportunity to hear language spoken and to acquire comprehension of it. If there is any question of a limitation in hearing and if the report of the parents has not revealed enough useful information in the area of hearing and language, the examiner should elicit from the mother at the time of the interview detailed and precise data. It will depend on the particular mother whether this is best accomplished before the interview, perhaps while the child is occupied with the "warm-up" toy, or after the examiner himself has undertaken a systematic check-up on the hearing behavior of the child. A mother who shows an understanding of the problem and who appears to be a good observer and reporter might suitably be questioned prior to the examiner's check-up. Her findings will permit the examiner's measures to be more specific. A mother who appears unaware of anything amiss or unable to grasp the serious implications of a hearing defect in her child might more fittingly be questioned after the examiner has himself checked the child's hearing and has made a tentative appraisal of the problem, if one exists. The mother's answers will then contribute to a confirmation of the findings during the check-up. In either case, the specific questions can be formulated along these lines:

1. At what age did the child turn toward you or show in some other way that he knew you were calling him by name?

2. When he was quite little, was he easily frightened when people spoke in a loud voice or when he heard a door slam?

3. Did he use any toys that made a noise, like a squeaky rubber animal, a music box, xylophone, or a bell or rattle, and how did he use it? If he could not hold it himself, did he show you that he wanted you to produce the sound for him?

4. How did he let you know when he was awake in the morning?

5. How did he let you know when he wanted to come out of the playpen or carriage?

6. Did he like it when you sang to him; does he seem to like it now?

7. What is his favorite song? Does he have a victrola? favorite records? Does he like to listen to the radio? music? stories?

8. What is his favorite story, book, or nursery rhyme? How often does he want you to read to him or tell stories? How long can he sit and listen?

9. When he plays by himself, does he ever hum? Does it sound like a tune? Which one?

10. When he plays with little cars or dolls, does he mimic sounds, like making the noise of a motor for a car or the sound of crying or of sucking a bottle while playing with a doll?

11. Does he like horns and drums to play with? Did he ever attend a child's birthday party and what did he like best? What did he seem to dislike about it?

12. What does he do when you open a familiar box, such as crackers or potato chips, that is wrapped in crackling paper, in his presence, but in such a way that he has not seen what you are up to?

13. Does he pick up objects dropped on the floor (if he is physically able)?

14. What does he do when the telephone rings? Does he become annoyed when you use the vacuum cleaner, or when the washing machine or the frigidaire makes noise?

15. Does he show an interest in airplanes when he is outdoors and a plane flies overhead?

16. Does it frighten him when a dog barks?

17. Does he seem to recognize his father's step even before the father enters the room? Does he look expectantly at the door?

18. Does he seem to recognize the voices of some of his favorite people, perhaps a grandmother or an aunt? Does he show signs of anticipation even before they enter the room?

19. If he likes to listen to the radio, does he want the volume not as loud as you wish it, louder, or the same?

20. Does he ignore the radio?

21. What is his favorite television program? For how long does he like to watch?

22. Do you ever have to spell words that he is not supposed to overhear when you speak to somebody?

Used in conjunction with the data available in the child's developmental history, the answers to these questions should help to establish a gross estimate of the child's ability to hear. Many of the items are well within the range of children who have no capacity to produce speech, and some are involuntary reactions to sounds. The formulation of the questions aids the mother in recalling typical behavior. What may have appeared to the parents as disinterest or retardation may actually indicate an unawareness on the basis of lack of hearing or of sufficient hearing. Discrepancies between adequate reactions to gestures and inadequate reactions to verbal commands are important observations. Appropriate reactions to inanimate sounds, such as the crackling caused when the mother opens a familiar food box, a familiar step or the sound of airplanes, in the absence of equally appropriate reactions to verbal communication are significant findings. They would confirm that the hearing is intact and that the basis for failure to react to the human voice must be searched for in an area other than that of auditory acuity.

As has been pointed out in the description of visual impairment, so also in this area there are variations in the ways in which children adapt to impairment. The degree of hearing loss, the resourcefulness of the individual child, and environmental factors all play a role in creating the pattern which results when there is impairment in auditory functioning.

A gross test of the acuity of auditory functioning is provided for in the Evaluation interview. The sound blocks, consisting of a series of graded, matched sounds, which are used in items 14 to 16, are useful for children of two years of age and older for a gross check-up, and for children from four years of age and up for further probing of acuity. The carefully worked-out but simple procedure will help establish whether hearing is grossly present or not.

The examiner may decide to use this item before presenting item 1 in the case of children with known hearing difficulties or with suspected severe hearing loss. If the severity of the difficulty is confirmed, the items then have to be presented with the modifications that make them suitable to a deaf child. Since language comprehension in a nonhearing child may be nonexistent or poor, a re-evaluation of the child should be planned for the time when his hearing has been corrected and perhaps after he has had the benefit of special training in language comprehension.

The examiner may wish to have a picture of the child's pattern of functioning and of the nature of his spontaneous adaptation to an impairment in hearing before the extent of the hearing loss is definitely demonstrated. The specific item to establish grossly how much the child can hear may then be presented in due time, while the first few items of the sequence would be utilized to inspect the manner in which the child organizes himself in order to respond. Too, a correct response by the child to the first item, using whichever way of responding is within his physical capacity, in itself demonstrates simultaneously that the child can hear (the request), comprehend (the verbal formulation used) and see (the items among which he selects his response).

If the first item is failed, the method of cross-checking and of retreating to lower levels of demand in the search for the weak area gradually eliminates suspected reasons for failure until the actual basis for the child's poor performance can be demonstrated and isolated. This approach is as valid in tracking down difficulties in auditory perception as it is in tracking down those in such other areas as vision.

Again, it is with caution and some misgiving that the author offers a description of some of the patterns of behavior observable when children try to adapt to, compensate for, or surrender to difficulties in auditory perception. The reservations are based on the experience that such descriptions can be received and utilized either dynamically or mechanically. An examiner who himself has spotted patterns of adaptation in various children will welcome the interpretations of another observer against which to check his own findings. An examiner who attempts to apply the suggestions in the manner of a check list, on the other hand, may be persuaded to depend too heavily on a literal interpretation of what he observes, rather than on his original investigation of the total behavior pattern of the child before him.

Proceeding with our fictional interview with the child with cerebral palsy, we now assume that the developmental history, the mother's report and our preliminary glance at the child during the warm-up period have led us to wonder whether the child can hear adequately. We assume further that no formal hearing examination has been conducted because of the child's young age and inability to cooperate, because the parents' recognition of a hearing difficulty has been too recent, or because they have hesitated to have the child undergo a psychogalvanic skin test at this time. In other instances, where a difficulty in this area may be milder or more subtle, perhaps no doubt about the child's hearing will arise until the sound blocks (items 14 to 16) have been presented and something has been revealed during the interview which prompts us to investigate more closely.

Some difficulties in adequate hearing may be noticed quickly. The examiner will spot, or soon learn to spot, the child who strains to catch his voice, who fails to hear a soft-spoken comment exchanged by the adults, or who asks for, or waits for, a repetition of a verbal request before responding. He may respond with an air of tentativeness, as if trying to judge whether he understood correctly by waiting for the reception which the examiner gives his response. By his willingness to attend and concentrate and by his obvious awareness of being addressed, he demonstrates that his hesitation is not based on incomprehension of the fact that people have a way of communicating by using sounds, as might be true of a child with receptive aphasia. He also appears to demonstrate a readiness to be contacted, which he would not feel or show if his hesitation or lack of response were based upon autistic features. The question then remains whether the problem is that he does not comprehend although he hears or whether he could comprehend if only he could hear the request more clearly. If he has shown some constructive occupation with the "warm-up" toy, giving a hint of a fairly adequate level of comprehension and attention span, or if by some other intelligent and resourceful act he has shown himself capable of simple reasoning, such as calling his mother's attention to some feature of the interview room (the armchair, the telephone just like the one at home, the blackboard, etc.), the examiner would be inclined to suspect that the trouble might be inadequate hearing. Further checking then would be directed toward confirming or ruling out this possibility.

A less obvious difficulty, but possibly one more detrimental to useful reception and acquisition of language, is the difficulty which results from a hearing cut-off in certain frequencies only. In such an instance the child hears many of the noises which are part of the daily environment and his difficulty may not be suspected because he reacts to them in a convincingly normal fashion. The child who has no physical impairment of the speech organs may give a clue to his problem by his faulty articulation. He will speak as he hears; if he fails to hear the high frequency sounds, such as t, k, c, p, s, f, sh, he does not reproduce them in his own verbal production. This may erroneously be ascribed to retardation and excused on that basis, or it may be considered a speech impediment rather than recognized as what it is, the consequence of an auditory difficulty. If the child cannot speak at all, due to physical involvement, it is even more difficult to detect such a partial hearing cut-off. Sometimes, the first hint the examiner receives during the interview, in the case of either the speaking or the nonspeaking child, is a reaction of selective hesitation or indecision, when the child is asked for the spoon or the shoe. He may be found to narrow down his choice to these two only, offering first one, then the other, trying to judge the examiner's expression as he does so, while the other objects may have been selected without hesitation. To him only the vowels may be audible, and "spoon" and "shoe" may both sound like "oo." In spite of mutilated reception of spoken words, by using a combination of reasoning, memory and visual cues, he may have learned to discriminate between similar sounding names by the context in which they are used. A quick cross-check with item 2, presenting the same four objects but describing them in terms of use instead of by their names only, may confirm a suspected difficulty of this type. There will be enough words that the child can hear partially or completely when the request is formulated as: "Give me the thing we use to eat our cereal," or "find the thing we put on our foot," for him to catch the general drift of the request and to determine from the context the object in question. A performance resembling this may also be characteristic of a partial aphasic difficulty, but with a difference; here the child whose problem is the recall of words or the connection of the word with the appropriate object will probably have difficulty with all four objects. It is the selective confusion, limited to objects whose names sound alike to a child with a high frequency loss, which provides a more specific clue to the nature of the difficulty.

Hearing impairment for which a child is trying to compensate by alert attention to the face, mouth and gestures of the speaker is especially difficult to spot in a nonspeaking child. His anxious attention to the speaker's face, coupled with the fact that he will react appropriately at some times but not at others, is too readily considered a sign of retardation or of distractibility or inattention. Since these attributes are considered to be so typical of the "brain-injured" child and the child with cerebral palsy, the true underlying cause for the behavior pattern, such as impaired hearing and an eager desire to detour the difficulty by using other faculties, may not be suspected and explored. The examiner should consider the possibility of partially compensated hearing loss when a child seems to "glue" his eyes to the examiner's face or mouth whenever he speaks, rather than getting ready to respond by beginning to turn his eyes to the available choices. Checking can be done by speaking inaudibly, without voicing, while the child watches. This can be cross-checked by speaking in a normal tone of voice but with the hand covering the mouth or by turning the face away from the child's field of vision. The child who continues to respond appropriately as long as he can watch the speaker's mouth and face, even though the speaker has made no sound, but who seems unaware of being addressed or unsure of what is expected of him or stops responding when he cannot see the speaker speak demonstrates his pattern of compensated, or partially compensated, difficulty. The pattern has then been isolated and hearing loss demonstrated.

But again the examiner must keep an open mind, because some children who have receptive aphasia also may spontaneously look for cues in the examiner's face. They may have learned that some particular situation is usually preceded by, or combined with, a certain expression visible on the mother's face. Without having an awareness of words and of the meaning of words, they may have learned to react to these visually received cues by suitable action. One such child, who liked above everything to go out in the car and to go to bed, had observed the two distinct and different mouth formations so well, the one a lip-pursing for "bed," the other an open mouth for "car," that he began to use a silent "b" to ask for bed and an "ah" with a rising inflection for car without showing any apparent awareness of the meaning of words nor of the fact that the sounds coming from people could convey meaning. This child was diagnosed as having receptive aphasia; his hearing was excellent.

The examiner may wish to check on the possibility of receptive aphasia during the initial presentation of the first item, while he is still trying to gauge the pattern of the child whom he is interviewing. Removing the comb unobtrusively from among the four objects and bringing it under the table or in back of the child without arousing his attention, the examiner can produce an insistent soft sound by running his thumb over the teeth of the comb. A child with hearing loss will fail to hear this sound unless it is made very close to his ear. A child without hearing loss but who may be aphasic will hear the sound and will search for the source of it. If he is physically handicapped, he will show by a questioning look or a turn of his head that he is aware of a noise. The use of the sound blocks (items 14 to 16) will then serve to confirm the findings.

It has been observed that hearing impairment affects children in different ways. While some children try to compensate for it, as described, or try to cover up for what they consider a fault for which they may be blamed, others surrender to the difficulty and give up trying to listen when listening is so unrewarding. They fail to develop any or much language comprehension, so that their initial difficulty is compounded by the effort of their submissive behavior. The degree of hearing loss may not be any more severe than that of children who meet the difficulty more resourcefully and defiantly. It is also possible that a hearing loss has become progressively more severe, perhaps in connection with colds and "running ears." Since the family may have observed the child's ability to hear moderately loud sounds, his indifference or inattentiveness to verbal communication may be ascribed to retardation or to an uncooperative attitude, the more so because the child may respond to his name spoken in a normal tone or when repeated once or twice. In a child who has no speech due to involvement of the speech apparatus and who has no means to demonstrate the adequacy of his intellectual level by performance, this pattern is particularly difficult to demonstrate. Every effort should be made to detect it, however, if it does exist, since correction with a hearing device and intensive language training may salvage a child who might otherwise be doomed to a life of isolation and resignation. Presenting such a child with the items of the Evaluation in a mode suitable for deaf children will reveal his level of development in nonverbal comprehension, although those items depending on verbal comprehension will have to be omitted and postponed to the time of a later re-evaluation.

Occasionally, it is desirable to attempt a preliminary differentiation between the two possibilities, retardation and pseudo deafness, before the items are presented as one would for a deaf child. This can be tentatively attempted by presenting some unstructured material which lends itself to nonverbal use; the ability to use it in a way commensurate to the chronologic age level or to imitate some demonstrated use on that level would rule out the assumption that the child fails to comprehend verbal requests simply because he is too retarded to understand them. His failure to comprehend could be assumed to be based on a more selective deficit, the failure to have developed language comprehension due to faulty listening habits, which in turn have been the result of hearing impairment. In chapter 9, modifications for such contingencies are described. The hundred-hole peg board is used for this purpose, and its use even with a motor-handicapped child, who can give his directions for placing the pegs to the examiner, is described there. Pencil and paper, or crayon, or the blackboard can also be utilized for this end, if the child has the use of his hands. A drawing on a level disproportionately higher than that of language comprehension would help to rule out primary retardation as the responsible factor.

Again, the examiner has to be on guard because an indifference to verbal communication in the presence of fair or adequate hearing is also characteristic of receptive aphasia, as well as of autism. The autistic child, however, shows a different and more severe kind of inaccessibility, while the aphasic child may perform differently than the child with pseudo deafness on items which have to do with concept formation and association. Such items, which can be presented by pantomime and without verbalization, are amount recognition by matching of pennies (item 26), sorting in a multiple choice and shifting from one concept to another (items 28 and 29) and understanding of the relationship of incomplete parts of a whole to each other (item 32; see also Fig. 1).

Frequently, mild impairment of hearing may be revealed only gradually during the interview by an uneven performance which will prompt the examiner to review the nature, meaning and possible basis for such a manner of performing. The effect of impaired hearing on language development and language comprehension varies with the nature of the impairment, the time of onset of impairment, environmental influences and the child's own compensatory reactions. A physically handicapped child will be more severely restricted in developing resourcefulness even if the mental development is entirely adequate. A chair-bound child cannot, like a more able-bodied one, follow his mother around and place himself so that he can watch her face as she speaks or so that he can remain within the range of her voice. The absence of verbal production can be so plausibly explained on the basis of physical involvement of the organs of speech that it may not be suspected that even given a sound vocal mechanism the child would not develop speech because he does not hear words and therefore cannot imitate them. The additional clue for spotting impairment of hearing by investigating faulty articulation is not available in the case of such a child.

The sequence of items provides, in addition to the specific gross test of functional hearing (items 14 to 16), the opportunity to observe comprehension of language of increasing levels of complexity. If auditory functioning is impaired in more subtle ways, the examiner will be alerted to such a possibility as discrepancies arise between the over-all level of functioning and the level of language reception and comprehension on specific items. Such a hint will then lead the examiner to search for the factor responsible for the discrepancy.

The interview has to be conducted with *two objectives* in mind; one, *to delineate the area of impairment;* the other, *to accommodate the impairment* by the mode of presentation.

In order to delineate the area of impairment, it is advisable during the presentation of the first item to avoid giving any clues by gestures and to avoid making the request more concrete, such as by introducing the doll. It is necessary to demonstrate the child's ability to receive and react to verbal communication alone. If the child performs poorly or with difficulty, the next step is a reduction of the intellectual demand by reducing the number of choices, but the request should still be made verbally, avoiding gestures. Depending on the suspected nature of the difficulty, the examiner must experiment by using those objects whose names sound unlike each other, perhaps hairbrush and comb versus spoon, and follow this up by deliberately using spoon versus shoe, whose names to the child with the high frequency difficulty would sound alike. Such an experiment would serve to confirm or refute the postulated nature of the difficulty. Restricting the initial maneuver to purely verbal communication helps to demonstrate whether it is hearing impairment or inability to comprehend intellectually which is at the bottom of the poor performance. A child who can perform correctly in response to verbal requests when choices are reduced to two, but fails when he has to choose among four choices, demonstrates that his hearing is adequate enough to respond to verbal requests. His earlier failure would then have to be evaluated as being on the basis of intellectual inability to comprehend successfully on the level of the standard sequence.

While successful performance on a lower level proves that hearing is adequate, unsuccessful performance does not necessarily prove that it is inadequate, but must lead to further probing. The child may function on an intellectual level where verbal comprehension is poor or nonexistent, or he may be uncooperative for other reasons while the ability to hear is not at all reduced. It then becomes the examiner's job to probe the intellectual functioning. The child is presented with the four choices of the first item and the doll is introduced. At this stage the ability to hear or the ability to comprehend the verbal formulation is not under scrutiny. The examiner would simply point to the doll's foot and indicate by gestures and facial expression that he would like to put her shoe on, then indicate the lined-up choices of objects and gesture a request for the child to assist in this game of dressing the doll. If the problem is inadequate reception of language due to hearing impairment, and perhaps an associated delay in the development of language comprehension, but not intellectual inability to understand the use of the four objects, the child will be able to perform correctly. If he is intellectually unable to comprehend, he will not, or will not adequately and readily, respond to requests given by pantomime. It may be useful to go directly on to the presentation of the picture of objects (items 4 and 5; see Fig. 9), if the child is two and one-half years of age or older, and let him apply the doll to the pictures or the pictures to the doll. The examiner may point to the doll's hair, or mimic brushing her hair, to ask for the picture of comb and brush. A child who understands will eye-point, reach for or point to the picture of comb and brush, or he may hold the doll to the correct picture or bring the picture to the doll's hair as if pretending to use the brush. This would be followed by similar performances, such as placing the doll's foot on the picture of the shoe when the examiner has asked in pantomime for something to put on her bare foot. The ability to respond to requests given in this mode of presentation, after having failed to respond to verbal requests, would conclusively show that it is not intellectual inability to comprehend but inability to hear adequately which caused the earlier poor performance. The difficulty has then been pinpointed and isolated. Especially convincing is the child's ability to go on to pictorial material. The attentiveness to gestured communication and the ability to go on to pictures would simultaneously answer an unresolved possibility, namely, that the difficulty in receiving the verbal request might be due to receptive aphasia rather than to hearing impairment. In receptive aphasia, an awareness of the fact that people communicate (by words *or* gestures) is frequently poor; the transition from concrete objects to pictorial material is sometimes delayed. Pictures are a symbolic representation of a concrete object and comprehension of symbolic representation may be affected in aphasia, while in the nonretarded child with a hearing difficulty, it would not be affected. The question of the possibility of a motor aphasia would not arise since verbal requests are received adequately in cases of motor aphasia.

Before continuing with the presentation of the items in the standard sequence, the sound blocks (item 14) should then be used to probe grossly the degree of hearing impairment.

The rest of the interview will have to be conducted in the light of the auditory difficulty, the mode of presentation being suited to the child's impairment. Pantomime, gestures, examples and demonstrations of using sorting rather than requesting the child to match will answer the needs. Specific directions will be found in chapter 9, which describes the modified use of the items. (See also Figs. 16 and 17 for examples.)

The level of development can be evaluated nonverbally in many areas. This will permit tentative conclusions about the over-all level of functioning. Specific items testing language comprehension may serve to give clues to the present limited level achieved in that area; a re-evaluation will have to be planned for a future time, after correction of the impairment and exposure to language training.

The implications for comprehension and acquisition of language of a defect in hearing acuity need to be studied carefully; this may require repeated sessions, until the examiner is in a position to understand all the ramifications of the impaired functioning.

The planning for the child will call for early medical examination of hearing to define, confirm or rule out hearing loss, to establish the severity of the impairment and to provide corrective measures. Educational planning will have to be based upon the child's needs and will have to be arrived at mutually by the medical specialist, the examiner, speech therapist, and school personnel. Early therapeutic and training measures are essential in order to take advantage of the natural stages of language development. Appropriate schooling can begin as early as at two and one-half or three years of age in a specialized nursery school program for children with such difficulties. The levels of readiness to communicate can then be utilized while there is a dynamic drive to maximum growth and development and before resignation or poor habit patterns result from the child's impairment. The habit of communication and the adapted means to receive verbal communication and to produce speech, if speaking is physically possible, should be well established by the time the child reaches elementary school age.

In the report of the findings of the Evaluation, the examiner needs to describe the effects of auditory impairment on school activities, both for the child who is hard of hearing and the one who has a frequency cut-off in high frequencies. The teacher can then share these findings and adapt her approaches to the child, where adaptations are necessary and desirable. An accurate description of the pattern of hearing behavior, of spontaneous adaptations and difficulties as observed during the interview, will enable the teacher to seat the child most advantageously in the classroom and to be receptive to his other needs. A description of the level and the nature of the language comprehension, as it is influenced and limited by the hearing difficulty, will give the teacher information about the need and the readiness for a specific language building program.

Where a high frequency cut-off exists, a description of the child's very subtle and specific difficulty will make it possible for the teacher to understand his difficulty in reading and spelling. The child will need very understanding special instruction, even though he can remain in a regular classroom, by a speech therapist working together with the teacher. He has to learn to become aware of those sounds and the letters representing them in his reading words and spelling words which he does not expect to be there, because to him they are and have always been inaudible. For him, a printed word like "see-saw" will not automatically summon up the picture or image of a see-saw on the playground, because what he has heard it called, and has called it himself if he can speak, was "ee-aw." Fortunately, it is sometimes possible to foster a better understanding of speech as it is normally produced, by the introduction of the printed word. Visual impression can supplement the impaired auditory perception or reception as the child becomes aware of his difficulty and is ready to be guided in the use of looking, remembering, and thinking in addition to listening and pronouncing.

The child who has re-enforced his inadequate hearing with automatic reading of expressions and some lip-reading will probably become quite adept when provided with some special training and may possibly be able to remain in a regular school setting. The report should explain his attempts at adaptation and also the effects of the inadequate intake of verbal communication on language development. Limitations to the effort of listening, combined with looking, means that in a group setting he cannot quickly discover who is speaking, since, if he cannot see the speaker, he does not really hear him. A resourceful teacher might accommodate this difficulty by having the child seated facing the group and by having each speaker give a sign, such as raising his hand, to enlist the child's attention to the change in speakers. This is especially important when the child is physically so involved that his spontaneous mobility is severely restricted.

The child who has given up listening to verbal communication will need intensive and specific correction and instruction, probably in a special program, until his poor habit pattern is overcome and corrected, some language acquired, and a return to a regular school setting possible, albeit with continued attention to his problem and his tendency.

Impairment of auditory functioning is not limited to our fictional child with cerebral palsy but will be found to exist also in nonhandicapped children, in children with brain lesions but without motor handicap, and in retarded children. A thorough knowledge of patterns of hearing behavior, of kinds of impairment in auditory functioning, and of the manifestations and ramifications of deviations is invaluable for any examiner of young children. It will help him in spotting subtle difficulties early. The importance of this aspect of the Educational Evaluation cannot be stressed too much. Unlike adults, who have known normal functioning in a given area, children who are handicapped from birth, cannot be expected to be aware of a lack or a deviation in their functioning. They are not yet able to realize that not everybody has the same difficulties. It is the responsibility of the examiner to detect the difficulties by the use of the items of the Evaluation and by his educated observation. That is why it is not enough to note the correctness or incorrectness of a performance alone, without noting the functioning pattern of the young organism as he mobilizes himself to respond.

The interrelationship of limitations in various areas, such as auditory-visual or auditory-motor interaction, must not be ignored if one wishes to evaluate the child's total potential for functioning and developing. An illustration will suffice to make the examiner aware of the possibilities: the inability to raise the eyes above a certain level will limit or prohibit the use of them for lip-reading whenever the speaker's face rises above the level of the child's eyes; the effect will be a proportionally limited or fragmented intake of verbal communication. The inability to hold up the head or to turn the trunk appropriately, as may exist in cerebral palsy, will likewise effectively terminate the child's chances to supplement his insufficient hearing with lip-reading whenever the speaker moves outside of his very restricted area of vision. The additional inability to voice a protest and thus call the speaker's attention to the predicament may let such pernicious chain-reactions of interacting limitations go unnoticed. If they are known, such cumulative obstacles can be accommodated and functioning can be improved accordingly. Since the child is not in a position to report his problem, it is the examiner's responsibility to be on the alert and to inform the professional workers concerned with the child's progress.

Other, less frequently met, deviations in functioning in this area are an integral part of the description of the modifications (chapter 9) and will be found there.

The *tactile sensitivity* of the child is tested with the materials of item 38. While very gross impairment in this area may become obvious during the manipulation of such objects as the pellets or the push-button table bell (items 22a and 23), it cannot be confirmed conclusively and accurately until this specific item is used. Children functioning at a level below four years of age cannot cooperate readily on this item and it can be omitted, unless there are specific reasons why an investigation of the area is desirable.

The area is important mainly for two reasons. One is the implication which impairment in tactile sensitivity has for manual dexterity. The other is the fact that impairment in this area generally stems from some, perhaps unsuspected and undiagnosed, pathology of the brain; it therefore is a revealing finding when present in a child who shows no obvious motor handicap and in whom no gross neurologic signs have been demonstrated in a neurologic examination.

Impairment of tactile sensitivity is selective. Many children with cerebral palsy have no impairment of tactile sensitivity at all. Some children have been tested who had unimpaired tactile sensitivity in one hand, while the other hand was found to be affected. Sometimes, but not always, such a finding is made in a child who also has pincer grasp of the "good" hand and palmar grasp of the other hand; not all of these findings are confined to children with cerebral palsy. Manual awkwardness can exist in any child without simultaneous impairment of tactile sensitivity, but impairment in this area will certainly affect dexterity adversely.

Negative findings in the area of tactile sensitivity are noted in the report in order to confirm that all is well, and in order to have this finding on record, should a change be found on a later evaluation.

Positive findings are to be used as follows. When made in the evaluation of a child who is not diagnosed as having a brain lesion, the findings must be brought to the attention of the child's medical supervisor for their possible meaning. The findings and their demonstrated or postulated effect on manual performance, both of the child with known brain lesion and the one with unsuspected or undiagnosed brain damage, must be described in the report of the Evaluation in such a way that the teacher and therapist concerned with the child will be assisted in their understanding of the child's problem. Suggestions would include the training of the child to supplement his impaired tactile funtioning with alert awareness of his specific difficulty and with increased attention to the function of his fingers by using his eyes, his memory and his intelligence. Activities affected will be use of crayon, pencil or pen for printing, writing and drawing; unbuttoning and buttoning, lacing and tying and perhaps other dressing activities; grasping of small or thin articles, such as the handle of spoon or fork, hairpins, thumbtacks.

An investigation of the intactness of tactile sensitivity may help to reveal the true basis of the difficulty in the case of a child referred for an Evaluation because he presents a problem in writing, drawing, sewing, or self-dressing or perhaps because the teacher feels he is careless and always drops things. No neurologic basis for his poor behavior or performance may be suspected, either by the family or the school. In the interview, auxiliary materials may be used (see Fig. 19) in order to study the extent of the resulting difficulties more closely. Such materials would include pencil and paper tasks, scissors, peg and peg-board tasks, shoe-lacing, buttoning and even such simple acts as dialing a telephone and turning a light switch and a key. (The child's own clothing presents ever available auxiliary materials.) Sometimes, an improved way of dealing with his problem can be suggested to an older child during the interview. If he is just becoming aware of his difficulty, he may be grateful at being shown ways to help overcome some of the effects. He may learn to use his eyes to inform him of what his fingers do not feel adequately: the child may not feel it when the slant of his pencil changes as he writes if he is intent on the correctness of his spelling. He may have difficulty tying a bow although intellectually he can comprehend the motions involved. His difficulty might be in the unreliability of perceiving with his fingertips just how to secure a loop.

While positive findings will be helpful in proving a point, the examiner must remember that negative findings do not necessarily disprove it, if an undiagnosed and unconfirmed brain lesion was postulated. The Evaluation is not a diagnostic tool, but it can provide extremely helpful and suggestive data. These should never be permitted to remain lost in a record, but must be conveyed to the medical specialist.

Modifications are possible down to a very low level of functioning. These are described in the chapter on modifications (chapter 9). For children who function below a four year level, they are used mainly when additional information about neurologic intactness or the lack of it is sought. Sometimes, this is the case when a hyperactive child is to be tested. Modifications are valuable also in the evaluation of a blind child or one with severe visual impairment. The intactness of tactile sensitivity must be investigated as early as possible in a blind child because so much of what he will be able to learn will have to be learned through the touch of his fingertips. By using modifications of the item (chapter 9, see also Fig. 19) it is possible to test for tactile sensitivity children who are as young as, or who function as low as, eight to ten months of age. The implication of impairment in this function for later learning of reading Braille is obvious.

In the education and training of children who are mentally retarded, manual dexterity is considered one area in which retarded children may be able to function on a par with nonretarded ones. This fact is utilized in prevocational guidance and training. But manual awkwardness is not uncommon in a number of retarded children. This area is, therefore, one in which the findings possible by means of the Educational Evaluation assume added importance. If the tactile sensitivity is found to be not intact in a child who is mentally retarded, the description of his impairment will enable those responsible for him to set goals and plan his training program realistically. Utilizing existing potential, rather than providing prevocational training along more general lines, will prevent futile and discouraging attempts at job-training requiring accuracy and speed, for which such a youngster would have little aptitude.

The description of the fictional interview with the child with cerebral palsy should have served to provide the user of this manual with insight into many aspects of functioning, those of intact functioning as well as deviations, and of the manifestations of functioning on significant developmental levels. It should be possible, on the basis of this detailed, vicarious experience, to learn to conduct the interview with young handicapped children. The examiner should now know how to elicit responses even from nonspeaking children, and the need for constant, educated observation of the total behavior while a child mobilizes himself to respond to presented items should have become obvious. The author has offered substantiation of the important and direct connections between observable behavior patterns and their implications for developing and learning, both at home and in school settings. This was undertaken in the hope of persuading the examiner to make full use of the Evaluation to assess the potential of the child and to convey the findings to those in charge of his education and training. By constant references to the meaning of the possible findings, the examiner should be able to interpret them in his report in a manner most useful to those using his reports.

Once the ability to receive instructions and impressions and the manner of responding have been determined, the interview can proceed as directed in chapter 8. Special needs which may call for modifications in the presentation of items will have become apparent during the beginning of the interview and can be accommodated by the examiner as directed.

The Evaluation, because its scope is not confined to an investigation of intellectual adequacy, aims to gain insight into the potential for adapting and adjusting. The behavior pattern is appraised as the child responds to each item, and even children with manual difficulties are given an opportunity to assist the examiner in collecting and putting away materials after use, so that habits of orderliness, helpfulness, and dependability are disclosed. The degree of self-awareness of a physically handicapped child becomes clear, as does his attitude to his limitations by his cheerful attempts to utilize what he has or, conversely, by an attempt to display or flaunt his disabilities. The stamina of the child is revealed by how untiring is his struggle with his unruly body in his attempts to react to the items. A sense of humor or a solemn attitude, an ability to relate with confidence or a guarded, suspicious attitude can be recognized during the self-absorbed occupation of the child with the materials.

The examiner probes with special interest and attention the child's ability and willingness to take suggestions, to imitate, to ask for help or explanations and to carry a task begun to its conclusion. If they are interfered with by something in the child's personality structure, the prospect of maximum development of the potential becomes proportionally poorer. Resistance to or grudging acceptance of suggestions, inability or unwillingness to imitate, refusal or reluctance to finish a task are obstacles to developing and learning which are difficult to surmount or remove. Suitable motivation during the interview may help to make the session fairly fruitful, but the effects of such negative attitudes are not limited to the brief interview session. They are an integral part of the elements which make up a child's potential.

Two other areas have to be surveyed and studied, that of the *concept of self* and that of *self-help functions*.

Because the Evaluation has been developed in a form which makes possible its use with severely handicapped children, the level of awareness of the body image cannot be routinely explored by having the child produce a drawing of the human figure. Experimental material used by the author has demonstrated that the growth of insight in this area, as in all others, parallels that of nonhandicapped children. It has additionally provided some hints about the need for an opportunity for self-expression and self-exploration with suitable materials, even for the most severely impaired child, perhaps especially for him. As children form their image of the human body, they become aware of their own. The recognition that the handicap is a permanent condition develops only gradually. As the child lives through the stages of recognizing his difference from the nonhandicapped, his own reactions and attitudes need to be known so that he can be guided wisely. Ready-made, easily movable parts of the body that can be pushed in any direction by even a handicapped child will make it possible for him to project his idea of the human figure. His readiness for therapeutic training may be revealed by his performance. If he is troubled or puzzled about his condition, his fears or wishes may be reflected in his figure building, especially if he performs in an atmosphere conducive to coming to grips with his handicap.

Using such experimental material, children have, at more confiding moments, portrayed themselves as emphasizing or omitting an affected limb; wishfully adding an extra limb to help out the useless one ("God gave him an extra leg, for when he gets tired"); encasing the figure in braces as in a suit of armor, especially after just having been given new braces; carefully covering fingers with a layer of "muscles" which have to be brought under control like strings on a puppet; and have contributed other revealing material.

At present, the Evaluation interview includes no specific items to test this area, although the examiner can obtain a drawing of a person if drawing is physically possible for a child. In young and handicapped children the level of body awareness is evaluated by inference. If the child is too handicapped to be able to point to his eyes, hair, ear or nose, his reaction to a doll will demonstrate whether he accepts the doll as a replica of a baby or child. Appropriate application of objects in the daily routine (shoe, spoon, cup, hairbrush and comb) shows an essentially adequate orientation in this area. Adequate response to the pictures portraying children's activities (item 7, see also Fig. 10) and successful performance in using the wedgie figure (item 30) are evaluated as a demonstration of appropriate awareness and recognition of the human body image. On lower levels the child's response to the direct offer of the spoon, shoe or comb and brush will show whether or not he has a beginning orientation toward an awareness of his body. The reaction to the image of himself or of his mother in the mirror, or, on a four months level, the reaction to a mask placed over his mother's face, will make clear whether he is capable of this degree of awareness of persons.

In the report, a description of the reaction will give information about the level on which he can react. This information will be helpful to therapists, physicians and teachers.

A survey of the levels achieved in self-help functions, obtained from the report of the developmental history and confirmed by personal observation during the visit, must be made, especially in the case of young and handicapped children. Their eligibility for a school setting frequently depends on adequacy or independence in this area. Some observations will be possible by observing the child as he employs the materials of the Evaluation, such as trying to comb his hair or bringing the spoon to his mouth. Other observations can be made simply by taking the child to the bathroom at the end of the interview and observing his ability to use the toilet himself, in washing and drying his own hands, in taking an offered drink of water and feeding himself a cookie, and finally his level of independence in getting dressed when ready to depart. The physically able child is observed on the stairway before he leaves, both ascending and descending. It is noted whether he alternates his steps or needs two steps per tread and in what manner he uses the rail, especially if he has one poor hand.

These observations are important for the record because they denote the level of competency and resourcefulness of the child. In addition, the attitudes of mother and child during these routine activities, coming at the end of a structured session, can give glimpses of overdependence on the part of the child and overprotection on the part of the mother or else show the understanding attitude of a mother and the habit pattern of a child who has been trained wisely. When indicated, suggestions can be included in the report which may subsequently be useful in the guidance provided to the mother by the social worker, therapist or teacher, to foster the training of the child if he is considered ready for greater independence in this area.

The final part of this chapter will deal with suggestions about the conduct of the interview with children who present special problems.

Difficulties which stem from impairment of the sensory equipment and from interference with the reception of language, making necessary adaptation of the presentation in order to accommodate the particular handicap, have been discussed in the foregoing. Modifications of items are expected to meet such eventualities. The difficulties which remain to be discussed are those which prevent direct contact with the child because the child is rendered more or less inaccessible by his condition.

The first question that arises is why one should insist on subjecting a child to an Evaluation interview if he is emotionally disturbed, inaccessible or completely negative and evasive. The answer is that it is necessary to evaluate a child not in spite of his being upset, inaccessible or negative, but because of it. The Evaluation may contribute to a clarification of the child's problem and may make possible a more suitable management of him. Sometimes, also, children are transported at great expense in time and money to a clinic from an outlying district and it cannot simply be suggested that the child be brought back when he is in a more favorable frame of mind. A knowledge of some useful approaches is therefore advantageous. No experienced examiner expects to present every item of a scale to a child under circumstances which make direct contact impossible. But by a combination of free field observation, tactfully introduced standard items, and sensitive and flexible management, a baseline can be demonstrated. This baseline will reveal the minimum level on which the child can function, and any higher performances which the examiner may be able to elicit sporadically during the interview may give a clue to the maximum performance of which the child might be capable if he could cooperate and apply himself without restriction.

The more frequently encountered difficulties are conduct disturbance, autism and schizophrenia, and hyperactivity.

The problem of testing the very disturbed child starts with the question of how to induce him to enter the interview room. The room itself should be prepared with most of the material out of sight and reach, preferably on a high shelf. A preliminary conference with the mother of such a child can serve two purposes. It should give the mother the assurance that the examiner is willing to follow any suggestions she can offer from her own knowledge of her child and that he welcomes her flexible cooperation, both inside and outside of the interview room. It should give the examiner all the information he needs about known fears and preferences of the child, such as fear of doors, left open or closed; of light, left on or turned off; of being placed on a table or of being placed on chairs; of certain toys, such as dolls; of men; of women; of being spoken to, looked at or touched; of noises; of having his hat and coat removed anywhere but at home. Likes and preferences might include: mirrors; water in a basin; music; spinning tops; looking out of windows; sitting under a table; hiding in a closet.

Armed with such information, the examiner rids the room of articles the child fears so that no disturbing factor will intrude inadvertently later on if some fragile contact with the child should have become possible. The child's fears are respected. A first interview is not the time to start retraining, although toward the end of the session the examiner may wish to probe the severity or validity of reported fears. This can be accomplished by deliberately committing some little "indiscretion," such as matter-of-factly closing a door if this should happen to be a sensitive point. Sometimes, a child proves to be more robust than the well-trained parent, who has learned to cater to his needs, has suspected.

The examiner can try to meet the child with a music box (item 23), which he might play as he approaches the child; or he may place the milk bottle set (items 24 and 25) somewhere between the child and the door leading to the interview room, with a few single bottles spread out, as bait, ever closer to the room. Under most circumstances, if the child is greatly disturbed, it will be simplest to have the child led to the room by the mother, with the examiner remaining in the background. The child may cling to his own toy or book and carry it with him. A toy or two can be displayed in the room. The milk bottle set frequently is very well liked; the hundred-hole peg board with just a few pegs inserted and a few more placed alongside sometimes catches a child's eye and he will start to use it. If the mother succeeds in leading the child into the room, the examiner must judge whether to remain outside, an oblique spectator, while mother and child inspect the room or while the mother engages the child in some game. After the child appears to feel a bit at home, the examiner can attempt to enter the room and immediately become occupied with something on his desk, neither ignoring nor contacting the child but presenting a positive air of co-existence. If the child can tolerate this degree of proximity, the examiner may use the music box, if the child is reported to like music, or the spinning top, if he is reportedly not afraid of moving objects. After briefly using the toy, he can leave it matter-of-factly within convenient reach of the child, returning to his former position behind his desk and waiting unobtrusively for the child's reaction as he pretends to be busy with his papers.

If the child is not afraid of dolls, the examiner may next busy himself with the first four objects (item 1, see Fig. 3) and the doll, either silently or speaking softly to the doll, and again leave the objects within reach of the child and retire to his desk, leaving the field open for the child. If the child is afraid of dolls but likes mirrors, the four objects, which include comb and brush, can be placed near the mirror and left there. The mother can be instructed to suggest to the child that he fix his hair. The examiner will be able to observe, if the child accepts the suggestion, whether the child is able to select correctly the described object from a choice of four and if he can apply it correctly.

Unless the child begins to scream every time the examiner approaches, it may be possible for the examiner gradually to join the mother in her attempts to provide the child with "something nice to do." This quote is placed here not because that is what one tells the child, but because that is what it should look like to him. His experience may have included visits to relatives who tried to entertain him with toys, objects or pictures; if the interview can approach this experience, it will look less formidable to him. If the peg board has not been used by the child at first, the examiner might use it near the child, placing a box of pegs conveniently, and again retire to his desk, leaving the peg board with the child. His way of using it will give some information about his level. From the age of three years up, an attempt to organize the pegs rather than placing them at random can be expected. Organizing includes filling one or part of one row systematically, either horizontally or vertically, or using one color selectively but without attention to placement.

It is possible to present many of the items silently by using a mixture of pretended self-absorbed occupation with them and a polite willingness to "let the child play too" after the examiner has enjoyed the playing.

The pictures of objects may be presented, either in the stand or placed on the table (item 4, see also Fig. 9). Either with the doll or, if the child cannot tolerate dolls, by directly applying them to himself, the examiner can pantomime the use of each picture. He can pretend to pick the spoon off the picture and bring it to his mouth; or he can bring the picture of the shoe near his own foot, lifting the foot and pretending to step into the shoe portrayed on the picture. The pictures are then replaced but their position is changed. The field is again left to the child, with the examiner preoccupied near his desk. It will then be possible to observe, if the child tries to imitate or if he decides to share this new game with his mother, whether he can apply each picture appropriately. This would show that he can see and recognize the pictures and that he can select among a choice of three.

The pictures of children's activities (item 7, see also Fig. 10 and 16) can be "played with" as for deaf children. The spoon and piece of red cloth are placed, as if the examiner is undecided, between the two pictures. If the child does not spontaneously use the spoon to "feed" the children seated at the table, or use the cloth to cover the children sleeping in their beds, the examiner "plays" this game, reverses the position of the pictures and materials, and again wanders away, leaving the child free to help himself. If the child will play, the correct or incorrect use of object applied to picture will show whether he can recognize a picture of this degree of complexity and understands the activity portrayed. If it is desirable to check, so that accidentally correct choices are not assumed to be conclusively correct, one picture can be removed but the spoon and red cloth left near the other picture. Now the child must decide once more which material to apply to the picture and thus he will demonstrate his actual comprehension, or lack of it. If the child can speak and if he verbalizes to the mother or himself about the pictures, one can sometimes observe whether he understands them even if he does not apply the materials. Occasionally a child will pick up the picture of the sleeping children and hum "Rock-a-bye baby" or he will kiss them goodnight. These are correct responses and demonstrate that the child recognizes the pictures.

Depending on the child's age, the cut-out forms (item 9) or the square cards with symbols (item 10) can be "presented" next. The examiner can scatter the cards on the table and then sort them with studied effort, making sure that the child can observe that choices are to be made and that it is not just a set of cards to be stacked. After sorting them and leaving the three small piles exposed for a while, face up, the examiner can leave a row of three cards exposed (square, circle, triangle) and scatter the second set, which he hopes the child will sort by matching each card to a similar one. If the child tries this "game" the examiner has an opportunity to evaluate his ability to discriminate between and to match simple forms.

In such a cautious, impersonal but entirely polite and friendly manner, it often becomes possible to present many of the items, omitting, because any attempt to present might break the fragile rapport, all those where direct verbal requests are necessary, such as recall of missing picture from memory (item 6), recognition of the time of day (item 8), finding forms or symbols from memory (item 11). With some disturbed children, a working relationship of this type can be maintained as long as the examiner respects the child's reserve and keeps his distance. If the child gradually permits proximity and direct contact, all the items within his chronologic age level can be attempted. The flashlight item (item 33) should be given with caution and discontinued the moment the child's reaction indicates fear. Testing of tactile sensitivity (item 38) should be omitted since it requires more cooperation than can be expected from the first meeting with a vulnerable child.

If the child resists or ignores direct contact steadfastly, reacts to proximity with screaming, ignores any material placed near him consistently, or is so completely out of reach that no progress can be made, nothing is gained by insistence. It is sometimes helpful if the child can be left in the room alone, or with the mother, with the examiner observing through the door or a one-way vision window without the child's knowledge. Experimental materials can be placed on the table, such as form boards, nest of cubes, crayon, pencil and paper, a box of crackers or lollipops. Before the examiner leaves the room, he might "accidentally" spill the form board and the nest of cubes and leave without restoring them to their former order. Left alone, such a child is sometimes discovered to use materials meaningfully, put forms back in the form board, show his level by his ability or inability to fit the nest of cubes, show his resourcefulness by opening the box of crackers or else display a lower level of comprehension by using materials in a very primitive fashion, such as chewing the forms of the form board, the crayon or the paper, or flinging everything within reach to the floor.

The examiner can base the Evaluation tentatively on observed reactions to the items which could be presented or to which a child reacted at any time during the interview. Where responses could be elicited, the child's performance will reliably demonstrate that he can function on the level of development necessary to respond to those items. The estimate will have to be considered minimal. The form of interview should be described briefly in order to sketch the pattern of the child's behavior in a semi-structured situation.

Not all children who are emotionally disturbed will remain extremely reserved nor will all become accessible to calm, impersonal, noncommittal persuasion. Some will begin to cooperate after the first half hour or so and may even begin to cling and seek physical contact. Others may become increasingly agitated or refuse to remain in the room. In one such extreme case, testing was finally attempted with fair success by using the father to present the items. The examiner, watching through a one-way vision window, observed the child's responses to the items, which one after another were given to the father by the examiner with instructions as to how to present them. The child returned to a preoccupation with a spinning top after responding each time, and the father and examiner used this recess to confer about the next item in the hallway. The device of returning to play with a favorite toy, between brief periods of cooperating, works with some children, and can even be initiated by the examiner if the child seems to cooperate more comfortably when allowed to withdraw every few minutes. Sometimes the child will even be willing to "trade" his toy, letting the examiner "mind" it for him, while his own hands are busy figuring out the "school work" which the examiner keeps presenting to him and then welcome it back when he has "finished the school work."

One might speculate whether such a pattern represents an attempt on the part of the child to preserve a barrier between himself and the outside, which makes demands on him, by using the object almost in place of a symbol. But for the purpose of evaluating the developmental level, whatever the reason for the child's need of the object, one utilizes the tendency to further the course of the interview.

This tendency must not be confused with the well-known pattern of normal young children to become extremely attached to a certain toy or piece of clothing, at some stage of growing up.

With patience, ingenuity and a calculated disregard of the expenditure of energy and time, it is possible to be occupied with the child sufficiently intensively to gain some insight into his way of functioning and to arrive at a tentative estimate of his minimum potential.

Some extremely remote and upset children have been induced to establish a grudging or conditional sort of working relationship through approaches arrived at by trial and error and evolved just for the individual child. A description of such attempts may help the examiner to utilize his own ingenuity when the need arises.

One three year old girl was brought to the interview red-eyed and hoarse from screaming since the moment she had been put in the car an hour earlier to be transported to the clinic. She was reported to flee to her crib whenever possible at home. The examiner turned the big table on its side in the manner of an improvised playpen (see Fig. 4A). A table mat was placed inside the space on the floor. Since this child's mother felt that her presence would only result in the continued agitation of the child, she remained outside. The child reportedly liked pull toys. For a good ten minutes, examiner and child both pulled musical pull toys from the waiting room to the interview room, only to have the child balk at the entrance each time. Finally, the author pulled her toy into the playpen arrangement and seated herself there. A minute later the child wandered in too and inspected the enclosed space. The author, leaving the toy on the mat, moved to the far corner of the room, ignoring the child. The child installed herself in the playpen, turned on her side and put her thumb in her mouth. The author remained seated at the desk for a few more minutes, but hummed softly a repetitive nursery song. Then she placed the doll and a doll nursing bottle on a low chair next to the playpen. The child took the bottle and inserted it in her mouth. The author placed the first four objects (item 1, Fig. 3) on the chair near the doll. The child flung the bottle to the floor, reached for the comb, combed her own hair, then the doll's hair, then undressed the doll, then took off her own shoes and socks and tried to put her own foot into the shoe of the test item. The author quickly and silently placed on the chair three colored socks, red, yellow and blue, removed spoon, cup, and hair brush and comb, and, in passing, dropped the second red sock. The child put this sock on her own left foot, inspected the three socks displayed on the chair, selected the second red one, flung the other two to the floor, and put the second red sock on her right foot. The author then made a bridge of three blocks and left five more blocks in a pile next to the bridge on the low chair, placing the undressed doll near the bridge. The child pulled herself up to a standing position, regarded the bridge, pushed it off the chair and made a tower of five blocks. The author made some sounds in a complaining voice and pretended to speak for the doll, saying: "I want my house. Make me a house." The child hestitated, then using three blocks taken off her tower, made a bridge of three blocks, after some difficulty with the width of the space between the base blocks, and flung the doll to the floor.

Without being aware that she was being tested, this girl demonstrated within the first fifteen minutes of the interview her recognition of objects and knowledge of their appropriate use; her ability to discriminate between and match primary colors and a beginning awareness of numbers (two socks for two feet, three blocks for a bridge of three); her ability to perceive a structure on a three year level and repeat it from memory; her ability to undress (the doll and her own shoes and socks) and put on socks.

It was possible by using devices and without addressing the child directly to gain a tentative estimate of her developmental level and to demonstrate that she was not seriously retarded, if she was retarded at all. Her emotional-social adjustment and her language development were the major problems.

One twelve year old girl was reported to become completely inaccessible whenever brought to clinics, offices or school. Over the years, attempts had been made to assess her eligibility for school placement, but she remained silent and immobile during each session, so that testing was not possible. She was reported to play with dolls at home, speak, help a little around the house and dress herself completely. She refused to visit even relatives and never left the front porch of her house except when taken by her parents.

After a telephone conference with her mother, in order to enlist the mother's cooperation, the child was visited at home. The testing material was carried in two shopping bags so as to disarm the child and to gain access to her house in the guise of a friend of the mother dropping in for a chat.

While the author and the child's parents conversed in the kitchen, she refused to enter, remaining in the hall for more than an hour but peeking through the open door occasionally. Her sixteen year old sister, a high school senior, then entered and cleared the table of breakfast dishes. She commented on the fact that the only brother had just been drafted into the army, and she offered the information that the child usually set the table. The author, who noticed out of the corner of her eye that the child had followed the sister's comments with interest, asked, addressing the room in general, "Where does your brother sit when he is at home?" The child pointed to his place at the table and said distinctly, "Over there." Here the author made the mistake of looking at the child and thanking her for the information; she immediately burst into tears and ran upstairs, where she remained for another hour. The author then unpacked some of the test material, placed it on a table and proceeded to show the sixteen year old "what nice things she had bought for her children." The child could be seen leaning over the stair rail and watching. She was not addressed by either the author or her sister and gradually approached the table, with a guarded expression, as if ready to fly away any moment. The author and the sister seated themselves next to each other behind the table with the materials. The author placed the first four objects before the sister and asked, "How do you like the comb and brush I bought today?" The sister, acting on a whispered instruction, pretended to hover with her hand over the objects, as if undecided. The child then seated herself shyly next to her sister, on the side farthest from the examiner, and, taking hold of her big sister's hand with her own left hand, guided it to the comb and brush.

After this, the rest of the items were presented ostensibly to the sixteen year old, who pretended uncertainty but held her hand conveniently ready. The child "helped" her after each request to make a choice by guiding the sister's hand with her own. By this method, although persistently unable to be contacted directly, the child was led fairly rapidly through twenty-five of the items. The pellets were omitted. She failed the color blocks except for matching the three primary colors, failed to grade circles by size, was able to select three milk bottles but failed with four and above. She listened to the story, but after selecting the two bears, she failed to select the two beds.

The author had to be careful to avoid at all times looking at her or thanking her for her answers, praising instead the sixteen year old for finding the answers. The child, too, began to praise her sister after she had "helped" her to make a selection, impartially and unself-critically praising each response regardless of correctness.

It was possible to establish tentatively that, at age twelve, the child functioned not higher than on a three and one-half year level. She rewarded the author with a shy, "Come again."

Although this session took all of one morning, not counting traveling time, it is worthwhile to invest such time and effort rather than inspecting the child once a year and, after spending a fruitless hour each time, concluding that she is inaccessible and will not cooperate. The Evaluation is a helpful contribution to the medical diagnosis. The advantage to the parents is that they can plan for their child with greater confidence rather than having to wait year after year for a definite explanation of the child's behavior and status.

Some children appear not so much agitated as completely shut off, seemingly unaware of or indifferent to the environment and to the presence or absence of the parents. It is frequently possible to evaluate the level of development of such children by an observation of the level on which they use materials. They may be able to use the inanimate environment without qualms or hesitation, often similarly making use of people's hands as if they were tools. They may take someone's hand and guide it to their untied shoe lace. When a music box is demonstrated, they may lift the examiner's hand back to it when he stops winding it and push his hand in a circular direction. Again, the examiner has to gauge the child's ability to be addressed directly or whether requests must be conveyed silently, by inference or through oblique observation on the part of the child as the examiner demonstrates. The child may imitate in a detached manner the demonstrated use of materials. Sometimes, too, a hesitation or unwillingness to touch objects with his own hands can be detected. If the examiner places his own hand conveniently, he may discover that the child will guide it to the correct choices with an impersonal, indirect attitude. The interview can then proceed on these lines, with the examiner "lending his hand." An examiner who has had experience in the testing of children with cerebral palsy, although the underlying reasons are entirely different in this type of child, will be ready to conduct the interview in a way tailored to the special needs of such a child. A quietly hummed tune of a simple nursery song, continued all through the session, frequently has a tranquilizing influence on the child. It also gives him the illusion of having his reserve respected, with everybody more or less living in his own world, the examiner with his song and the child preoccupied with inanimate objects.

A different problem is presented when one attempts to test hyperactive children. The examiner has to have many facets to his nature. From the stealth and silence required to watch a shy, frightened, little bird, when testing the above described children, he has to shift to the stamina and resilience needed to withstand the onslaught of a small human steam engine, when meeting up with a hyperactive child.

How to persuade the hyperactive child to enter the interview room may be not so much of a problem as how to keep him there, and off the window-sill, table and desk. The room has to be emptied of anything that can be spared. The test material is kept on a high shelf or in a closed closet, and each item is obtained when needed. The work table, which the child may be persuaded to use eventually, is pushed flush against the wall to cut out any distractions. If the child seats himself, he faces the blank wall, the table surface, the test item and nothing else (Fig. 4B), providing maximal conditions for him to apply himself to the task. The examiner remains beside or in back of him. The recording form may be tacked to the wall or a bulletin board, where it will be available to the examiner but may pass unnoticed as a part of the room fixtures as far as the child is concerned.

Is is usually preferable to take on a hyperactive child without having the parent in the room. The fewer distracting elements present, the greater the possibility of creating an atmosphere which will aid in calming down the child for brief moments of attending and responding to a task.

The examiner must cultivate an attitude of imperturbable, matter-of-fact, convinced firmness. He must succeed in conveying to the child the idea that a job has to be done and a routine followed. Rather than creating the impression that it is the examiner who decides arbitrarily that the child must do his bidding, the child must be impressed with the fact that both of them, the examiner and the child, have to tackle this job together. This by no means implies that the examiner should not be in control of the situation or let the child do as he pleases. But it serves to remove the onus of authority from the examiner and thereby frequently robs the child of an object for his teasing, resistive, erratic defiance. Once he begins to accept the idea that the examiner will do his best to help him get through with the mutual task, he may become receptive to suggestions on how to settle down.

A child who functions at or above the four year level can sometimes be won to cooperate for ten or fifteen minutes at a time by starting him with an appealing task, such as the milk bottle play (item 24, see Fig. 11). The examiner can go about it in this way : the item is presented as directed, even though it serves a play value primarily and tests the amount concept only secondarily. Then, if the child just has to jump up and move around, the examiner can turn this need into an acceptable part of the task by having the child carry the stand to various points of delivery around the room. If he needs to manifest his protest about being made to comply by throwing, dropping or rolling the bottles rather than handing them one by one or lining them up, he can be instructed to deliver them all by rolling them to a certain spot (rather than letting him continue to throw and endanger the examiner and the windows), but he should be thanked politely for delivering them and paid with imaginary money or real pennies (borrowed from item 26). By a bland expectation that this milkman game is what he likes to do and an affable overlooking of his challenging form of delivery, he can be helped to adopt nicer ways of handing them over when he learns that he did not create a turmoil. After the milk bottle play is finished, the examiner can attempt to start a routine. If the child is not seated, he may be placed in a friendly and firm way on his chair and ordered to close his eyes while the examiner finds another game for him. Done in the right spirit of fun and firmness, this works very well. The child will try to peek from beneath his hands, and the examiner will keep reminding him that it is not fair to peek until the next item is lined up. What happens is that the child becomes so engrossed in trying to peek without being caught at it that he quite forgets to jump up and run around; by the time he remembers, the next item holds his interest. A rapid change of items and an appreciative attitude will enable him to keep up this tempo for a while. In fairness to the child, who is driven by internal impulses beyond his control, this routine must be interspersed with a series of brief recesses, such as a look out of the window or the pellet item, during which he can move around and jump up and down. The child should be given the entire responsibility for putting used items away, such as replacing the color blocks in their box, cards in their envelopes and the sound blocks in the closet. This cooperative activity helps him, one, to let off steam, two, to feel that he and the examiner are both intent on getting the job finished.

The hyperactive child who is not retarded or who is only mildly subnormal frequently actually welcomes a firm hand and a structuring of activities for him, because something in him would like to pursue an occasional interest and deplores his constant flitting of attention. Sensing that outside structuring helps him to organize himself, he often will be found to return of his own free will to such a device. He may even remind the examiner to make him sit down and tell him when to close his eyes, while he then gleefully awaits the next item.

The child who is hyperactive and moderately or severely retarded cannot be persuaded by such an approach. Depending on his particular circumstances and the degree of hyperactivity and of retardation, several approaches are possible, and a series of approaches may have to be tried until one is found which wins the child's maximum compliance. Where the hyperactivity is relatively mild, regardless of the degree of retardation, restraint by implication will be found helpful. The chair of the child is backed up to the wall, with the table pushed in front of it and held in place by the examiner sitting opposite the child. If an armchair can be used for the child, it makes it difficult for him to get up without a great deal of effort (Fig. 2), and he may settle down to work rather than continue his effort to puzzle out how to leave the chair. Either cooperating maximally or responding to prodding, he can then be presented with the materials. Where the hyperactivity is more severe or the child resents the implied restraint and cannot be induced to sit still for brief moments of "home work" or "school work," with longer periods of ball play wedged between tasks, he may simply have to be tested while he wanders around. The materials then are placed around the room, as suggested for other contingencies, although here the underlying reason for the approach is a different one. When it is recalled that the one important consideration is: does his performance reliably demonstrate whether he can function appropriately in response to the request, it will then seem appropriate to the examiner to use that motivation which may lead to a response, whether or not the form of response is unconventional.

The hyperactive child who is not destructive can be challenged to see how fast he can find the requested choice. The hyperactive child who is competitive can be challenged to show whether he or the examiner can find the requested choice first. The hyperactive child who is mildly destructive can be given the sparkler toy (item 33) to use as a make-believe gun and can be challenged to shoot the requested choice. With hyperactive children who are very destructive, the test material may have to be replaced with copies of the cards, such as symbol cards, configuration cards, drawn on comparable pieces of paper, while the child watches or lets off steam by playing by himself. The child can then be asked to find the requested choice and if he tears or crushes the paper, it will not matter; some very aggressive children may even be challenged to see how fast they can find the requested choice and tear it up. Possessive children can be challenged to find the requested choice by permitting them to keep it if they can find it.

Such ruses make it possible to observe the correctness or incorrectness of the selection and to evaluate the developmental level of the child's intellectual functioning. The Evaluation interview is just that, an interview to find out how the child can function. Therefore, the motivation has to be adapted to the particular handicap of the child, whether the handicap is physical, mental, emotional or social. The interview is not the time or place to start retraining of a child with such deepseated difficulties.

The report of the findings must contain a description of the behavior pattern of the child as observed during the interview and of the approaches used to elicit his responses, in addition to the inventory of the developmental levels. If suggestions can be offered which will contribute to an effective educational management of the child, they should be specific and substantiated by examples. In that way, the teacher will be able to translate them into her classroom situation and utilize them in planning for the child.

The very young hyperactive child can sometimes be successfully confined to the improvised play pen (Fig. 4A). If the table, which is turned on its side, is not solid enough to withstand vigorous pushing by hands or feet without falling over, it should be braced. Or perhaps a triangular corner of the room can be enclosed by placing the table across it, with the table legs toward the room. The advantage of keeping the child confined is that he can apply himself more successfully when an outside agency provides the controlling factor than when he must cope with his vulnerability to constant inner and outer impulses alone. That is the reason why there is seldom any real resentment against the restraint or the restrainer, if it is accompanied simultaneously with an opportunity to play. The emphasis is on the play, or the attention received from the examiner while playing, and not on the confinement. The child responds to the offer of play, his cooperation is won and sustained by continued play; thus, the presentation of the items must be made to look to him like playing. That he happens to have been placed within a given space is then not regarded by him as confinement or punishment, but just as a part of the examiner's way of playing with him.

The very young child who functions below a two year level will have to be evaluated using modifications. Even if he is hyperactive, by the use of the modifications it will become possible to establish whether he can function in the areas investigated. The sensory areas are explored by the use of items scaled down to meet his level. It is important to establish grossly whether there is any serious impairment in the visual or the auditory area. Such impairment, especially that of hearing, sometimes renders a child hyperactive, inaccessible and driven. Attention to the impairment, measures taken to correct it, and provision of special training will then greatly alleviate the hyperactive behavior.

The author is aware of the danger of selecting these particular special problems. They are discussed only because they are met not infrequently by examiners of young and of handicapped children, and because it is possible to conduct an interview with children presenting special problems if one can find the workable approach for the particular child.

Those children who, to varying degrees, fit into the one or other category do not represent a clinical entity. The only characteristic which they have in common is that they are not, or not readily, accessible. Since accessibility is an important point when one wants to conduct an interview, this characteristic had to be highlighted and suggestions offered as to how to circumvent the problems involved in testing a child to whom one has no direct access.

The sequence of items which serve to investigate intactness in various significant areas needed for developing and learning explores so much more than intellectual adequacy that deviations in functioning become revealed during the interview. Such deviations may also be present in children who are not readily accessible. It is important to establish intactness, or discover impairment of intactness, in the less accessible child as well as in the more accessible one. Impaired functioning in one or another area may contribute, aggravate, and perhaps even be responsible for the behavior pattern of some of the children who have and present special problems.

The Educational Evaluation is not intended to diagnose or to serve as a basis for speculation about whether a given behavior pattern is organic or not organic. But there are innumerable patterns which an examiner learns to recognize because the children exhibiting given deviating patterns will in turn demonstrate a test behavior which follows a distinct and recognizable pattern. This makes it sometimes feasible or obligatory to report that a certain child displays behavior reminiscent of, or observed frequently in, children who have been diagnosed as autistic or schizophrenic; as having chronic brain syndromes with hyperactive behavior, or with overdependence on the mother, or with difficulties in the use or the reception of language symbols; and similar descriptions.

The examiner must learn to remain simultaneously cognizant of the areas of functioning and their possible impairment, which he has been shown vicariously by means of the fictional interview with the child with cerebral palsy, as well as of the various ways in which young and young handicapped children may act. Only then will he be able to conduct the interview and exercise the quality and quantity of educated observation which alone will lead to a complete evaluation of the child's developmental potential.

8. The items and directions for their presentation

II-0 — VI.

1. RECOGNITION OF CONCRETE FAMILIAR LIFE-SIZE OBJECTS.
   a) when named.

Level: 2-0 and up.

Main areas:	Other areas:
language comprehension; object recognition.	hearing and vision; orientation in the environment; body awareness; awareness of more than one.

MATERIALS: spoon, cup, comb and brush, shoe (Fig. 3).

PROCEDURE: place all objects on the empty table, starting with *shoe on child's left, then spoon, comb and brush, cup.* Leave six to eight inches of space between objects. For child with involuntary arm motion and for hyperactive child, place objects out of reach toward back of table. Use the verbal formulation most suitable to the child's way of responding, e.g.: "Look at," "Give me," "Show me."

In this order ask for: *spoon, comb and hairbrush, shoe, cup.*

Replace objects in their original order after each response. It is permissible to say to a shy or immature child: "Give to mother."

If child fails, see chapter 9 for modifications; *use them now.*

II-0 — VI.

2. RECOGNITION OF CONCRETE FAMILIAR LIFE-SIZE OBJECTS.
   b) when described in terms of use.

Level: 2-6 and up.

Main areas:	Other areas:
language comprehension; body awareness; incipient ability to generalize.	if given after 1., ability to shift; communication; hearing and vision; eye motion; handedness; orientation in the environment; awareness of more than one.

MATERIALS: same as 1. (Fig. 3)

139

PROCEDURE: same as 1.

Ask: *"Which one does mother (mommy) use to fix your hair?"*
"Which one do we eat with?"
"Which one goes on your foot (on a baby's foot)?"
"Which one can we use to drink our milk?"
Replace objects in their original order after each response.

(*Caution:* Children raised in institutions and bedridden may not know shoes.)

If child fails, use modifications, chapter 9.

II-0 — VI.

3. RECOGNITION OF SIZES IN CONCRETE FAMILIAR OBJECTS.

Level: 2-6 and up.

Main areas:	Other areas:
language comprehension;	hearing and vision;
incipient mathematical concept;	awareness of three;
ability to recognize differences in sizes.	willingness to follow verbal request;
	ability to judge by use of visual cue.

MATERIALS: two teaspoons, one doll spoon.

PROCEDURE: Place the three spoons parallel to each other, horizontally to the side of table nearest child, with the doll spoon in the middle; leave at least two inches between spoons.

Pointing to each of the spoons in turn, say: *"See the spoons? Look at this one and that one. Show me the tiny little spoon."* Then ask for a big spoon.

Replace all spoons in their original order after each response.

Holding out your hand, say: *"I will put them away. Give me all the big spoons, please."*

(As described in chapter 7, the mode of presentation is adapted to the handicap of the child, so that in the case of a child, who cannot use his hands, one asks: "Show me" or: "Is this . . .?" instead of: "Give me . . .".)

II-0 — VI.

4. RECOGNITION OF LIFE-SIZE FAMILIAR OBJECTS IN IMAGE, WHEN NAMED.

Level: 2-0 and up.

Main areas:	Other areas:
picture recognition;	vision and hearing;
language comprehension;	awareness of three;
ability to accept visual symbol in place	eye motion;
of concrete object;	communication;
ability to perceive an integrated image.	pattern of problem solving;
	reaction to unfamiliar procedure.

MATERIALS: pictures in color, life-size, of spoon, shoe, comb and brush, 8½ x 7 inches. (Pictures are shown in Fig. 9.)

PROCEDURE: place the pictures in the wooden stand, one to each row. Picture of comb and brush to child's left in top row. Take care that pictures do not overlap.

Explain casually: *"See, I put them in here so that you can see them better."*

In the usual form, (depending on the child's physical ability to respond by manual reaction, verbal response or by eye-pointing or by giving his sign for affirmation and negation) ask for: *spoon, comb and brush, shoe.*

Replace pictures in their original position after each response if child has removed or changed them.

If child fails, see chapter 9 for modifications.

II-6 — VI.

5. RECOGNITION OF LIFE-SIZE FAMILIAR OBJECTS IN IMAGE WHEN DESCRIBED IN TERMS OF USE.

Level: 2-6 and up.

Main areas:
language comprehension;
picture recognition;
ability to relate a visual symbol to an imagined act;
incipient ability to project into past or future situation.

Other areas:
hearing and vision;
eye motion;
handedness;
communication.

MATERIALS: same as 4. (See Fig. 9)

PROCEDURE: same as 4.

Say: *"Listen carefully. Show me the picture of the thing we can use to eat our cereal."*

"Which thing does mother need to fix your hair?"

"Can you find something that goes on your foot?"

If the child names the object without pointing it out, repeat: *"Show me . . ."*. Avoid carefully the naming of any of the objects or pictures yourself, but nod in a friendly manner if the child names it. Indicate by your manner that you expect him to *show* you the picture under consideration.

Concretely functioning young children frequently begin to *fail on this item.* Use the appropriate modifications in chapter 9 immediately, before going on with the next item.

III-6 — VI.

6. RECALL OF MISSING PICTURE FROM MEMORY.

Level: 4-0 and up.

Main areas:	*Other areas:*
immediate recall of mental image;	frustration tolerance;
memory;	sense of humor;
presence of mind.	awareness of three;
	visual intactness—grossly.

MATERIALS: same as 4 and 5. (Same pictures as in Fig. 9.)

PROCEDURE: place pictures in the stand, setting the picture of the shoe in the left upper corner as seen from child. Make sure pictures do not overlap.

Pointing to each picture in turn, say: *"Now we are going to play a new game. I want you to remember what you see. Here is the picture of a shoe, here is the hairbrush, here is the spoon. I am going to hide one of them and you must tell me which one I took away. Close your eyes."*

Screen the stand with the fiber board and remove the picture of the *shoe,* placing the picture of the comb and brush in the left upper corner instead. Expose the stand and say: *"Which one did I take away?"* Be careful that the removed picture is not visible on the table or on your lap; if possible hide it in back of the stand.

Children without speech may look at their own or the examiner's shoe meaningfully. This is a suitable response.

Give a second trial, placing the pictures so that the comb and brush are in the right upper corner as seen from child. Make sure pictures do not overlap. Repeat the instructions to look at each picture, pointing to each in turn and naming them slowly. Then say: *"I am going to hide one of them. Let's see if you can remember and tell me. Close your eyes."* Screen the stand with the board and remove the picture of the *spoon,* placing the picture of the comb and brush in the place formerly displaying the spoon. Expose the stand and say: *"Which one is gone?"*

Children without speech may gesture with the hand to the mouth or may make a lip-sound indicating eating. This is a suitable response. If the child merely points toward the emptied space, tell him that he is to tell you what the missing picture shows. Give plenty of time for him to study the two remaining pictures and perhaps by a combination of his verbal recall and his visual after-image to arrive at the correct solution.

Make a mental note if a child of four or over had unusual difficulty with visual recall.

II-6 — III only.

(*Caution:* if item 8 is to be presented, item 7 must *not* be given. The practice given would invalidate the response to 8.)

7. RECOGNITION OF ACTION IN IMAGE (PORTRAYED ACTION).

Level: 2-6 to 3

Main areas:	*Other areas:*
interpretation of pictures;	ability to perceive an integrated
language comprehension.	picture;
	vision;
	possible clues to feeding and sleeping
	problems.

MATERIALS: two pictures of children, 10 x 6½ inches, in color, sleeping in beds and eating at a table. (See Fig. 10.)

PROCEDURE: place both pictures in the stand, or, if child indicates a preference for this, place them next to each other on the table in front of him. Allow time for leisurely perusal, making sure that the child looks at each in turn. Do not describe pictures except to encourage the child to *"Look at these nice pictures."* If he offers any comment, accept it with friendly silence.

Then say: *"Where are the children sleeping in their beds?"*

Next say: *"Show me where the children are eating their dinner."*

Failure may be due to several different reasons. Be alert to the nature of the response. See chapter 9 for modifications *if child fails.* Also see *modifications* for children who *do not comprehend or hear language.*

III-0 — VI-0

8. ORIENTATION IN TIME AND ACTION IN IMAGE (TIME OF DAY).

Level: 3-0 to 3-6

Main areas:	*Other areas:*
interpretation of pictures;	vision.
orientation in time;	
language comprehension.	

MATERIALS: same as 7. (See Fig. 10.)

PROCEDURE: Place both pictures in the stand, or, if child indicates a preference for this, place them on the table next to each other. Say: *"Look at these two pictures. See what they are doing here and here?"* In turn point to each picture and make sure the child looks at each of them at his leisure. Accept any comment with friendly silence.

Then ask: *"Which one tells you (or "makes you think") that it is night time?"*

No further trial is needed if the child can conclusively select the correct picture. *If he has failed,* present the item as described in 7. After he has succeeded on 7, give a second trial with the item as presented in 8. If child has required practice with 7, but then has succeeded on a second trial with 8, make a notation or a mental note about the need for practice.

II-0 — III only.

9.   RECOGNITION OF SYMBOLS AND FORMS.

Level: 2-0 to 2-6

Main areas:
ability to perceive visually and to discriminate intellectually similarities and differences in symbols.

Other areas:
language comprehension;
awareness of more than one;
ability to follow a verbal direction.

MATERIALS: two sets of cardboard cutouts, two inches in diameter, yellow, of triangle, circle and square. (Visible in Fig. 18.)

PROCEDURE: place on the dark board (if the table top is dark, no board is used) a square, then a circle, another square and another circle, in a row, with not more than two inches of space between cutouts. Pointing to each in turn and making sure that the child looks at all of them, say: *"See what I have? Look at the balls."* Point to each of the circles as you say it, repeating *"Ball"* each time. After the child has looked at all the cards at his leisure, pick up the *circle* at the end of the row, hold it up for the child's inspection and say: *"See the ball? Find another ball."*

If the child points to or looks at only the circle held by the examiner, say: *"I can see another ball. Where is it?"* and indicate the row of cards on the table.

If the child still hesitates and seems uncertain about what is expected of him, place the circle clearly visible in the mother's hand or on the doll's lap (whichever is more suitable or available), and say: *"Mother (the dolly) likes the balls. Give her another ball."*

The child with involvement of hands or arms may indicate his choice by fixing his eyes on the correct card in the row. It may be necessary to tilt the board or the table slightly to enable some chlidren to see all the cards if they cannot voluntarily bring their eyes down to the surface. In some instances it may be helpful to hold the sample card next to each card in the row and invite the child to give his sign of negation or affirmation, as he decides on his selection. Some children may wish to place the circles on top of each other. This is permissible.

After the child has matched the circles, the cards are returned to the row on the table in the former order. Then say: *"Now look at this one."* Hold up for the child's inspection the first *square* in the row. If the child offers a name for it, such as block, box or window, accept it silently. Then say: *"Give me one like that."* Use the approach suggested above if the child seems better able to respond in that way.

After the child has correctly selected circle and square, add one triangle in the exact center of the row and the second triangle at the end of the row. Say: *"Look what I have."* Point to each card in the row in turn, making certain that the child looks at all cards. If the child volunteers a name for the triangle, such as hat, boat, house, accept it silently. Pick up the *triangle* at the end of the row, hold it up for the child's inspection, and say: *"Find one like that."* No other trial need be given if the child succeeds.

If the child fails, remove all cards. Then place one circle and one triangle on the table. Hold up the second triangle and say: *"I can see one just like that. Can you?"* and indicate the two cards before him.

If he can select the correct card in a choice of two, add the square in such a way that the triangle lies in the center of the row of three cards. Holding up the other triangle, say: *"Let's do it again. Find one like that."* No further attempt need be made if the child can select the triangle in a choice of three cards.

If he fails, go on to the next item for his age level and return to form-recognition toward the end of the interview by using the suggestions for modifications in chapter 9.

II-6 — VI.

10. RECOGNITION OF SYMBOLS AND FORMS.
    a) matching.

Level: 2-6 and up.

Main areas:
ability to perceive visually and to discriminate intellectually similarities and differences in symbols;
ability to perceive a solid figure against a background;
eye motion.

Other areas:
ability to follow verbal directions;
awareness of three;
language comprehension.

MATERIALS: two sets of cardboard cards, 4 x 4 inches each, with solid red symbol, 3 inches in diameter, of circle, triangle and square. (Visible in Fig. 18. See also Fig. 6.)

PROCEDURE: place one set of cards in the stand, adapting the placement to the child's individual ability to regard material; the circle is placed in the center. If the child does not spontaneously look at each card, point to each in turn, saying: *"Look at all of them."*

Then hold up the second *circle* for the child's inspection and say: *"You have one that is just the same,"* indicating the stand, *"Show me your card that looks like my card?"*

If the child hesitates or points to the card held by examiner, repeat: *"You have one just like it. Which one is it?"* If necessary, hold the sample card over each card in the stand in turn, saying each time: *"Does this one look just the same?"* Observe the child for his way of agreeing or disagreeing with the choices offered.

After the child has correctly selected the circle, ask in turn for *square* and for *triangle* in the same way.

If the child is slow in getting the idea, it is permissible to name the first card (a "ball") and to ask for the *"ball"* among the cards in the stand. Once he has understood clearly, no further help is given. Give a second trial for each card if the child has had difficulty catching on. Make a notation or a mental note, if this modification had to be used.

It is important to observe closely the child's attempt to solve the task. Especially note whether he seems to understand the verbal directions. Does he offer any card? Does he succeed with the circle but consistently confuse triangle and square?

If the child fails, remember the directions given in chapter 7 and look under modifications in chapter 9. Present a modified version probing the same faculty, either immediately or at a later opportunity, depending on the child's awareness of and reaction to having failed. Young children are usually not self-critical. Four to six year olds frequently are more self-aware.

III-6 — VI.

11. RECOGNITION OF SYMBOLS AND FORMS.
    b) finding from memory.

Level: 4-0 and up.

Main areas:	*Other areas:*
ability to recall a visual image from memory;	language comprehension; probably incipient ability to categorize; awareness of three.
perceptual intactness;	
systematic eye-sweep.	

MATERIALS: same as in 10.

PROCEDURE: place one set of cards in the wooden stand, in the way most suitable for the individual child. Permit time for leisurely inspection, making certain the child looks at each card. (Fig. 6.)

Say: *"Now we will play a new game. We will play hide and seek."* Shield the stand from view with the board, hold up the card with the *circle,* and say slowly: *"Look at this one. Remember what it looks like."* Expose it for ten seconds counted from the moment the child focuses his eyes on it. Remove the sample card, expose the stand by removing the card board so that the original three cards are visible.

Say: *"Which one did I show you?"* indicating the cards in the stand. If the child hesitates, say: *"Which of these cards looks exactly like the one I showed you?"*

At the first trial it may be necessary to permit a second glance at the sample card, after first screening the stand from view again. This is indicated when it is apparent that the child has only gradually comprehended the nature of the task. Once the child has reliably understood the task, no repetition of showing the sample can be given. An incorrect response must be accepted once it is certain that it is inability to recall and not lack of comprehending the task which causes the failure. After the child has succeeded with the circle, ask in the same way first for the *triangle,* then for the *square.* No further trial is necessary if the child has succeeded with each symbol.

If the child succeeds with the circle but *seems to confuse* or *fail to see* a difference between square and triangle, giving either one of these two cards (but not the circle) when asked for the square, it may mean that he only compares the baseline of the symbols. This may be true even after in direct matching (item 10), he was able to succeed. When he is called upon to remember, he cannot make a complete mental note of the fact that one symbol has three sides and one four. His awareness of amounts may be only three or less. He may limit himself to noting the most striking difference, namely, that between roundness and straightness or angularity.

Since our aim is to determine if he can function in this area, we reduce the demand. Insert in the stand the card with the circle and the one with the triangle. Invite the child to: *"Take a good look so you can remember them."* Then shield the stand and show the sample card of the *triangle* for the child's inspection. Say: *"Try hard to remember it."* Remove the card and expose the stand immediately. If he succeeds, ask for the *circle* next in the same way, to exclude the chance of an accidental success.

Then remove the circle from the stand and, while the child watches, insert the square, so that the stand contains just two cards, triangle and square. After the child has regarded both cards for a while, say: *"I bet you can remember them now."* Screen the stand from view, hold up for the child's inspection the card with the *square,* reminding him to take a good look so that he will know it again later. Remove the card, expose the stand immediately and ask: *"Which one looks like it?"* If he succeeds, ask for the *triangle* next in the same way.

If the child still fails to differentiate reliably between square and triangle after this reduction of difficulty, place the three cards in the stand and invite the child to name them by asking him: *"What do they look like?"* If the child cannot speak, suggest names, such as *"ball or apple"* for the circle, *"box or window"* for the square, *"boat, hat or funny clown's hat"* for the triangle.

If the child can succeed in selecting from memory the correct cards among a choice of three after this device is used, a brief notation of it is made.

If he fails again, the next step is to let him trace or to help him trace the outline of each card with the index-finger of his leading hand. Observe whether he looks at it closely while doing so or whether he appears to memorize the sensation of the motion executed with his hand instead. When he indicates that he is ready, offer a new trial, using only the cards with the square and the triangle. After holding up the sample card for his inspection, remove it and immediately expose the stand. Observe the child closely to detect, if possible, his attempt to utilize the mode of recall which seems to serve him best, namely, tracing of the outline with his hand in the air, on the table or even on the respective card itself; or repeating to himself the verbal designation of the card in question, or concentrating by closing his eyes while his finger experiments with remembered motor experiences of outlines. Note down what you were able to observe. Give a new trial using the three cards and observe further his way of recalling the after-image.

If he still fails, go on to item 12. Return to this area at the end of the interview, using the suggestions in chapter 9.

II-6 — VI.

12. DISCRIMINATION OF COLORS.
    a) matching.

Level: 3-0 and up.

Main areas:	*Other areas:*
color recognition;	ability to follow verbal directions;
language comprehension;	awareness of more than two;
incipient ability to abstract (the quality of color from the concept of similar forms).	ability to inhibit (the impulse to use blocks for play).

MATERIALS: six pairs of wooden blocks, red, yellow, blue, green, orange and purple.

PROCEDURE: hold the box containing the blocks on your lap out of sight. Place on the table in front of the child and at the distance required by his physical needs one red and one yellow block.

Holding up for the child's inspection the *red* block (from the box on your lap), say: *"Show me one like that."* If the child points to the block you are holding, say: *"You have one just like that. Which one* (indicating the blocks in front of him) *looks just the same?"* If necessary, hold the red block in turn over the child's yellow block and then over his red block, saying slowly: *"Does IT look exactly the same? Is IT the same color?"* Make sure the child watches. Then ask once more: *"Which one of yours looks the same as mine?"*

The child's individual way of indicating his choice will have become plain during the earlier items, such as picking up, pointing to, eye-pointing or giving his sign for affirmation or negation as the examiner points to each possible choice in turn.

If the child gives the wrong color, place the red block on top of the child's red block and indicate that this is how they go together, then place the second yellow block on top of his yellow block and point out that they both look the same. Remove the red and yellow sample blocks once more and repeat the original request by holding up your *red* block and asking the child to find one like it.

If he fails, remove all blocks and use the procedure described under modifications, chapter 9. Use the appropriate *modifications* also if the *child is deaf, hard-of-hearing or seems to have aphasic difficulty;* this also is described in chapter 9.

If the child succeeds, display in turn the *yellow* block and ask him to match it as directed above. If he succeeds with these two colors, add the blue block to his row of blocks, call his attention to it, and ask for the RED block once more in the form directed above, then ask for the *blue* one in the same way, namely, by holding the second blue block up for the child's inspection and asking him to find one like it or to show you his block that looks just the same.

If he succeeds, add the green and orange blocks. Insert them in his row so that the green is placed next to the blue and the orange next to the yellow and red blocks. Ask for the *orange* block in the form directed earlier. If he succeeds, ask for the *yellow* one to check the reliability of his response.

If he succeeds, ask for the *green* block by holding up the second green block for his inspection as described above. Once the child has comprehended the task, it is frequently sufficient just to hold up the blocks to be matched and to wait for his response.

If the child begins to make errors by indicating near-likeness, such as selecting blue instead of green or yellow instead of orange, arrange his row of blocks in such a way that warm and cold colors are alternated: red, green, orange, blue, yellow. If needed, hold the sample block slowly over each block of his row in turn to facilitate visual comparison.

If errors still persits, they may be due to an inability to handle a number of choices, which is probably an indication of his limited amount concept and of his intellectual functioning rather than of color recognition. Therefore, the difficulty of demand is reduced by removing the blocks and leaving in front of the child the red and the green blocks only. Repeat the matching process in the directed form. If he can succeed with this reduced degree of difficulty, remove red and present blue. Then repeat the request for matching by asking first for *green,* then for *blue* in the usual form. Repeat the same process by using orange and blue only, and, if successfully responded to, present only orange and yellow. Ask him to match each color as directed above.

It is sometimes possible then to go back and present the child with the row of five colors and to make a quick check for *green* and for *orange.*

After the child has succeeded with the five colors, either immediately or eventually, add the purple block, placing it next to the blue and green blocks if the child has had no difficulty but between the red and yellow ones if he has had trouble. Ask in the usual form first for *blue,* then for *purple.*

This item offers many opportunities for observing the child's way of functioning in addition to his ability to discriminate between colors. As discussed in chapters 6 and 7, the Educational Evaluation is intended to reveal learning difficulties and sensory as well as physical-mechanical limitations. By observing his eyes, the examiner may sometimes spot a reason for failure: the child may be unable to lower his eyes sufficiently to see materials below his eye level. This reminder is placed here to insure the examiner's full utilization of the procedure as described in the two preceding chapters. At the same time, there is no point in persisting with devices if the child is immature or simply fails to comprehend or is disinterested.

If child fails, see chapter 9 for downward modification.

III-6 — VI.

13. DISCRIMINATION OF COLORS.
   b) when named.

Level: 4-0 and up.

Main areas:	Other areas:
association of colors with their correct names;	ability to shift from one set of demands to another;
discrimination of colors.	verbal comprehension;
	eye-sweep.

MATERIALS: same as 12.

PROCEDURE: place before the child one red and one yellow block. Say: *"See these blocks? Now we are going to play a different game."* Whether he can speak and spontaneously names the colors or whether he cannot speak, allow a moment for him to digest your comment.

Then say: *"Which one is red?"* If further help is needed, say: *"Show me (give me, look at) the red block."*

If he succeeds, ask for the *yellow* one in the same way.

If he fails, pick up the red block and say: *"This is the red one."* Then point to the yellow block and say: *"This is a yellow one."* Casually reverse the position of the two blocks and observe if the child smiles, frowns or in other ways signifies that he has noticed the change. Then ask: *"Now you show me the* RED *one."* If he succeeds, ask for the *yellow* one.

After the first two colors have been identified by name, no further practice is given. Add the rest of the blocks, placing them before the child so that orange is between yellow and red, and purple between green and blue. Place the whole row at the distance most suitable for the child. Say: *"Now show me (give me, look at) the blue one."* In turn, ask for *green, red, purple, blue, yellow, orange.* Observe how the child goes about his task, whether he needs to let your verbal direction sink in for awhile before responding, whether he guesses wildly, whether he tries very carefully to compare some colors, as blue and purple, orange and yellow, blue and green. Note if he names some colors himself.

Purple and blue are frequently confused even after the age of four. If a child uses designations, such as "like an apple" for red, "sky" for blue, make a mental note for later recording.

If the child fails, it is worthwhile to lower the demand by presenting only two or three contrasting colors at any one trial, such as red-blue-yellow, or green-orange-purple, placing them in that order. If he can find the correct block as it is named for him in a choice of three and under favorable contrast conditions, he demonstrates that he can associate the correct name with the corresponding color. The difficulty may be intellectual or, possibly, in language assimilation.

II-0 — VI.

14. SOUND BLOCKS AND RELATED SOUND ITEMS.

a) hearing.

Level (not to be omitted on any level): 2-0 and up.

Main areas:	*Other areas:*
hearing acuity;	interest span;
ability to attend to auditory stimulus.	spontaneity of interest;
	ability to shift or tendency to perseverate.

MATERIALS: three pairs of hollow wooden blocks, green, containing small amounts of, respectively, pebbles, rice and sand. Other sound makers: noise-maker cricket, bell with handle, table bell with push button, music box.

PROCEDURE: in preparation for this item the material should be handy but concealed, perhaps in the examiner's pocket or in a small box under the table out of the child's view. While still occupied with the removal of the previous materials (color blocks), gently ring the *handled bell* under the table with your other hand.

Observe the child for his reaction. If he has conclusively heard the sound, show him the bell and offer it to him. If the child is motor-handicapped, assist him in grasping it. Observe how he uses it (investigating, experimenting or disinterested).

If he conclusively fails to hear the bell when it is rung under the table, offer it to him as above. Suggestions to elicit reactions to auditory stimulus are given below. *Use them now.*

If it has been demonstrated that the child has reacted to the sound of the hidden bell and while he still plays with it, present the *table bell with push button.* Allow a few moments for the child to figure out how to make it ring. If he fails to do so by himself, demonstrate the method by hitting the button and invite the child to imitate. Remove the handled bell if it can be done without protest.

While the child is still exploring and using the table bell, step in back of him very casually, keeping his (and your visible) interest concentrated on the table bell. *Shake the softest sounding block* (sand) in back of the child's head, 10 to 12 inches distant, being very careful not to let him see your arm move. In the intervals of his possibly producing sounds with the table bell, *shake this block persistently* and watch for his reaction. The younger child may pause and listen and then return to his preoccupation with the bell. The older child may turn around and look for the source of the sound.

If the child reacts in a conclusive way, give him the block in question and while he tries to shake it himself or while you help the motor-handicapped child in doing so, *shake the medium loud block,* again hidden in back of the child's head. If he reacts to it, offer him this block also and invite him to use it.

Remove the table bell casually and place it out of sight.

It is not necessary to try the same procedure with the third sound block, since it is assumed that the child can hear if he has reacted appropriately to the other two degrees of sound. *Offer the third block to the child without shaking it. If he does not* spontaneously try to shake it, *demonstrate* by *shaking it* and call the child's attention to the fact that these blocks make noise.

If the child has failed to react to the first sound block or even to the first two, the testing has to continue by using the *loudest sound block* as above, namely, shaking it in back of the child's head.

If he reacts to the third block only, *offer it to. him* and demonstrate it. Give second and third *trials with the medium loud sound block,* again in back of the child. If necessary, keep the child occupied and his visual exploration focused on a toy, such as a ball or crayon and paper, while you continue this testing of his hearing, until it becomes evident that he does not perceive this degree of noise or until he perhaps shows by a concentrated expression and a cessation of playing that he does faintly perceive the sound.

Invite the child to use all three degrees of loudness, regardless of whether he has reacted conclusively to each of them or not. If necessary, help him to shake them and encourage him to listen.

It is not regarded as conclusive evidence of the child's ability to hear the sound if he indicates by his response or his shaking it persistently that he knows there is something *in* the block, even the medium loud or softest sounding one. He may only have a tactile perception of the material moving in the block and may keep on playing with it for that reason. On the other hand, it is regarded as fairly reliable evidence of his ability to hear the medium loud one if he returns the softest sounding one to the examiner, indicating that it does not work, but retains the loudest and the medium loud ones.

If the child is mature enough to participate, hearing can be investigated further by explaining to him that he is to listen carefully so that he can tell you *where* you are making the noise. Tell him not to look and step in back of him. Shake the *loudest* block first, behind and to one side of him. Show him how he is to indicate where he thinks he hears the noise by raising his arm on the side where he hears the noise. Care must be exercised so that he does not spy any movement. Each ear can be tried separately. *Each degree of sound* must be tried over and over.

Go on to the next item if the child has demonstrated that he can hear.

If the child failed to respond to the bell with handle when it was sounded under the table, offer it to him and help him to shake it. While he is occupied with it, sound the *cricket noise-maker* underneath the table, again avoiding carefully having the child catch your motion. If he reacts to the cricket, show it to him and help him to snap it to produce the sound.

Offering the *table bell with push button* next, remove the handled bell and the cricket. Let the child explore the table bell as described earlier and, walking casually to the greatest distance permitted by the limits of the room, sound the *cricket noise again,* keeping your hand hidden from the child's view. Observe the child's reaction. If he indicates that he has heard it, show him your two hands, one holding the cricket, the other holding the handled bell and have him show you which one he thinks has made the noise. If he indicates correctly the cricket, it can be tentatively assumed that he can hear this degree of sound at the distance of the room.

The *loudest sound block* is then shaken in back of the child's head persistently but so that the child does not see what is going on. It may be possible to focus his attention in front of him by slowly rolling a ball or little car back and forth noiselessly on the table top. If he responds to the loudest sound block by a conclusive reaction, such as turning his head and searching for the source of the sound, he should be handed *two handled bells, one with the tongue removed, one intact,* and be invited to play with them. If he discards the one with the tongue removed after a while but retains the sounding one, it can be tentatively concluded that he may hear it faintly.

He should then be handed the *loudest and the medium loud sound blocks* and invited to play with them. His reaction to the medium loud one may be complete disinterest, while he may persistently play with the loud one. Or he may show by a puzzled expression that he expected to hear the same noise from both blocks and is surprised that this is not so. Either of these reactions would show with fair reliability that he can hear the loudest one.

It will be worthwhile to make a trial with the *music box,* again playing it hidden underneath the table. If there is no reaction, it may be shown and demonstrated. If the examiner, after a few bars, stops actually turning the crank while visibly continuing the circular motion, the child's sudden reaction may show that he has noticed the cessation of the music. Wait for him to demand his own chance to use this toy. If he indicates this wish, let him, or help him, turn the handle and observe his reaction at the point when the tune is ended and there is a short pause. If he looks puzzled or displeased, he probably has been able to hear some sounds while the tune played and this can be checked by continuing the playing and observing his reaction when the tune is resumed again.

Medical study of the hearing of a child is indicated if on the sound block test he shows a degree of hearing loss.

Before going on to the next item for a child with a suspected hearing loss, *demonstrate the table bell by hitting the button and invite the child to imitate this,* or assist him to do so. This bell is used to test recall later on.

As described in chapter 6, if hearing loss is found to exist, or is suspected, the presentation of the rest of the items must take this into. consideration. Both the presentation and the interpretation of the gaps possibly existing in the child's language comprehension will need revision in the light of this finding.

If further exploration of hearing appears indicated now, look for modifications, chapter 9.

OMIT *items 15 and 16 for the child with suspected hearing loss.*

III-6 — VI.

15. SOUND BLOCKS.
    b) matching.

Level: 4-0 and up.

Main areas:	*Other areas:*
hearing acuity;	ability to abstract, namely, the quality
ability to discriminate between sounds of varying degrees.	of sounding from the similarity of blocks;
	ability to shift or tendency to perseverate.

MATERIALS: same as in 14: sound blocks. Other sound-makers are not used.
PROCEDURE: place the three pairs of sound blocks on the table. If the child starts to shake them, allow him to do so for a few moments. If, however, he starts to build a tower, stop him gently (noting in passing his manual pattern of building his tower and making a mental note of it for later recording), and say: *"Listen carefully. Let's play a new game."* After his attention has been secured, shake in turn the loudest, medium loud and softest sounding block. Push toward the child one block of each pair, keeping the others near your side of the table.

Say: *"Each one makes a different noise, doesn't it? See if you can find the one that sounds real loud like this one in my hand,"* at the same time picking up the *loudest* sound block and shaking it repeatedly. Indicating the three blocks in front of the child, say:

"Shake each one until you hear one that sounds real loud exactly like mine. If you can find it, give it to me." Hold out one hand to indicate that you expect him to go ahead and *repeat sounding your loud block once in a while* so that he can remember how it sounded. If he simply hands you a block without shaking it, ask him to make sure he finds the one that *sounds* the same.

The child with a tendency to perseverate may find it hard to regard blocks in terms of sound after having regarded them recently in terms of color. Since the sound blocks are all green, he may simply match *any* green one to yours. Sometimes a child will even insist that, "It *does* look the same." The child with a motor handicap may undergo the same difficulty and it is therefore necessary to wait for his intention to be indicated before offering to help him manually.

It may be necessary to repeat a few times that they all *look* the same but they make *different* kinds of *noises*. If indicated, *repeated demonstration of each of your or his blocks by shaking them briefly,* or by asking him to shake each, can be given. Then ask again for the loudest block.

Say: *"Now let's find one that sounds as loud as this one."* Shaking your loud block once in a while to remind him of the sound and the task, help him to take each of his blocks up in turn and shake it, if necessary simply moving his hand holding a block by holding it lightly with your hand, as if taking for granted that this is what he wants to do. This can be done even for and with the child who needs no help manually.

After the child has made his choice, place your loud block and his selection on top of each other and move them to a remote corner of the table, out of his reach. Then say: *"That was fine. Now let's find the one that makes a tiny little bit of noise, like a little soft kitten walking."* While shaking for his inspection your *softest sounding* block, unobtrusively *bring back one of the loud sound blocks* from the corner of the table and place it among the blocks before the child so that he has to choose among three degrees of noise again. If necessary, guide him again in the process of picking up each block in turn and shaking it. Assume an attitude of concentrated listening yourself. If needed, remind him that he is to find one like the real quiet one and periodically demonstrate this *by shaking the softest sounding block* you are holding.

After he has made his choice, place his selection on top of your softest sounding block and move them to the corner of the table out of his reach as before.

Next say: *"Now we must find one that sounds just like this."* Shake repeatedly the block with the medium loud sound. Say: *"Hear it? It's not so loud as the real loud one and it's a little louder than the very, very quiet one, it's a middle loud one."* Again while shaking your *medium loud block* repeatedly for the child's inspection, unobtrusively *bring back one of the softest sounding blocks* and place it among the child's choices so that the selection has to be made among three degrees of loudness.

After the child has made his choice, place it again as before on top of your medium loud block, or invite the child to do so.

Although this task is difficult even for many four year olds and requires much practice and time, *the information it gives on the child's hearing acuity,* if he succeeds in comprehending and in correct pairing, *is important enough to make the time and effort spent a worthwhile investment.* It is equally revealing if the problem presented is conclusively comprehended by a child but the child by his selection shows that he is unable to distinguish between the medium and soft sounds. It also shows up the difficulty in hearing, which in usual communication may not have been detected, if a child believes that the softest sounding pair makes no noise at all and pairs them confidently, indicating, "These make no sound," or "Nothing," shaking his head to signify that one hears no sound coming from them.

Unlike school children who may be seated far back in a classroom and have to strain to hear, preschool children as a rule are never physically far removed from those in whose care they are and a *slight hearing cut-off may go undetected. Detecting it during the Evaluation interview provides an opportunity to suggest medical confirmation so that appropriate help can be given early.*

Many children will be able to cooperate without difficulty on this item. Some will spontaneously begin to compare the blocks and shake them all in turn, including the second set, in order to make their choices. This is encouraged.

Demonstrate in pantomime for children who hear but do not comprehend language or English.

IV-0 — VI.

16. SOUND BLOCKS.
   c) grading.

Level: 4-6 and up.

Main areas:	*Other areas:*
auditory intactness;	ability to keep a leading idea in mind;
language comprehension;	ability to carry through alone after
ability to listen for and recognize	verbal direction;
minor differences in degree;	capacity for insightful learning.
ability to learn to understand the concept of ascending or descending serial relationships.	

MATERIALS: same as in item 14: sound blocks.

PROCEDURE: pushing all the sound blocks left on the table after the last item into a heap nearer your side of the table, say: *"Now we will play one last game with them. Listen carefully and watch me."*

Shake the loudest block with one hand and then *in turn the medium and soft sounding ones* with the other hand, visibly comparing them by ear. As you shake the *softest* sounding one, say: *"Hear the very soft noise it makes?"* Lower your voice to a whisper and shake a few times *in turn the loudest* and *the softest* sounding blocks. Then indicate with emphasis a spot on the table, on the child's extreme left; place the *softest sounding block there, shaking it once more* as you place it, and say: *"The softest sound we will put here. And here we will put the loudest one,"* placing your hand on the child's extreme right on the table with emphasis. *Shake the loudest block* with one hand, *then the medium loud one with the other hand,* indicate the loudest one and say: *"Hear the loud noise it makes?"* Raise your voice in a playful manner to underline the loudness. Place this block on the spot on the extreme right end of the table as seen from the child. Holding the block with the *medium loud sound* in one hand, *lift the loud one up but keep your hand with it at the spot where it belongs.* Then *shake in turn a few times each of these two blocks.* Say: *"This one is not as loud as the loud one, is it?"* Invite the child to help you listen and shake the two blocks alternately, watching for the child's reaction. After he indicates that he has heard the difference, say: *"That one goes here, in the middle."* Hold up the *medium loud* block over the spot in the center of the table, *shake it once more* as you place it to impress the sound on the child's memory or awareness, then place it on the spot.

Say: *"See, now they go like that."* Lifting up briefly and shaking it, proceed from the child's left, and sound briefly each block in turn, *soft, medium, then loud.* If the child wants a repetition, repeat. If he expresses a doubt as to the correctness of the placement of the soft and medium loud blocks, indicating that you did not compare them, oblige by shaking each briefly to help the child detect the difference and clarify his doubt.

Removing one of the sets of blocks, push the other set in front of the child, scrambling them as you do so. Say: *"Now let me see how well you can listen. Make your ears very sharp. Remember, the soft one goes here,"* patting the spot on the table to the child's extreme left, *"the middle loud one goes here,"* patting the spot in the center of the table, *"and the loud one goes here,"* patting the spot at the extreme right of the child. Say: *"Go ahead."*

Help the physically handicapped child if he needs assistance in picking up and shaking the blocks. Avoid looking at the correct spot for any block until the child himself conveys his intention. Then help him place it. Repeat until he has placed them all to his satisfaction. Make sure that any child, motor-handicapped or not, shakes the blocks and listens. Some children succeed in memorizing slight irregularities in some of the blocks, such as chipped paint, and attempt to place them without listening.

Observe the child's pattern of performing the task. Bright children and older ones may immediately place correctly any block they happen to pick up and shake, without having to compare them and without being rigid in their adherence to the gradual placing. Others need to compare many times and will spend much effort on finding them in order of placement, sticking more rigidly to the rules and to the left-to-right progression. Some may show meticulousness in placing them at exactly right angles or in a perfectly straight line. Some children will seek constant reassurance from the adult, saying: "Am I doing it right?" or "That way?" before every decision.

Some few children seem incapable of inhibiting a tendency to shake both hands simultaneously, each holding a block, with the result that they cannot hear the difference. Watch closely to find out whether it is a simple intellectual backwardness which keeps the child from learning that auditory comparison must be done in time sequence or whether the child has in other activities the same pattern of unknowingly aping the motions of one hand with the other. This can be found out by watching his other hand when he uses scissors with one hand, or taps the table in a simple beat in imitation of the examiner, with one hand. It must be observed whether lateral dominance has been established yet or not. On this task, it is permissable to assist such a child by gently holding his one hand still and encouraging him to listen hard to the sound the block in his other hand produces.

A notation or mental note must be made of performance patterns observed during this item.

Demonstrate in pantomime for children who hear but do not comprehend language or English.

II-0 — VI.

17. SPATIAL RELATIONSHIPS. (Same area as item 36.)

a) fitting two halves of a circle.

Level: 2-6 and up.

Main area:	*Other areas:*
orientation in space;	understanding of twoness of things; probably ability to revisualize a whole from its components.

MATERIALS: two half-circles, 7 inches in diameter, green card board. (Material is visible in Fig. 18.)

PROCEDURE: place the *two half-circles* next to each other on the table with the straight sides parallel to the horizontal side of the table directly in front of the child.

Say: *"Look what I can do. I can make a ball."* Push the two halves together to complete the circle, leave them in this position for the child to study.

Say: *"Do you want to make a ball?"* and push the two halves back in their original positions.

Help the motor-handicapped child by holding firmly in place the half which he first pushes into a vertical position until he can push the second half into an approximately correct position.

Give a second demonstration if the child fails, repeating the above instructions.

The intention of the motor-handicapped child usually can be observed quite reliably by observing his manipulation in combination with his visual attempt to fit the two parts. If necessary, steady his hand while permitting him to push the pieces in the position he decides upon. It is not required that the straight sides meet exactly; any performance which brings the straight sides opposite to each other to form a rough circle is acceptable.

The most frequent inadequate performance is to place the two pieces on top of each other or to simply push them away.

Placing both halves in a vertical position but so that the straight sides both face in the same direction, or away from each other, is sometimes observed. If the child leans back to indicate that he has finished, leaving the material in this position, it is advisable to *give a second and even a third demonstration* until it becomes evident that he fails to understand the task. For him, the two pieces may not yet have assumed a relationship.

Observe the child's way of performing. Some children succeed unwittingly by simply imitating the motor performance of the examiner. This is acceptable at this level.

II-6 — IV only.

18. Recognition of Sizes in Small Black Outline Circles.
     a) big and little.

Level: 3-0 to 4-0

Main areas:

rudimentary mathematical thinking;
language comprehension;
ability to differentiate by visual com-
    parison;
ability to perceive outline drawings.

Other area:

flexibility: since given after item 17,
    "big" here is a relative concept.

MATERIALS: set of seven cards, 2½ x 3½ inches, with outline drawings of circles, one circle on each card, graded in size from ½ inch diameter to 2 inch diameter. (Material shown in Fig. 8.)

PROCEDURE: place in the stand the cards with the *smallest* (½ inch diameter) and the *largest* (2 inches diameter) of the circles only. Allow a few moments for the child to take in the material. Call his attention to the cards by saying: *"Look at the two round balls. See this one and that one?"* After it is certain that the child has studied both circles, say: *"Show me the BIG ball. Which one is the BIG one?"*

The child may look at it steadily, point to it or lift it out of the stand. After he has succeeded, replace it as before and say: *"Can you look at the tiny LITTLE ball? Where is it?"*

IV-0 — V-6 only.

(*Caution:* if item 21 will be presented to the child, this item must NOT be presented to him. The practice given would invalidate the response to item 21.)

19. Recognition of Sizes in Small Outline Circles.
     b) grading by size.

Level: 5-0 to 6-0.

Main areas:

beginning understanding of non-
    numerical relationships;
ability to perceive outline drawing;
ability to make finer visual compari-
    sons;
carry-over of earlier learning: the
    principle of ascending serial.

Other areas:

language comprehension: the relativity
    of meaning of similar words;
adaptability to an unfamiliar mode of
    performing.

MATERIALS: set of seven cards, 3½ x 2½ inches each, each bearing one black outline drawing of a circle. Sizes: in diameter: ½ inch, ¾ inch, 1 inch, 1¼ inch, 1½ inch, 1¾ inch, 2 inches. (Material shown in Fig. 8.)

PROCEDURE: spread the cards on the empty table at random, then holding up one after another, say: *"Look what I have. I have a lot of circles* ("balls" is permissible). *See, THIS is a TINY LITTLE one* (show ½ inch circle). *And here is a BIG one* (show 2 inch circle). *And this one is a LITTLE BIGGER than the TINY one* (hold ¾ inch circle next to ½ inch circle). *And this one here is just a LITTLE BIGGER than IT* (holding the 1 inch circle next to the ½ inch and ¾ inch ones). *Watch what I do, and afterwards I will let you do it too."*

After his attention has been secured and while he watches closely, *insert the cards in the stand, in the order of sizes, starting with the smallest one.* Start in whichever row is easiest for the child to see. *Start at the extreme left* of the row. If the child has demonstrated earlier any difficulty in spotting material visually, the whole stand may be moved so that the material comes into the child's field of vision. This adjusting must be done before the task is demonstrated.

Then *insert the cards slowly one by one.* In order to fit all seven cards in one row for easier display, they will have to overlap slightly. Be careful that overlapping does not result in covering up any part of any circle.

Let the child see that you have to compare and judge, even exaggerating your effort a little or waiting for him to advise you on your selections, as this will provide opportunity to observe whether he understands the task.

If the child has no difficulty surveying materials placed on the table in front of him, hold cards next to each other in order to compare the sizes. If he has difficulty, insert the cards at random in the stand and hold them in turn next to the last one each time inserted in the row and to one close in size to show the child how you compare them.

After all seven cards have been inserted, allow enough time to study the result and the arrangement, until the child indicates that he is ready.

If the child prefers it, he may do the task with the cards placed on the table. If he prefers the stand, or has to use the stand on account of his motor handicap, offer to insert his cards as he indicates which one comes next.

Insert the first three cards as before, with slight overlapping. Displaying the other four cards at random either in the stand (see Fig. 8) or on the table, be sure that the fourth card (1¼ inches) does not lie directly in line with the started row. Say: *"Go ahead. Now it's your turn."* Help the motor-handicapped child by holding the unplaced cards next to each other so that he may decide which one comes next. Be careful to show no reaction if he selects them incorrectly. Place them as he directs.

After a child has completed the task, tell him to look it over to make sure it is correct. *If the child has made some errors,* wait to see if he discovers this by himself and allow as many changes as he needs to or wishes to make until he indicates that he is finished.

If he fails, remove all cards and present only the ½ *inch, 1¼ inch* and *2 inch* cards. Insert them in the stand in that order (or place them on the table if the child prefers). Invite him to look at them. Then scramble the cards, pick up the *smallest circle* and place it at the beginning of a row. Say: *"Which one comes next?"* Display the *other two cards* and let him see them next to each other until he makes a choice. Then finish the row for him at his direction with the last card and allow him to study the result. If he wishes to make any changes, let him do so until he indicates that he is satisfied.

If he then should express a wish to do the whole set over again, it is permissible to let him.

Note down the performance pattern of the child. See chapter 9 for *modifications if the child cannot seem to get the idea of this task at all.*

IV-6 — VI.

20. DISCRIMINATION OF COLORS.
    c) grading shades within a color.

Level: 5-6 and up.

Main areas:	*Other areas:*
finer visual discrimination;	language comprehension;
carry-over of learning: the principle of grading.	ability to abstract: the fact that various shades can mean the same color;
	completion of a task on one's own.

MATERIALS: two sets of cards, each set consisting of five graded shades of color: pink to dark red and light blue to dark blue.

PROCEDURE: place *all cards* of the *red set* at random before the child, either in the wooden stand or on the table, depending on the child's need and preference. Allow a moment for inspection. Then say: *"What do you see?"* If the child says: "Red" or if he says, "Cards," point out that they are all of one color but of different shades, like pink and dark red. If he says, "Different kinds of red," praise him. Pick up the *pink color* and place it at the child's left side (table or stand).

Say: *"Let's put them all in a row, from the lightest one to the very darkest one. Remember, first the very light one, next to it one just a little darker. Then the next darker one and so on until the very darkest one comes at the end."* If the child is motor-handicapped, ask him to look at the one he wants you to place for him. It may be necessary to pick up the pink card and hold it next to each of the other four cards in turn until the child signifies his choice. Return the pink card, place the second selection briefly next to it for the child's benefit, then repeat holding the second card next to the three ungraded ones in turn so he can make his choice. After he has decided, place the second card, insert the third one briefly for the child's benefit, then, using the third to compare, continue as before, until the task is completed to the child's satisfaction. The nonhandicapped child may need a little assistance until he, too, begins to compare the cards one by one.

After a child indicates that he is finished, allow a few moments for him to survey his job. *If he has made any errors,* wait to see if he discovers them. Allow as many changes as the child desires. Accept whatever he offers. Then say: *"That was fine. Now here is another color."* Again place at random the cards of the set (*blue*) convenient to the child. Offer no further instruction except to say: *"Go ahead. Do them the same way."*

Do the manual part of the job for the physically handicapped child as above.

Allow *sufficient time* for self-corrections, if desired.

If the child fails, make a notation of the nature of his performance, as: piles cards, reverses order, etc.

V-6 and up.

21. RECOGNITION OF SIZES IN SMALL OUTLINE CIRCLES.

  c) insight into the principle of ascending serial placement.

Level: 6-0 and up.

Main areas:	*Other areas:*
capacity for learning by insight;	resourcefulness;
capacity to carry-over from one situation to another one resembling it in some respects;	visual discrimination; awareness of more than five.
ability to perceive small outline drawings;	
non-numerical mathematical concepts;	
attention to detail.	

MATERIALS: same as in 19. (Fig. 8.)

PROCEDURE: if the child has been given item 19, omit 21. Place *all seven cards on display* at random, either in the stand or on the table. After the child has inspected them for a few moments, remove the cards. Then place the *first three sizes, ½ inch* diameter, *¾ inch* diameter and *1 inch* diameter to the extreme left of the table or in one row of the stand to the child's left, with not more than ¼ inch of space between cards. Adjust the position of the stand to the child's visual needs if necessary. *Display the other four cards* at random, in the other rows of the stand or on the table depending on the child's needs. (See Fig. 8.) Say: *"Which one comes next?"* Indicate with one hand the ungraded cards and with the other point briefly to the three graded cards with emphasis on each one from left to right.

No further directions are given. Help the handicapped child by offering to place them for him after he tells you which one he wants you to put in. Tell him to look at the one he thinks comes next.

Whether the child understands or not, let him experiment at his leisure. If the child without manual ability indicates that he cannot make up his mind about which one is smaller or bigger, thereby showing that he is beginning to get the idea, ask him to point in his way to the ones he wants to see better; then hold them next to each other so that he can decide.

If a child asks for help, silently point again in sequence and with emphasis to the *first, second* and *third* graded cards. Say: *"Think."*

If the child fails, say: "That was a hard one. You are a good worker." See chapter 9 for modifications.

II-0 — VI.

22. PELLETS AND BOTTLE.
    a) dropping pellets in bottle.

        Level (not to be omitted on any level): 2-0 and up.

Main areas:	*Other areas:*
manipulation;	visual difficulties;
handedness;	awareness of more than one;
tactile sensitivity;	ability to inhibit.
awkwardness.	

MATERIALS: clear bottle, about 3 inches high, neck about ¾ inch wide, broad base desirable. Candy pellets, about ⅜ inch in diameter, red (cinnamon pearls). (Visible in Fig. 19.)

PROCEDURE: on the empty table place directly before the child the *empty bottle;* on *both sides of it place about 10 pellets.* Wait a few moments to see if the child automatically begins to drop the pellets in the bottle. *If he does not start spontaneously,* pick up one *pellet* with *your left hand* from the heap *on the child's right side,* drop it in the bottle, then *repeat* this with *your right hand* on *his left side.* Then say: *"You do it."* and look at him expectantly. *If he hesitates,* say: *"Let me see how you can put them all in. That's a good boy (girl)."*

To the older child, if he hesitates, it is sometimes advisable to say: *"I want to see how fast you can put them in."*

For the *severely motor handicapped* child *OMIT* this item. For the moderately and mildly handicapped child, give help by steadying the bottle, the child's arm and in other ways. It is not important for the motor-handicapped child to put in all the pellets.

If further encouragement is indicated, use appropriately the following:

"It's all right to use both hands." "You can use your other hand too." "Put them all in."

Very young and immature children will drop only a few pellets and then perhaps try to dig in or dump the bottle to get them out. Some children will be so quick at shoving some pellets into their mouth that all you can do is reassure the mother that it is all right because they are candy. And most children will not care for the taste and will expel them again.

Observation has to be accurate and needs to be made quickly, since the whole act takes only a few moments.

The following characteristics are to be observed:

handedness? type of grasp? same grasp on both hands or not? accuracy of aim in inserting pellets? all inserted? many spilled? pronounced awkwardness? subtle awkwardness? finally, inhibits eating pellets on verbal command or not?

   b) finding dropped pellet on floor.
   Level (not to be omitted): 2-6 and up.

Main area:
visual intactness, gross.

MATERIAL: one red pellet.

PROCEDURE: when child is almost finished dropping pellets in the bottle, manage to *drop one to the floor.* Whether the child has noticed this or not, say: *"Oh. One fell down. Do you want to pick it up for me?"*

Help the physically handicapped child to get off his chair and hold him securely while he searches the floor. If he is unable to grasp it himself, have him point out where he sees it and pick it up for him. All other children can walk or crawl by themselves until they find it.

If the first pellet has rolled out of *your* sight, too, manage to *drop a second one.*

Observe very closely: any difficulty? needs to bring eyes very near floor? feels around with his hands? peeks out of one corner of his eyes? turns head in any unusual way? fumbles when picks it up? reaches directly? spies it in shadow? eats it? steps on it? intent?

II-0 — VI.

23.   PUSH-BUTTON TABLE BELL, MUSIC BOX.
      Level (not to be omitted on any level): 2-0 and up.

Main areas:	*Other areas:*
manipulation;	memory;
difficulty of it.	awareness of more than one or two;
	hearing;
	handedness;
	possibly vision.

MATERIALS: table bell with push-button; music box with hand crank that works both ways without coming off. (Visible in Fig. 19.)

PROCEDURE: on the empty table place before the child the *table bell.*

Observe whether the child remembers how to make it ring or whether he tries to pick it up and shake it like the handled bell. Since demonstration was given on item 14, child may recall it.

Demonstrate, after the child's attention has been secured, how you can hit the button *with every fingertip,* starting either left or right and either with thumb or pinkie, but systematically hitting the bell clearly and at fairly regular intervals. Say: *"Now YOU do it,"* and push the bell into the best position for the child to use it. Unless he holds it himself with one hand, steady it with your hand. *If he hits it only* with index finger, thumb or palm and then stops, say: *"Use every finger." Demonstrate once more with your own hands* and return the bell to him.

The aim of this item is to reveal motor awkwardness. It is *omitted* in testing the child too involved to use it since his difficulty need not be revealed. *Help him* to *hit the bell button a few times* with any part of his hand since the bell is utilized with the next item in another connection and the child must be familiarized with it now.

Young and immature children, or retarded ones functioning at a level under three years of age, will not be able to understand the task very readily. *Observe* them for: can learn to hit button? can contact button with fingertip without fumbling? uses palm instead of fingertip? picks bell up by button and shakes it? turns bell over and explores it? which hand used more frequently or with greater ease, if any? does other hand ape the motion of the occupied hand?

After three and a half or four years of age, children will readily imitate. Many of this level have no difficulty using every finger for the bell. If they forget one or another finger or use the same finger twice, this may be on the basis of the number concept, which is less than five and therefore less than the number of fingers. *Observe* them for: uses second joint of finger rather than finger tip? unable to move finger in vertical direction singly? turns hand to approach bellbutton? brings two or more fingers to button simultaneously? forgets thumb? forgets other hand unless reminded? apes motions of one hand with other hand? prefers which hand? fumbles for button? takes a hold of his hand with the other hand and guides each single finger to the button in turn? repeats with other hand? looks closely? gives up in disgust and uses palm of hand? or thumb only? appears to understand the task intellectually better than he can perform it manually? appears to have no difficulty manually but intellectual limitation causes him to omit some of his ten fingers?

Five and six year olds usually have no difficulty in comprehending what is expected. Therefore, any unusual performance is noteworthy. *Observe* them for: uses second joint rather than tip of finger? holds finger extended stiffly, moving whole hand rather than finger individually? turns hand to approach button? fumbles for button? misses it frequently? prefers which hand?

Remove the table bell and place the *music box* on the table. Say: *"Look what I have."* Start turning the handle in clockwise direction (to the right) and produce the tune until the child indicates his wish to try it. If he does not do this, simply push the music box toward him on the table and say: *"You do it."* It may be necessary to steady the box while he turns it.

Help the handicapped child and also the young child to grasp the handle and turn it in a clockwise direction. Loosen your grip on the child's hand while still supporting his hold on the handle and *watch* in which direction he tries to push. *Watch* to see if he gives the handle a half-turn and then swings back another half-turn the other way. Or if he completes a whole circle in circular motion. If interrupted, which hand does he offer next?

Observe the nonhandicapped child for: clockwise or counterclockwise motion? interchangeable? handedness? completion of circular motion or, by way of least resistance, hesitation and changeover to return motion? grasp on handle? firm, uncertain? tries to push it up and down? turns box on its side and does better turning handle vertically?

II-6 — IV-0 only.

24. AMOUNT CONCEPT.

   a) "one only" and "more than one."

Level: 3-0 to 3-9

Main areas:	*Other areas:*
concept of amounts;	ability to make believe or role playing;
ability to conceptualize in general;	language comprehension.
spatial orientation.	

MATERIALS: wooden milk-bottle stand with six bottles (Fig. 11).

PROCEDURE: prepare for this item by keeping the table bell handy and placing the doll within your reach but not within the child's sight in the event modifications will be needed. Place the *milk-bottle stand* on the empty table near the child's leading hand. Say: *"Do you want to play Milkman with me? You must be the milkman and I will be the lady (man) who wants to order some milk. All right?"* Give the *table bell a few rings* and *hold your hand up to your ear* in imitation of telephoning. Say: *"Hello, Milkman."* If the child does not spontaneously bring his hand to his ear, say: *"Pick up your telephone. I am calling you up."* Help him to bring his hand to his ear or his ear down to his hand. Place a suitable small object in his hand to serve as a telephone receiver if he cannot pretend to telephone with his hand empty (small box, eraser, tightly rolled up piece of paper). Also, make a mental note of his need to have a tangible make-believe object.

After he is ready with his "telephone," *ring the bell again,* holding *your hand up to your ear* very firmly, and say: *"Hello, Milkman."* Nod at him encouragingly and expect him to answer. If he has no speech, expect him to indicate by nodding his head that he is listening. Then say: *"How are you today? Do you have nice fresh milk today?"* Wait for his nod or verbal reply before going on. Then say: *"I want to order ONE bottle of milk today. Just ONE bottle. Can you please bring it right over?"* Wait for his nod again. Then say: *"I will be waiting for you. See you later."* Put down your hand as if indicating that the call is finished and observe whether he will put his hand and object down appropriately. If he begins to pick up a milk bottle with one hand while the other one is still held to his head, guide it down gently and say: *"Put your phone down."* Make a mental note of it if he perseverated in this manner.

If he cannot manually manage to remove bottles himself, help him to lift out one bottle, then wait poised and ready but looking to him for the decision. If he indicates the bottle as if terminating the task, accept it and thank him. If he makes a motion toward the stand to get another bottle, help him to lift it out and wait for his next decision as before. Remove as many as he decides to remove in this way. Then say firmly: *"I want ONE bottle of milk, just ONE."* Look to him for the next move. He may push one bottle toward you and terminate the task correctly. If he continues to give you bottles after the first one on *this second chance,* accept them and thank him.

The nonhandicapped child may perform much like the description just given.

For some reason, many children like to empty the whole stand before they are ready to perform by responding to the original direction. The second trial should be given as described, by repeating the request after the stand is emptied, in order not to mistake the child's correct response.

After the child has responded and only if he was able to stop after giving one on one of two trials, pretend to drink the milk in your bottle, return it to him and say: *"That was good. Here is your empty bottle back. Put it back in the stand."* Help the handicapped child to return the bottles. Observe how the child goes about putting back the bottles. The stand is placed so that one row of bottles is toward the child (Fig. 11). After he has filled the front row, observe whether he is aware that there must be another row for the rest of the bottles or whether he tries to solve the problem by substituting those in front with the unplaced ones, which will again leave him with three unplaced ones. The manually helpless child may make the same errors, directing your hand, which is helping his, again and again to the front row, suggesting that you squeeze in the extra bottles. Make a notation if the child performs in this way. If he is aware of the back row, he will indicate this by filling it or having you fill it with the other three bottles. Now, using the above described telephone routine, order *TWO bottles*. In the same way as before, await the child's decision as he brings his bottles. If he stops reliably after giving two bottles, thank him, share a pretended drink with him and return the bottles to him to put back in the stand.

A response of giving more than one, but not two, or giving two for *"two"* at one trial and three or four for *"two"* at the second trial is an indication that the child's concept of amounts is emerging gradually but is still fluctuating. Giving all of the bottles for *one* and for *two* indicates that the child has not yet formed a concept of amounts.

Use modifications, chapter 9, to probe the level *if the child has failed.*

III-6 — VI.

25. AMOUNT CONCEPT.

   b) separating a stated number of objects from a larger group.

Level: 4-0 to 6-0 and up.

Main areas:	*Other areas:*
concept of amounts;	left to right progression in lining up;
spatial orientation.	role playing and capacity for imaginative play;
	cooperativeness;
	ability to share.

MATERIALS: same as 24. (Fig. 11.)

PROCEDURE: prepare for this item by keeping the table bell handy and provide yourself with 20 pennies or plastic chips in case they are needed. Place the *milk bottle stand* on the empty table near the child's leading hand. Say: *"Do you want to play Milkman with me? You must be the milkman and I will be the lady (man) who wants to order some milk. Here is my house. You can deliver the milk bottles here. All right?"*

Place the *cardboard* to your left or right on your side of the table, depending on the child's handedness, so that he will be able to place his bottles there. Repeat: *"Here is my house."* Point to the cardboard and make sure he understands. Then say: *"I am going to call you on the telephone. Listen."* After his attention is secured in this way, *place your hand to your ear* in an attitude of telephoning, *ring the table bell* a few times and look at him expectantly. If he does not spontaneously pretend to hold a receiver and say: "Hello," say: *"Pick up your telephone, Milkman, I am calling you."* Note whether he can pretend immediately or whether he looks unconvinced or even looks meaningfully at the real telephone, indicating poor ability to imagine. Say: *"Let's make believe."* If necessary, give him a small object to hold and guide his hand to his ear with it.

Ring the bell again, hold *your hand to your ear* with emphasis and say: *"Hello, Milkman. Is that the milkman?"* Wait for his sign that he has gotten the idea, such as a nod in the child without speech or such as some appropriate word. Then say: *"Do you have any milk today? I want to order TWO bottles of milk. Can you bring TWO bottles over to my house right away, please?"*

In the usual manner, help the motor-handicapped child in the manipulative part of the task but be completely passive and leave your hand at his disposal to carry out his decision. Be careful not to make any sign of surprise or hesitation if he arrives at incorrect answers.

Note the child who "forgets" to lower his hand and begins to lift milk bottles with one hand while holding the other to his ear. It is advisable to pretend to terminate the telephone conversation if this delay is observed, because instead of being perseverative, the child may actually be living his part. In such an event, the basis for the delay would become clear by his response to you. Say: *"Ring my bell when you come to my house. GOOD-BY NOW."* Put down your hand with emphasis and observe his reaction. By watching him in the same situation at subsequent trials, it will become clear whether he truly perseverates or not.

The correct response is removing two bottles only, even if they are not handed to the examiner. If the child can stop after just two, indicating conclusively that he has finished, accept his answer and thank him.

After making suitable motions of using the milk, hand him back the bottles and tell him that they are now empty. If he does not replace them in the stand, tell him to put them back. Observe whether he hesitates slightly because they are "empty," and reassure him that it is all make-believe. Then say: *"Watch. I am going to order some more."* Repeat the telephone play as described above and say: *"Today I need FOUR bottles of milk. Can you give me FOUR bottles, please? Bring them over to my house."*

As he places the bottles on the cardboard, observe whether he lines them up in a row or just places them at random. If he gives the correct number, thank him, pretend to use them or share a drink with him, and return them to him.

Observe closely his way of solving the problem of placing bottles in the back row of the stand as he puts them away.

In the same way ask for *three,* then *five,* then *four,* then *six* bottles, as long as he can arrive at correct answers, until the limit or extent of his amount concept becomes clear.

Many observations can be made during the child's responses to this item. Difficulties in space perception may be revealed by his performance in placing the bottles back in the stand. This must not be confused with the intellectual immaturity of being unaware or having forgotten the spaces in the second row. Manual awkwardness of the not obviously motor-handicapped child will be revealed in his handling of the material. The presence or absence of the habit of systematic lining-up of similar objects when counting and the direction of the pattern (left-to-right or right-to-left) can be observed. The eye-motion of the child, as he surveys his selection to check the correctness, can be observed by the examiner sitting opposite him: left-to-right, right-to-left, at random. Nonintellectual areas, such as distractibility during a task, meticulousness, perseveration, rigidity, insecurity, good social adjustment, uncooperativeness, hostility, extreme concretization, will be revealed by observing the child as he goes about this task.

The very concrete child will try repeatedly to open the wooden milk bottles without learning that they are just solid wood. He will be unconvinced and unconvincing in his telephone play. Some children cannot bear to give away or share. They may be toy-deprived children or there may be a new sibling in the family. *Such children must be given the chance to show what they can do by accommodation of their difficulty.* They may be willing to put the bottles in their "own frigidaire," or they may be tested by being "permitted" to take away from the examiner. Their amount concept can be tested if they are told they may have *TWO, FOUR, THREE* bottles and by offering them the stand to help themselves.

If the child fails with *two,* use modifications, chapter 9.

V-6 — VI and up.

26. AMOUNT RECOGNITION.
   c) matching a row of similar objects by amount when number names are not used.

Level: 6-0 and up.

Main areas:	*Other areas:*
actual amount recognition with or with- out knowledge of number names; ability to take away or add without use of number names.	eye-motion; left to right progression in placing.

MATERIALS: 30 pennies or plastic chips. If the table top is dark, have two large pieces of light cardboard ready on which to place the rows of pennies. Secure child's cardboard to table with Scotch tape.

PROCEDURE: secure the child's attention. While he watches, *place before him on his side of the table,* slowly and with emphasis and making sure you are going from his left to his right side of the table (right to left from examiner's side), *two pennies,* not more than two or three inches apart. Immediately *place the same amount before yourself,* going from your right to your left.

Prevent the child from picking up his pennies. Point to his and your rows of pennies with emphasis repeatedly. Then indicate the child and yourself with emphasis, to let him know that he and you have the same amount. Remove the rows. Wait a moment and repeat the demonstration in the same way, using *four pennies* for each row. Remove after the child has regarded both rows and has had a chance to compare them in his way. At the *third demonstration, begin placing the pennies on your side* of the table, using *three pennies.* Then *wait* instead of going on and observe whether the child anticipates a row for himself. If he does, *place three pennies in front of him* and leave the two rows exposed for about 20 to 30 seconds, repeating the gesture of indicating yourself and your row, and the child and the similarity of his and your rows. It is permissible to explain verbally that both of you have the same, but it is usually not necessary or expected by the child.

Place the pile or box of pennies within reach of his leading hand (a pile is easier to use for children with motor difficulties), remove the six pennies in the two rows, return them to the pile. Then place *four pennies* slowly and with emphasis in a row in front of you (from your right to your left), indicate the pile of pennies and invite the child to make his own row. If he succeeds, help him to push your and his rows back to the pile. Praise him matter-of-factly.

Place *seven pennies* before yourself and invite him to imitate it. If he can succeed with seven, remove the pennies as before and demonstrate slowly *one row of five, leave a space,* which should be about in the center of the table, then *make a second row of five.* Indicate the row of ten without especially emphasizing the space in the middle. Invite him to match it. Observe whether the child places ten correctly, whether he leaves a space after the first five, or whether he ignores the space but arrives at the correct amount. If he finds it difficult to keep track of your pennies, it is permissible to push your two rows nearer to him to facilitate matching.

If he has succeeded with ten, remove the rows. Do not neglect to praise the child so that he understands that he is on the right track. Next place *five* in a row, have him match it, then ask him to watch what you will be doing. While he watches, *remove the two pennies at the left end of your row as seen from your position,* push them to the pile and wait for his response. If he follows and removes two of his, even if he takes them off anywhere else (middle, left end, right end), praise him again. Next, with three pennies remaining in each row, secure his attention and while he watches, *push four pennies more* to your row to make a *total of seven.* Invite him to imitate. It is advisable to push the four singly rather than in one handful because the child may not be able to pick up with his hand. He may hesitate to imitate because of this difficulty rather than because of noncomprehension of the task.

Observe the child's pattern of performing. Help the motor-handicapped child in the usual way. Be cautious not to betray by facial expression or a slight hesitation any indication that the child has made an error. Be passive, observant and just lend your manual assistance.

The child's performance can usually be divided into:

a) attempts to ape and begins to fail by using more or fewer pennies than required but spreading his row to match it in length;

b) matches penny to penny and begins to fail when the row consists of seven or ten, probably due to inaccuracy of comparing back and forth; may discontinue his effort when the examiner takes away and adds, probably because he more or less can only adhere to a more rigid lining-up and becomes confused with the introduction of a different demand;

c) succeeds with all tasks, either by counting aloud or silently, or by seeing groups, or by a combination of matching, comparing back and forth, counting and imitating;

d) some children will push away their row of pennies instead of imitating taking away and adding. Give the child time to respond and watch whether he then proceeds to place anew the pennies required to match the row. While this may indicate a mild degree of rigidity, it is acceptable if the final result is correct. If he fails to place his row once he has pushed it away in response to your demonstration of taking away (two from five), it may indicate that he has stopped comprehending the various changes you have demonstrated and their significance.

Observe also the child's eye-motion, the direction taken in lining up his rows (left-to-right, right-to-left, at random), his manual ability in handling small objects while simultaneously under the impact of a guiding idea for their use. Some children like to slip a few pennies teasingly into their pockets.

V-6 — and up.

27. FAMILIARITY WITH NON-NUMERICAL MATHEMATICAL TERMS.

Level: 6-0 and up.

Main area:	*Other areas:*
correct understanding of less familiar words used in school activities.	language comprehension; hearing; listening habits.

MATERIALS: wooden milk bottles as in 24; thirty pennies as in 26.

PROCEDURE: place before the child a row of four milk bottles, then place one bottle in front of your place. After the child has looked at them, say: *"Who*

has *MORE, you or I?"* After he has reponded, say: *"Who has LESS?"*
Either the correct person or the correct group must be indicated by the child.
Remove the milk bottles.

Next say: *"How many shoes are a PAIR of shoes?"* If he hesitates, say:
"How many do we need to make a PAIR?" If he still hesitates, say: *"Who
put your socks on you today, mother or you yourself? Is it a new PAIR?"*
If he wants to look at his feet, let him. Either "two" or an appropriate
intentional pointing out of his two feet is accepted.

Next put all of the pennies except three to the child's left, put three
pennies to his right. After he has regarded both groups, say: *"I see a great
many pennies and I see where there are just a few. Can you see where there
are a great MANY?"* If he hesitates, say: *"Look at them."* Next say: *"And
now show me where you see just a FEW."* A common error is for a child
to indicate that all of the pennies on the table are "a great many." If he, on
the second trial, correctly singles out the row of three pennies for "just a
few," he shows that he is beginning to get the meaning.

Walking casually around the table, say: "I want to try something. Watch
what I do." Hold your arm, bent at the elbow, horizontally, in front of the
child at about the height of his chest and about three to four inches distant.
Then, say: *"I want to see if you can put your arm ACROSS mine. See if
you can do it."* If he just places his hand on your arm or if he holds his
arm parallel to yours, say: *"No, I mean ACROSS. Put it ACROSS my
arm."* DO NOT DEMONSTRATE. Any angle roughly between 45 and 90
degrees is accepted.

Next say: *"Tell me something. Is it MORNING OR AFTERNOON?"*
If he hesitates, say: *"What time of day is it AFTER you eat your lunch,
MORNING OR AFTERNOON?"* Ask the nonspeaking child to give his
sign for negation or consent as you use the two words *(MORNING,
AFTERNOON).*

III-0 — VI and up.

28. MULTIPLE CHOICE COLOR-FORM SORTING.*

a) sorting.

Level: 3-6 and up.

Main area:
concept formation.

Other areas:
color recognition;
form recognition;
incipient recognition of amounts;
work habits.

MATERIALS: cardboard symbols, three inches in diameter, of three circles,
three squares, and three triangles, one each of blue, red and yellow.

---

* This item was suggested by Dr. J. Meerloo, New York.

PROCEDURE: screen the table from view with the board, tell the child to close his eyes while you "fix a surprise." Place the *nine cards* at random on the table, not in a row, avoiding direct proximity of more than two that have direct similarities. (Do not place three of one form or of one color next to each other.) Remove the screen and tell the child to open his eyes. After he has looked at the material, say: *"I want you to put all of those together that go together."* If he hesitates, repeat: *"Put them together the way they belong together."*

For the young and immature child, it is permissible to *hold up one card for his inspection* and to start him off by saying: *"Which ones go with this?"* If he still hesitates, *hold up another card,* indicate all the material on the table with an inclusive motion and say: *"I can see some that look like it. Look around."*

The motor-handicapped child can show with his eyes which cards he thinks go together, while the examiner picks them up as the child directs. Be completely receptive to his signs and avoid placing them unless he directs you to. Just as will the nonhandicapped child, he, too, may reveal his way of solving the task, which may include placing cards in certain patterned designs. *If a child asks* whether he is to put all the colors together, say: *"Put them together the way you think they go."*

After the child has completed the task, present item 29.

The following reactions have been observed:

a) Sorting is done with dispatch and assurance; the child seems able to hold one concept in mind long enough to resist being swayed by the intrusion of the other common quality.

b) Sorting is done by color, and immediately after one set is collected, the child proceeds in arranging the three cards in some design. He collects the next set and again makes a design, similar or different, in juxtaposition to the first design or not. He may ignore or resist a suggestion that it is not necessary to bother. He may insist on completing the task by again making a design with the last set. It is possible that sometimes it may be a verbal misunderstanding, with the child believing he is to put the cards in a suitable pattern "the way they belong together;" more often, it may be playful use of material, and sometimes it may be perseveration, with the child going on in a disinhibited way. *Since a similar design cannot be made when the cards are sorted by form, his performance on the next item will reveal on what basis he did his first sorting.*

c) An interesting finding is that while retarded children are more likely to sort by color, very young children (under three) often sort by form. Color recognition as a conscious awareness of a quality, the conceptualizing of color, or possibly the perception of color may be undeveloped or incompletely developed at this stage, while the other concept, that of form, may be dominant. Since the intellectual insight at this level is not mature enough for the child to comprehend the next item, it is difficult to determine conclusively what is at work here.

d) Among retarded children, including mongoloid children with mental levels of four and above, sometimes a performance will show how the two concepts fluctuate. The child may sort two squares: he may happen to spot a triangle of the same color as the square that happens to be on top of his collection and place this triangle on top of the square. If he then chances to spot next another triangle, regardless of the color, he will match it to the card on top of his collection. His next selection may be a circle of the same color as the triangle now on top of his collection, to be followed by another circle. *He shows his poor ability to keep a guiding idea in mind, and this will be demonstrated conclusively on the next item, where he will be unable to change this pattern of step-by-step and short-lived planning* and be unable to gain a definite awareness of what he does and why he performs in that way. He may reveal that he is a plodder, that he wants to finish an assignment and has developed work habits in spite of intellectual limitations.

e) It is possible that the more intellectual child may sort by form rather than color. Very bright children will offer both possibilities, sorting first one way then scrambling the cards and sorting them in the other way, then collecting all to indicate they have finished, and handing them to the examiner.

f) Some children sort the cards in pairs and resist the addition of the third card. They may not be fully capable of understanding the verbal direction or may not yet have an awareness of more than two. Sometimes, such children will reveal their way of thinking by happily using two circles in imitation of mother powdering her face with compact and powderpuff, perhaps using a square for a mirror and a triangle for a hat. While their form perception appears adequate, their delightful but immature performance *reveals that conceptualizing is beyond them at the moment.* This ability to imitate and to make-believe with conviction in the absence of good concept formation has been observed in mongoloid children rather than in children retarded for other reasons.

g) A reaction of inhibition or "freezing" when faced with this task may also be observed; if the child feels pushed too far, the next reaction may be completely disinhibition, spreading to a "catastrophic reaction," such as scattering the cards, running out of the room or in other ways revealing inability to deal with what to the child represents an insoluble problem or a task of unstructured demand. This reaction will be observed also in some children with sensory aphasia and with sensory-motor aphasia, but not in those with a predominantly motor-aphasia. It may also be observed in some children with cerebral defects without gross motor handicap and with or without language impairment. More rarely, it also may be observed in children with cerebral palsy.

While this item gives much information, it will be found to be most valuable in combination with the next item, which can be used if the child can be expected to cooperate comprehendingly. His attempt to solve item 29, even if he is unsuccessful, will offer clues to his thinking.

IV-6 — VI and up.

(*Caution:* Item 28 *must* precede item 29.)
29. MULTIPLE CHOICE COLOR-FORM SORTING.
   b) ability to shift.

Level: 5-0 and up.

Main areas:	Other areas:
ability to abstract above the level of identity;	presence of:
conceptualization;	rigidity,
ability to shift.	perseveration,
	forced responsiveness.

MATERIALS: same as item 28.

PROCEDURE: after the child has completed the task in item 28, screen the table from view and *present the cards* as directed in item 28. Say: *"Now I want to see if you can think of another way in which you can sort them."* If the child does not understand what SORTING means, say: *"Another way in which you can put those together that are alike."*

If the child sorts them in the way opposite to his former performance, ask: *"Can you tell me how this is different from the first time?"* Note whether he knows the difference in a conscious way or only dimly.

Give three trials, if the child performs at first in exactly the same way as he did in item 28. It is permissible to say: *"Is there another way in which they look the same?"* If necessary, say: *"Is there something ELSE about them that makes them look alike?"*

If for any reason it seems desirable to go on with this area, the *cards may be placed in three rows of three,* such as:

red circle	blue circle	yellow circle
red square	blue square	yellow square
red triangle	blue triangle	yellow triangle

and the child may be given as many trials as he wishes.

The discussion at the end of the former item indicates that there may be various factors at work when a child has difficulty on this task. Some of the reasons may be other than intellectual.

II-0 — III-6 only.

(*Caution:* if item 31 is to be presented, this item is omitted.)

30. RECOGNITION OF WEDGIE DOLL AND MINIATURE TOYS.

Level: 2-6 and up.

Main areas:	*Other areas:*
ability to accept various replicas as representations of real things; body-image awareness.	language comprehension; vision; imagination; negatively: concretization.

MATERIALS: wooden wedgie man, rubber horse, plastic car. These objects form part of the story test, item 31. (Fig. 12.)

PROCEDURE: prepare the material in a way which prevents the child from seeing the eight objects in the box. Place on the empty table the *car, horse, man,* leaving about six inches of space between objects. Observe the child's immediate response, verbal or nonverbal.

If he names them spontaneously and correctly, no further directions are needed. He has succeeded without them. If he hesitates or looks disinterested, say: *"Look what I have."* After he has inspected the objects, say: *"You make the DADDY fix his CAR."* Be sure he can reach the materials; if they need to be moved closer, move all three. Help the handicapped child in the usual way and be careful to avoid looking at the correct object exclusively or to anticipate the correct next move until the child himself initiates it.

It is sufficient to bring the car to the man or the man to the car. No further manipulation is needed. If necessary, repeat: *"Make the daddy fix his car."* Picking up either or both of the correct toys without bringing them to each other meaningfully is not a conclusive response.

After the child has succeeded, say: *"Put the MAN on the HORSE (horsey)."* If he hesitates, say: *"Like a cowboy."* It is sufficient to bring the man near the horse or the horse near the man and no further manipulation is needed, but picking up either or both without bringing them together meaningfully is not a conclusive response.

If for any reason *a first response was missed,* such as by an accidental dropping of a toy, *give another trial.* For the motor-handicapped child or for nonhandicapped, shy children, *a further trial* may be given by holding the man and either one of the other two toys up for him to see, far enough apart to make his response conclusive, and to say: *"Look at the man (daddy)."* *Repeat with the second toy.* Give at least *two trials with each pair.* The man must always be one of the paired toys, e.g., man versus horse, man versus car. *Reverse the position of the two toys for each trial* to check the correctness of the response.

Observe carefully when a child seems to show interest in the toys but fails to follow verbal requests. If he shows by his use of a toy that he recognizes it conclusively, accept it.

Examples of acceptable meaningful usage are:

a) kissing the man or holding it upright and smiling or regarding the face; holding it in an approximately upright position and showing it to the mother or examiner with a meaningful expression; looking at it and saying either: "Man" or "Daddy."

b) pushing the car back and forth or rolling it across the table; showing it to mother or examiner meaningfully; looking at it and saying: "Car" or "Go car" or "Bye bye car."

c) holding the horse in an upright position and making it hop along the table; showing it to the adult meaningfully; naming it.

If he uses the toys meaningfully but fails to heed directions, observe hearing and language comprehension.

Negative responses are: piling the toys disinterestedly, throwing them away; putting them in his own mouth; placing the wooden man horizontally on the table like a building-block; turning the car upside down and manipulating the wheels.

If child fails, use modifications, chapter 9.

IV-0 — VI and up.

31. STORY COMPREHENSION.

Level: 4-6 and up.

Main areas:	*Other areas:*
language comprehension;	ability to listen to a continuous story;
understanding of a story;	can help tell the story;
recall of some pertinent factors of a story;	ability to accept replicas as representations of real things;
ability to assemble objects related to a story by multiple choice method.	projects own attitudes relating to his family.

MATERIALS: one copy of the story, "Goldilocks and the Three Bears." Set of eight toys: two bears, two beds, one man, one horse, one plastic car, one wooden boat. (Fig. 12.)

PROCEDURE: prepare by keeping the box with the set handy but out of sight. Leave this box closed. Keep also on hand a cardboard to screen the table from view. Use the book or tell the story without a book. The latter is definitely preferable. Say: *"Now we are going to do something you will like. I am going to tell you a story. You can sit back and rest up a little and just keep your ears wide open so that you will hear all of the story. Remember, listen hard. When I am through, I am going to show you something in this box"* (hold up closed box for child's inspection), *"something that has to do with the story. I will ask you about the story, so listen hard."* Remove box.

See that the child is really comfortable, encourage him to lean back or to rest his elbows on the table. Look relaxed yourself. Then *tell or read the story.* Encourage the child to help tell it, either by helping to repeat the repetitive phrases or, if he volunteers, by telling it in his own words if he is familiar with it. Follow his recital carefully in this latter event. If he skips parts or changes the story, the correct version must be substituted. *Observe* also whether, in repeating phrases, he uses them appropriately or not. *Note* carefully if a child tends to parrot words without obvious comprehension.

After the story is told, screen the table from view and inform the child that you are getting ready for him. Place the objects in this order: from the *child's left to his right; boat, little bear, big bed, man, horse, little bed, plastic car, big bear.* (Fig. 12.) *Before* exposing the display, say: *"I am going to let you look at these toys. Some of them GO WITH the story I have just told you. SOME of them DON'T GO WITH IT AT ALL. They don't BELONG to the story. We don't want THEM. You pick out ALL THE TOYS THAT GO WITH GOLDILOCKS AND THE THREE BEARS."*

Expose the toys. Leave the *cardboard* on the table nearest the child's leading hand. *Remove the box.* Then say: *"You can put them here."* Point to the cardboard. *"Remember, you are to pick out the TOYS THAT GO WITH THE STORY of Goldilocks and the Three Bears. DON'T take the wrong ones. We don't want THEM, do we?"*

Help the handicapped child in the usual way. If it becomes necessary to point to each object in turn, so that he may give his sign for negation or consent as he selects his responses, *avoid carefully use of the expression:* *"DOES THIS GO?"* Instead, say: *"Does THIS GO with the STORY?"* (Some children misunderstand and decide that you expect the things that "go." Since cars, boats and horses can go, the confusion is best avoided.)

Conclusive evidence that he understands the story is selection of two bears and two beds.

At four, many children add the wooden man, in the clear desire to have a daddy bear. *This is acceptable at that age.*

At five, most children are able to select the correct toys and to pass up the father figure knowingly.

At four years, six months, children who understand the story select first the four correct toys, then imply, verbally or by gesture, that they wish to include the man, although they know he is not a father bear. *At that level, this is acceptable.* It is not essential that the child remember to place his selections on the cardboard. Explain that he can use it to put those toys that go with or belong to the story together if his responses seem too ambiguous to evaluate conclusively otherwise. Do not use the box to collect his selections; he may misunderstand and put everything away.

An evaluation of responses shows the following:

a) The child understands the story as well as the directions. He confines himself to responding appropriately by immediate correct selection, appreciating the nature of the test situation.

b) The child understands the story and the directions, selects the correct objects and adds the man probably for reasons of emotional needs and the need for completeness. His awareness of the test situation may retreat a little before his personal need to have things the way he likes them.

c) The child understands the story and the directions, selects the four correct toys and adds the car "because the three bears took a little walk." Especially when coming from a nonwalking child, this response has its merits. If inquiry reveals that the car is meant to be used for the "walk," *this response is acceptable.*

d) The child understands the story and the directions but has difficulty in a multiple choice method. This is described as typical of some children with brain-lesions. Such a child may include several of the incorrect objects, seeing remote relationships which to him seem plausible. One must take care to differentiate this response from that of a child who selects incorrect objects because he fails to understand the story and/or the directions. This differentiation is made by asking the child: *"How does this go with the story?"* or *"Why is this in the story?"* His response will determine *whether he has understood the story and will illuminate the pattern of his thinking.* He may explain: car—"a toy for the baby bear" or "for the father bear to go to work;" horse—"his pony" or "it's his pet because he has no one to play with;" boat—"a bowl for the porridge;" man—"father bear." While he demonstrates that he understands the story, *his pattern of thinking reveals the difficulties he may meet* in a school situation if his tendency to go off at a tangent is not known, recognized, modified or accommodated in his educational management.

e) The child appears to understand the story, tends to ignore the verbal directions, but occupies himself immediately with the four correct toys, ignoring the incorrect ones or pushing them aside, perhaps acting out some recognizable part of the story. His *ability* to take directions and to cooperate intelligently in a group-situation *may be poor* but his *comprehension may be near normal.*

f) The child listens to the story appropriately, apparently understands the directions, but stops after selecting the two bears. He may be able to show that he recognizes the beds as beds, when questioned, but does not relate them to the story. His recall may be poor and he may be too inarticulate in inner language to figure out how they could belong. Less frequently, only the two beds are selected. The child may be able to explain his selection: " 'cause Goldilocks tried to sleep in the bed," but he may call the bear figures "Pussycat" or "Teddybear" and not relate them to the characters of the story at all. *These responses must be evaluated as insufficient.* They reveal limitation of comprehension, of recall and of the ability to make the transition from real things to the imaginary or portrayed representation of tangible things.

g) The child listens to the story with either rapt or only intermittent attention and to the directions with doubtful comprehension, occupies himself with several objects, but when reminded to pick out the ones that go with the story, hands all of them back to the examiner, perhaps saying: "All go in there," and indicates the box. He may refuse to give up the car. Responses of this and related degress of noncomprehension demonstrate the inability of the child to understand a story of this length and content. He may appear to understand, he may even anticipate the repetitive phrases with glee or spontaneously offer them or repeat them at the correct point in the story, as well as at inappropriate moments. This apparent appreciation of the story may be more of the nature of listening to familiar nursery rhymes, with partial comprehension of familiar words here and there. His repetitions may be parrot-like rather than comprehending. *His response is evaluated as insufficient.*

h) The child is unable to attend to the story without constant reminders to listen, interrupts, looks around the room, yawns, wants to see the things in the box. He hardly listens to the directions given after the story. He then may surprisingly select at first all of the correct objects, only to follow this apparently correct response with a hasty and impartial selection of the other four objects. It is often revealed that he does not listen to the radio, attends television programs only briefly, has never liked to be told stories or nursery rhymes and has never been told this particular story. Nor could it be assumed that he would have been able to sit through it or the reading of any story at any time. His behavior and reaction demonstrate his incapacity to listen or attend for more than a few moments, but hint at a possibility of unused and unrealized potential which could become available to him if he could be helped to organize himself and learn to resist distractions and disinhibition. *His response must be regarded as insufficient.*

i) The child expresses vocally or by signs an unwillingness to listen to the story. If he cannot be motivated at this interview, *the item should be omitted.* The history of early development, domestic behavior and his performance on items which test hearing and those which test language comprehension on lower levels *may reveal his reasons.*

j) The child listens attentively to the story and to the directions. He may select the correct toys and it may be possible to understand conclusively that he knows what is expected. He may then immediately begin to play out some action with such affect or with such an air of secrecy that it becomes reasonably obvious that he has projected himself in the story characters. He may become quite oblivious of the room and the persons in it and proceed to express in play some of his emotional problems, such as sibling rivalry, hostility or fear of a parent, fear of being left alone. Even nonspeaking motor-handicapped children may fling the father figure off the table with a telling facial expression, or have the mother bear scold the baby bear, or express a wish that the daddy would play more with the baby bear when he is home. *The performance can be evaluated for adequacy of story-comprehension if the child at first selected the correct toys conclusively.* The information revealed by his unexpected *performance of a projective nature is utilized by giving a descriptive report of it in the Inventory of Development.* This will enable those responsible for his educational care to help him to a happier adjustment.

This item has been found extremely useful in testing the level of language comprehension of nonspeaking children, especially those with cerebral palsy. It may reveal good comprehension where the severity of physical involvement has made the parents sceptical of the child's understanding; it may reveal inability to comprehend where the seemingly appropriate smile of the child when spoken to has made the environment overly optimistic. In both eventualities, it will make appropriate educational planning more realistically suitable.

In spite of the time the story-telling consumes, it is considered one of the most important items of the evaluation.

IV-0 — VI and up.

32. UNDERSTANDING OF RELATIONSHIPS OF PARTS TO A WHOLE.*

Level: 4-0 to 6-0

Main areas:

orientation in the environment;
ability to reconstruct a mental picture of a situation from details;
ability to select by multiple-choice method;
probably: alertness to the immediate environment.

Other areas:

memory;
language comprehension;
attention to details;
association.

MATERIALS: doorknob, faucet handle, electric plug, key, electric bulb, sink stopper. (Fig. 1.)

---

* The author is indebted to a bright youngster, handicapped by cerebral palsy, for this item, which originated from one of his helpful ideas expressed when he was a pupil and seven years old.

PROCEDURE: place before the child on the empty table from his left to his right: *doorknob, faucet handle and electric plug* in this order. Leave at least six inches of space between objects.

Say: *"See all these things? Do you know what this is?"* Hold up the *doorknob* for his inspection, let him manipulate it until he names it or points to the door. Return the doorknob to its original place and show the *faucet handle* next in the same way until the child indicates that he knows what the object is. Nonspeaking children will be able to indicate by mimicry of hand-washing. Return the faucet handle and show the *electric plug* in the same way. Non speaking children may indicate a wall socket or look meaningfully at the ceiling light. Return the plug to its original position on the table. Then place the following objects next to each other before the child, with only an inch of space between objects, from his left to his right in this order: *sink stopper, bulb, key.* Move the first three objects far enough back to stand out but close enough to the child to be within reach. (Fig. 1.)

Say: *"Look at the other things I gave you."* Let him study them for a few moments. Then say: *"With which of these things* (pointing out the first three objects) *does this one go?"* Hold up the *sink stopper* and let him handle it if he wishes. If he hesitates, say: *"Which one do we use it with?"* and again indicate the three objects placed first *(doorknob, faucet handle, electric plug).* If he correctly indicates the faucet handle or places the sink stopper with it, praise him, then return the sink stopper to the three objects directly before him in its original position. If he has removed the faucet handle while responding, return it to its original position. This is necessary to maintain the demand of the item.

Next hold the *key* up for his inspection. Let him take it if he wishes, and wait a moment to observe whether he spontaneously matches it to the doorknob. If he waits for your direction, say: *"Which one of the things up here does it go with?"* and again indicate the top row of objects. If he places it correctly with the doorknob, repeat as directed earlier, making certain that the six objects are returned to their original position. Repeat the same procedure with the *bulb.* If he does not clearly recognize it as an electric bulb, hold it up toward the ceiling light or a desk lamp and tell him: *"It's a bulb, an electric bulb. Which one do we use it with?"*

Common errors are:

a) Using the wire of the electric plug to push through the ring on the sink stopper.

b) Pairing the bulb with the doorknob, probably matching by form.

c) Trying to screw the key into the opening of the doorknob or of the faucet handle, evidently taking the directions literally and concretely ("go with, put together, use with"). *If the doorknob was selected, this performance is acceptable.*

d) Pairing plug and bulb and saying: "You need both for television." *This is acceptable.*

If the child does not arrive at the correct answer eventually, use modifications, chapter 9.

II-0 — VI and up.

33. FLASHLIGHT AND SPARKLER TOY.

Level (Not to be omitted on any level): 2-0 to 6-0 and up.

Main area:	Other areas:
eye-motion and vision, grossly.	motor awkwardness;
	comprehension;
	fear of dark, of flashlight and other anxieties.

MATERIALS: flashlight, sparkler toy (rotating toy with flint, which produces sparks similar to fireworks).

PROCEDURE: prepare for this item by checking battery and bulb of flashlight; examine windowshades or other means to darken the room.

This item is placed toward the end of the interview precisely for the reason that also demands a very cautious approach: the apprehension of children when faced with unfamiliar procedures.

After the child is used to the examiner, it may be possible with children over three to present this item without the mother being present, but under this age or if the child is an insecure, shy or remote one of any age, *ask the child to call his mother* so that she may watch the interesting toy too. Hand him the *sparkler toy,* without making it work, while his mother is entering the room. Then *demonstrate to* him and the mother how it makes sparks, encourage the child to manipulate it himself and help him to work it a few times. Then say: *"It looks even prettier when the room is dark. Shall we make it dark?" Observe* him carefully for signs of panic. If he feels more comfortable on his mother's lap, he should be seated there for the time being. *If he seems quite confident, ask him to help* you to pull down the window shades; it is wise to *maintain a pleasant conversation* while the room is getting dark and/or to let the child hold your hand if he so wishes.

The preparations can be done leisurely, but presentation of the sparkler toy should not be delayed once the room has been darkened.

With the child standing, sitting or walking and in whatever location he wishes to be, *move the toy slowly in wide circles.* The toy must be held so that the sparks can be seen easily from the child's position. If you start from the front (at least 12 inches from his face), move it to his left side about two feet away from him, continue on downward to about the height of his knees, bring it up on the right side, keeping about a two foot distance and continue on to a point directly above his head. *Do this a few times, observing* his eye-motion; if he stops following the toy, go back to the point where he still spotted it and try to guide his eyes along with the light. Go as slowly as he needs, then try to speed up a little. *Watch* if *he still follows it.* Then *change the direction of the circular motion.* Bring it up vertically in front, about 12 to 24 inches from his face, then continue on up so that he has to bend his head backward to keep it in view. *Observe* whether *he can do so.* (Steady him if he needs it.) Bring it forward again and *observe* if *he follows.*

Then *move it on his eye level,* keeping about 12 inches away from his face, slowly *toward the left* of the child, remaining all the time on his eye level. *Observe very carefully* whether he turns his eyes or his head or stops following and at what point he may stop. *Repeat* the same procedure *toward the other side,* starting from the front again.

After you have made certain that you have observed his eye-motion in all directions, including downward in front of him starting from his eye level, and that you have either seen that he has no restrictions in eye-motion or have found restriction and noted mentally in which direction he seems unable to follow, *switch on the flashlight while still moving the sparkler toy* for another moment.

Immediately *throw the beam of the flashlight on the wall* nearest the child, turning him gently if necessary so that he faces the wall and is about the distance of his arm away from it. While holding the beam there and moving it slowly left and right across an arc of about 24 inches, *put away the sparkler toy* and *pretend* yourself *to catch the reflection* of the flashlight on the wall by patting the wall. If the child does not automatically imitate, or has not initiated this catching game himself, *challenge him to try and see if he can catch it. Stand behind the child and throw the beam of the flashlight over his shoulders.* If he turns around, turn him back to the wall in the spirit of a game and move the beam up a little to "tease" him and back immediately so that you do not lose his interest.

The nonwalking child can be moved so that his chair faces the wall. If he cannot use his hands well enough to "catch" the beam, *observe* his eyes by standing next to him and holding the flashlight with a long reach from in back of him. Encourage him to *"spy"* it.

After the child knows how to "catch" the beam, or to "spy" it, bring it *high up* and *observe* if his eyes follow it, then *low down,* still throwing the beam on the wall, and *observe his eyes.* Always bring it back within his reach rapidly, so that he does not give up playing. Then bring it slowly *from in back of him to his far right* and *watch* if he sees it immediately, slowly, or not at all.

Repeat on the left side, keeping it at his eye level or a little below, until he catches it. *Note very carefully* any *delay* in spotting the beam during this check *of his lateral vision. Repeat* until you have demonstrated any restriction that exists or until you have satisfied yourself that he has no restrictions in eye-motion or in spotting the light in any direction.

While the *room is still dark,* take hold of his *chin* gently and *bring the turned-off flashlight in front of his face,* about 8 to 10 inches away. Say: *"What color eyes do you have, blue or brown?"* and turn on the light for a brief moment. *Try to catch* whatever you can of the pupils of his eyes before he closes them against the brightness of the light. *Observe,* if you can, the rapidity with which they contracted and whether both contracted equally fast. *Note* if they contracted slowly or unequally. With the older child, it is sometimes possible to try out *each eye singly* by holding a hand over the eye for a few moments and then quickly shining the light in it. *Repeat for each eye* until you have had a *chance to observe,* if the child is willing.

The whole item should not take more than two or three minutes. It can be done very quickly once the examiner has practiced the various procedures sufficiently. It should not be prolonged because children tire of it rapidly. The sparkler toy is used first to teach the idea of following the light; since it makes noise, simultaneous auditory and visual stimulation makes the learning process easier. The reason for the repetition with the flashlight is to make sure that *visual stimulus alone* causes the child to demonstrate conclusively *that he can follow with his eyes* in all directions; *spot* a light *laterally* on both sides even though he does not know where to expect it next; and *move his eyes* up and down without restriction. The reason for observing the pupils is to spot *irregularity in contracting* or *slowness of contraction.*

The reasons why such an eye-function check is included in the Educational Evaluation are:

a) young and immature as well as retarded children are generally difficult to test for vision;
b) this informal "flashlight game" is suitable for obtaining a gross evaluation of the child's visual functioning, if the examiner knows what to look for and has practiced before using it with the child;
c) children with cerebral palsy are frequently hard to test for vision, especially those under age three; yet, they may have difficulty in eye-motion or vision which it is important to detect.

Early detection of visual difficulties will facilitate early and appropriate medical attention, with the result that the child can receive the help he needs. The observations made during this item should be described in the Educational Evaluation. If either restriction in eye motion, or irregularity or slowness in contraction of the pupils on the approach of the flashlight after the eyes have become dilated in the dark have been noted, *this is reported. The Educational Evaluation is designed merely to observe the visual functioning.* Diagnosis is not within its scope, nor that of the examiner.

If it is observed during this item that the child has limitations in his ability to move his eyes, this finding must then be taken into account during the rest of the interview. If the child has failed earlier on some task requiring that he raise his eyes or that he scan an arc from one end of the table to the other, and if *it appears reasonable that he failed to see rather than to comprehend,* this new factor must be considered in evaluating his performance. Observation of eye-motion is recommended all during the interview on items affording the examiner this opportunity.

It is self-evident that *no child must be submitted to this item against his wish.* If it is impossible to gentle him into the situation, so that he is willing to go along with the game, it must be postponed.

II-0 — VI and up.

34. PREFERRED EYE.

> *Level (not to be omitted at any level): 2-6 to 6-0 and up.*

Main area:	*Other area:*
probably: dominant eye.	ability to imitate.

MATERIAL: cardboard tube, approximately one and one-half to two inches in diameter, about 12 inches long. Rolled up magazine will serve in an emergency; tighten it with rubber band; flashlight.

PROCEDURE: as soon as the materials of item 33 have been removed and the window shade raised, present the *tube* by using it to peek at the child. Say: *"I can SEE you. Can you see ME?"* Get down to the child's eye-level so that he may peek back at you through the tube if he wishes. If his mother is present, peek at her next and repeat: *"I can see MOTHER."* Continue two or three times, offer his mother a chance and *observe* what he does. *Stay within his reach.*

If he wants to take the tube and use it himself, *offer it to him* as if doing him a favor. *Observe* what he does. If he holds it appropriately over one eye and aims it until he can see his mother or you, play looking back at him through the tube. *Note* which eye he is using.

Then *move opposite to* the eye he is not using (if he is peeking with his right eye, go to his left side) and call him. If he turns to get you into focus, not changing the tube to the other eye, play peeking back at him as directed earlier. Then ask him for the tube and use it for a second or so. When you hand it back to him, make sure you place it in the hand *opposite* to the one he used. *Observe carefully* his use of the tube: does he now use it over the other eye? does he return it to the eye he used earlier? does he try the other eye first and then return the tube to the one he used earlier? *Note* also whether the *preferred eye* is on the same side or opposite to the *preferred hand*.

If the child makes no move to take the tube or to ask for it while you are using it, *offer it to him*. *Observe* as described above how he uses it and try to determine the persistent use of one eye or willingness to use the eye nearest to what he is looking at through the tube.

If the child is motor-handicapped and unable to hold the tube, *hold it conveniently* before his eyes and observe which eye he brings near it. If he is old enough to cooperate, *hold your hand near the farther end of the tube* and tell him to let you know if he can see it. Make it disappear and come back *a few times* until he lets you know whether it is there or not each time. Then *remove the tube* for a moment, *ask the child* if he wants to play some more and *hold the flashlight unlighted* at the other end of the tube before you bring the tube back to the child. *This time hold the tube directly before the eye he did NOT use* the first time. *Observe* his reaction. If he moves to get his other eye (the one used earlier) near the tube intentionally, *ask him* whether he wishes to use it for that eye and, if so, let him. It is not necessary or advisable to switch on the flashlight, unless the child asks for it. It is only used to disguise the change-over attempt to the other eye.

Note especially with the motor-handicapped child whether his preferred eye is on the same side as his preferred hand, or as his better hand if his hands are involved.

If desirable for any particular reason, footedness can be determined as well by letting the child kick a ball a few times and observing which foot he uses more frequently or more skillfully for this.

If a child demonstrates that he is too immature or too retarded to comprehend this item, perhaps by holding the tube over his nose, between his two eyes or by blowing through it, *terminate the task*. Then *hold the tube* yourself, *place the lighted flashlight* near or in the farther end of the tube and *hold it for him*. *Watch* whether this strong bait will motivate him to peek through the tube while you continue to hold it. *If he does, observe* which eye he uses. *Give a few trials,* trying unobtrusively to bring it *near the eye he did not use* at first. *Observe* whether he accepts this and peeks as contentedly as he did with the other eye, or if he tries to bring the eye which he used at first near the open end intentionally. *Observe* also whether eyedness, if demonstrable, coincides with handedness or not.

While the meaning of eyedness is not fully clear at this time, it seems to be *a factor* to be considered when, in a child with motor-awkwardness, the preferred eye and the leading hand are on *opposite sides*.

Children with cerebral palsy similarly need to be evaluated carefully on this item. Since the motor handicap may affect what might have been the leading hand, the child has to adjust to using his other hand for the leading hand. If his preferred eye, IF he shows any preference, should happen to be on the side of the poorer hand, this should be described in the Inventory. If he is so severely involved that he must give his body a half turn in order to bring his hand to the front, the preferred eye may be turned away from the front whenever he tries to use the preferred or better hand.

Some learning difficulties may have their source in a combination of difficulties of this nature.

III-0 — VI and up.

35. ORIENTATION IN TIME: SEASONS.

Level: 4-0 to 6-0 and up.

Main areas:	Other areas:
awareness of changes in seasons and recognition of regular repetition of seasons;	language comprehension; ability to recognize an integrated picture;
ability to take a clue from a pictorial representation and base a conclusion on it;	status of "believes in Santa Claus."
ability to perceive visually black and white illustrations.	

MATERIALS: two black and white illustrations, summer scene (apple tree with two children picking apples) and winter scene (men shoveling snow, house, porch, silo, hedge) (Fig. 13).

PROCEDURE: place *both pictures* in the stand or on the table next to each other. After the child has looked at them for a few moments, say: *"Which one makes you think of wintertime?"* If he hesitates, say: *"Which one tells you that it is wintertime?"* If he is still undecided, say: *"Which one makes you think of Santa Claus and wintertime?" "When does Santa Claus come?"* Do NOT mention the word "snow" at any time until the child has made his decision.

Observe carefully whether the child studies both pictures before responding. If the answer is not entirely conclusive, say: *"Look at this picture and that picture. Which one tells you that it is wintertime?"* If his indicating of the correct picture is done in a questioning manner, or if he points first to the summer scene, then to the winter scene, ask him: *"What do you see in this picture?"*

Common errors are:

a) pointing to both pictures and indicating on inquiry: "I see a Christmas tree (summer scene) and a chimney. Santa comes down the chimney (winter scene)." Further inquiry may reveal that the child believes the apples are decorations for a Christmas tree.

b) pointing to the correct picture but indicating the silo and explaining that Santa comes down here.

The child's response to the further inquiry should demonstrate that he recognizes the snow and *that he connects snow with the idea of wintertime, in order to be evaluated as acceptable.*

See modifications for *children who do not hear or understand language, chapter 9.*

III-6 — VI and up.

36. SPATIAL RELATIONSHIPS. (Same area as item 17.)

b) fitting two halves of a square, after demonstration.

Level: 4-0 and up.

Main areas:	*Other areas:*
orientation in space;	ability to perceive two-dimensional forms;
recognition of a square;	
probably, ability to keep mental image of square in mind until reconstruction.	understanding of the fact that two equal parts or halves make one whole.

MATERIALS: green cardboard square, five inches square, cut diagonally into two triangles. (Material visible in Fig. 18)

PROCEDURE: place the *two pieces of cardboard* next to each other on the empty table, both with the right angle to the left side so that the five inch lengths runs parallel to the long side of the table in front of the child. (See Fig. 18.) Invite the child to watch by saying: *"Look what I can make."* Hold *the piece on the left* of the child (your right) *fixed in its place flat* on the table with one hand and *rotate the other triangle* until the two diagonal sides meet to form a square, bring them together and say: *"See, I made a box."* (If child understands "square," or uses this spontaneously, use *"square,"* instead of "box.") *Return the triangle* which has been moved to its original position and say: *"Your turn. You do it."*

Hold the triangle on the left of the child *fixed in its place flat* on the table with your hand while he manipulates the other piece. If he wishes to pick up both or one of the pieces, just say: *"Fix it like I did,"* but *do not prevent him from* picking it up.

The motor-handicapped child may be able to push the second piece into place with his hand or wrist. Exact alignment of the square is not required as long as the two diagonals meet approximately. *Watch his eyes,* since he will reveal by his reaction to his manipulation and to the result of it his understanding of the task and his recognition of the correct result. If the piece does not come to lie the way he wants to place it, his facial expression will tell you of his awareness of the incompleteness of his effort. *If necessary, steady his arm or hand* while he experiments until he indicates he is finished.

Since both the back and front of each triangle are green, it does not matter if a child should turn a triangle over. The fitting can be done as well.

The child who understands the task and knows the result at which he is to arrive, but is unable to succeed, will express his awareness of failure. Give *as many trials as the child wishes,* until it becomes clear whether he can succeed eventually or not. *For each trial, the two triangles are placed in the original starting position.* It is permissible to *give a demonstration* at each new trial if the child wants it, but if he wishes to figure the task out in his own way, he should be permitted to do so.

The child who does not understand the task or does not succeed in remembering the sample performance will not be self-critical; he may call his result a boat, if he has placed the right angle against the diagonal, and declare himself pleased. *Give another demonstration* and say: *"See, I can make a box. You make a box like that."* Try: *"You put them like that"* if he appears unable to get the verbal designation of the "box" for what, to him, may just be snips of paper.

If a child places the two triangles on top of each other, give another demonstration in case he misunderstood the task. Say: *"Make a BIG thing like I do."* If, after repeated demonstration, he fails to change his efforts and continues to put them on top of each other, he demonstrates that he does not understand the task. *His failure would be on the basis of intellectual non-comprehension and not likely be on the basis of perceptual difficulty.*

Note carefully the performance of the child and *observe* whether he seems to be aware of failure if he either fails completely or fails the first few times. If he *verbalizes his problem,* he may give a *clue to the nature of his difficulty.* If he *can succeed* when you demonstrate the task *while next to him but fails* when you demonstrate while seated *opposite him,* this must be *noted.* He may be *able to learn from an imitation of the motor performance rather than from insight* into the process of constructing the square. *Note* which hand he uses and whether he looks at the material directly or sideways or in any other unorthodox way.

If he succeeds eventually, he can be presented with the next task of this area. If he fails, see chapter 9 for modifications.

A child found to have limitations in eye-motion or the visual field on the flashlight test and who fails on this item need not be presented with the next task until medical advice has been obtained. If a child four and one-half years of age or over fails on this item, his performance on other items of form recognition will need to be reviewed.

IV-6 — VI and up.

c) fitting four quarters of a circle, after demonstration.

Level: 5-0 to 6-6 and up.

Main areas:	*Other areas:*
same as under (b) ; amount concept of four.	possibly, ability to imitate ; ability to understand that four quarters make one whole ; ability to make use of concrete clues to solve the task without clear insight in its spatial properties.

MATERIALS: green cardboard circle, seven inches in diameter, cut into four equal pieces, each radius three and one-half inches long. (Material visible in Fig. 18.)

PROCEDURE: present the *four pieces* by placing them in a straight row, with the curved line to the left and the (straight) radius parallel to the long side of the table in front of the child. (See Fig. 18.) Invite the child to watch you by saying: *"Look what I can make with these."* While the child watches, *place the four pieces into a solid circle* and leave them there for about thirty seconds. Say: *"See, now we made a ball."* Trace the outline of the circumference with your finger while the child watches. Then *return them to their original position,* saying: *"I bet YOU can make a ball, too."*

As the child begins to place the pieces, assist the nonhandicapped as well as the motor-handicapped child *by pressing the pieces he has placed to his satisfaction firmly against the table* so that they will stay in place.

Proceed as before with the motor-handicapped child, watching by his eyes and expression his intent as he pushes the pieces into position. (The material has been found suitable for children with cerebral palsy with almost any degree of involvement due to its good size and its easy movability.)

For a response to be correct, accuracy is not required, but the four radii should roughly face in the correct direction and the curved line must be on the outside of every piece.

The most frequent type of inadequate performance of the child who understands the task but does not quite succeed: three pieces are placed correctly; the last piece is placed so that the one radius (straight line) meets one of the other radii already placed but the piece faces outward away from the circle and the curved line is nearest to the radius of a placed piece, toward which the radius of the incorrectly placed piece should face. *In a child under six,* this seems to be *due to immaturity of normal development* rather than to be a specific perceptual difficulty. It appears to be a delay found in nonhandicapped children of comparable ages as well.

There *may be other factors at work* as well in the construction of a solid circle from four quarters. The item is sometimes done successfully by retarded children with a mental age of around four years and over without any hesitation. Sometimes, but not in every case, the child will finish his performance and say matter-of-factly: "Birthday Cake," or "Pie." This may indicate that, seeing the pieces, as well as the end result, as a familiar, concrete and meaningful object, the child has no problem in reconstructing the form.

The attempt to introduce this clue in making the task more concrete to children who have failed it on the earlier trials has been made, but has not uniformly proved to bring such children any closer to solving the problem.

It is permissable to *give as many trials* as the child wishes and *to demonstrate not only when sitting opposite him but also by working next to him in the same direction he faces,* so that he may benefit from watching the *motor performance* of the examiner. *For each trial the pieces must be placed in a row in the original starting position.*

Observe very carefully the pattern by which the child tries to solve this problem, if he has difficulty. *Note* any comments he may make while working. *Performances which must be evaluated as inadequate need to be noted* so that a description of the child's performance and problem can be made in the Inventory, with suggestions for educational approaches.

Other inadequate performances are:

a) Placement of two pieces to form a half-circle without bringing two such half-circles into correct juxtaposition; both half-circles may face with the curved line in the same direction or the curved lines may face each other, the child being unsuccessful at learning to manipulate the final rotation which would complete the circle. *A demonstration of both his half-circles being* correctly *rotated* without taking them apart, and *letting him see the end-result,* should be made. After he has watched this, the *two half-circles* should be *returned to the position* he left them in, without taking them apart. *If he can learn* to imitate this, *give another trial with the four pieces returned to the original starting position in one row.* Note whether the practice has been successful in helping him to solve the task alone now. *If he succeeded after learning,* this must be described in the Inventory.

b) Piling the four pieces on top of each other may indicate that the child has misunderstood or not listened to the directions. *Return the pieces to their original starting position,* make sure he watches and *demonstrate again,* saying: *"Put them like this."* *Outline the circumference* first with your finger and *then help him to trace it with his finger.* Say: *"Round and around we go,"* while tracing it. Say: *"Now you do it."* *Return the pieces to their original position* and *observe* whether he makes an attempt to place some of the pieces appropriately or whether he again piles them, pushes them aside, or traces a circular line with his finger without further interest in the pieces. *If it becomes quite evident that he fails to understand* what is expected, *his performance must be evaluated as inadequate because of failure to comprehend the task rather than because of failure on the basis of perceptual difficulty.* His performance on this item must be evaluated against his other performances on items having to do with form-recognition and with amount-recognition. This may reveal the basis of failure.

If the child has failed after the various approaches have been given, see modifications, chapter 9.

IV-6 — VI and up.

37. AMOUNT RECOGNITION IN CONFIGURATIONS.

    a) matching.

Level: 5-0 to 6-0 and up.

Main areas:	*Other areas:*
ability to perceive similarities and differences in dot configurations;	ability to select in a multiple choice method;
amount concept;	eye-motion, especially for systematic left-to-right progression or other directions.
visual acuity;	
attention to slight but pertinent details.	

MATERIALS: fourteen white cardboard cards, $3\frac{1}{2}$ x $3\frac{1}{2}$ inches square, with black dots, $\frac{1}{2}$ inch in diameter. Two pairs of cards bear configurations from one dot to seven dots (part of material appears in Fig. 7). Three yellow cardboard cards, bearing configurations of five, six and seven dots, sizes similar, configurations dissimilar to those on the white cards. Wooden stand.

PROCEDURE: shield the stand from the child's view either by turning it toward yourself or by using the cardboard to screen it while you insert the cards. *Insert in an irregular arrangement one set of cards up to the configuration of six,* omitting the configuration of seven and the yellow cards (Fig. 7). Turn the stand toward the child or expose it by removing the screen and permit several moments for the child to look at the material. Observe the eye-motion he uses while scanning the material. *Make sure he can see all the cards* and experiment with the position of the stand until he and you are satisfied that he is able to spot any of the cards inserted.

This is important and must be attended to before the next step. *For a child who* glances habitually out of the corner of one or both eyes, who turns his head away from the material in order to be able to perceive it sideways, and for children with strabismus, adapt the position of the stand until the child can comfortably see the cards. *For a child with cerebral palsy and a diagnosis of ataxia,* hold the stand as far away as is suitable for him and screen the stand from view after *every* selection he makes. This will permit his eyes to rest before you present the next card to be matched.

Then say: *"See these nice cards? They have little dots on them."* Indicate the card with the two dots, point to each dot on this card in turn and say: *"See, here and here, just like two little eyes."* Indicate the card with one dot next, point to it and say: *"This has only one dot on it, hasn't it?"* Indicate the card with three dots and point to each dot in turn, saying: *"And here is one that has this many dots on it."* Indicate with an inclusive gesture all of the cards in the stand and say: *"You have a lot of cards here, don't you? Now we are going to see if you have sharp eyes. I will show you one of my cards and then you look around* (indicating the cards in the stand once more) *until you find one that LOOKS EXACTLY THE SAME. That is the one we will need. You show me. Ready?"* Present, in order, the cards with *two—one—four—three—six—five* dots on them for him to match. Tell him that it is not necessary to take his cards out of the stand. He can look at them and show you in that way, or he may point to them or touch them.

Observe his eyes for eye-motion as they move over the collection in his stand. Encourage him to take another look at the sample card in your hand if he has difficulty in making his selection.

As each card is matched, leave his six cards in the stand and if he should remove any or accidentally have pushed out any, *replace them as before.*

If he has succeeded with the first six, *add* the card bearing the configuration of *seven* in the stand, *not* next to five or next to six. Present *three* once more, then present *seven.* Give a *second trial* with each card, changing the sequence of presentation, *if the child has made errors. No second trial is needed if he has succeeded.*

If he succeeds with cards like two, three, one, six, but *confuses four versus five and four versus six,* remove the cards with six and five dots and *repeat* a presentation of the remaining cards. *If he succeeds, add* the *other cards again* and *repeat a trial* with a presentation of *five,* then *two,* then *six,* then *four.* Give *trials* also with *five* and *three* if he has made errors with these two cards.

If errors persist but the child is still willing to go on, *remove the cards which give him no trouble,* namely, those with configurations of one, two, and probably three dots, and *give a few trials with the higher configurations* only until it becomes clear whether he can match them or not. *If a child asks to hold your sample card so that he can see it better, or if he wants you to hold it next to each card in turn, oblige.*

Note also whether a child who fails appears aware of failure or is unaware of it. It is permissible to hesitate for a moment or to ask: *"Are you quite sure?"* if the child's selection was wrong but his expression or verbalized comment tells that he is not certain of his decision. DO NOT TELL THE CHILD TO COUNT THE DOTS. You are trying to find out his resourcefulness in solving his task and whether he uses matching of form-configuration or amounts to arrive at the solution. If he can select the correct cards after you have at first not accepted his incorrect selection, his previous failure may have been due to inattention to slight details or to a failure to comprehend the significance of such slight differences.

If a child points out cards at random, without apparently studying the dot configurations, *reduce the number of choices* to three and *try again,* then to two and give another trial. *If it becomes clear that he can perceive the configurations* and that in a situation of reduced demand he has no difficulty, try to *increase the number of choices* slowly until the basis of his difficulty is perhaps demonstrated. *Observe* his eyes very carefully and the way they work. Does he compare the sample card with each of his choices or not, and does he look systematically from one side of a row to the other to make his choice or does he look at random until his eyes fall upon a nearly matching card and indicate it without further attempt to check his choice once more with the sample card. *His difficulty might be a combination of inadequate attention to details or failure to realize their significance with an immaturity of effort to organize his attack on a task appropriately;* this may be on the basis of intellectual slowness or possibly of an unwillingness to cooperate in an effort which is as yet too abstract and meaningless to the child. *If his performance remains inadequate it is evaluated as such,* and if the basis of the difficulty becomes evident, a description of it is made in the Inventory.

If a child indicates any card, failing to notice the dot configurations as significant at all, *repeat the original instructions,* call his attention to the nature of the cards, and *try again,* with the *choices reduced in number* as explained above. If he fails again, you may *try turning a few cards around with the blank side toward him* and demonstrate to your own satisfaction that he matches each square card to what to him may appear to be just another such card. His performance will need to be *evaluated in the light of his other performances* on items testing the functional use of vision, amount concepts, and form perception.

See modifications if a child of 5-0 and above demonstrates difficulties disproportionate to the level of his functioning in other areas, *chapter 9.*

VI-0 — and up.

b) finding from memory.

Level: 6-0 and up.

Main areas:	*Other areas:*
same as under(a); also:	same as under(a); also:
ability to recall visual image after	pattern of memorizing for immediate
short exposure;	recall.
attack of work;	
rate of learning.	

MATERIALS: same as 37a. (Part of material appears in Fig. 7.)

PROCEDURE: insert the cards from configuration one to six, with the stand screened from the child's view as directed under (a). Then expose it and encourage the child to look at all of the cards by *indicating every card with your hand, starting with the one on the left upper side as seen by the child and going from left to right in that row (CAUTION:* this means from *your* right to *your* left), *continue on for the second row,* again starting on the left side and going to the right, *repeating in the same way for the last row.* Make certain that he follows your guided direction with his eyes. Repeat a row if you have lost him. Say: *"Look at every one of these cards because I am going to play a new game with you."*

Screen the stand from view with the cardboard. (Do not turn it around, since the child may have tried to memorize the placement of the cards and would experience possible confusion if he attempted to follow your rotation of the stand mentally in order to hold on to his image of the cards.) Hold up for the child's inspection a card from the reserve set that shows the configuration of *two.* Say: *"Take a look. Try to remember what it looks like."* After he has indicated that he is ready, *remove the card* and at the same moment *expose the stand* by taking away the screen. Say: *"Which one did I show you?"*

If necessary, repeat the direction that it is not necessary that he take the card out of the stand, that he may indicate it with his eyes or point to it. Present one after another the cards with *one—four—two—six—three—five —three—four.* Screen the stand from view each time before showing the sample card. *Return any card* he may have removed or which may have been pushed too close to another card *back to its original position.* After the first card with the configuration of two has been presented, try to *present cards for only as long as it takes you to give the verbal directions: "Take a look. Try to remember what it looks like."* If however that *imposes an undue hardship* because the child needs to adjust his physical position, regain his balance or rest his eyes after each trial, leave it exposed until the child indicates that he is ready. *You may ask: "Ready?"* and await his response by sign or sound before you remove the sample card and at the same time expose the stand. (In order not to create a sense of hurrying him, you may await his readiness to look at the card, withholding it until he indicates that he is ready to look. Then try to show it only for the time it takes to repeat the instruction.)

If he can succeed with the cards as they are presented, add the card with the configuration of *seven* and call his attention to the fact that you have added a card. Then present in the same way: *six—five—seven—four.*

Observe his eyes as he makes his selections and *try to gain insight* into his way of arriving at his solutions. *Observe* whether he appears to count the dots, or traces the form with his eyes, or perhaps closes his eyes after taking in the sample card in order to keep the image alive until he needs to find it again. Also *observe* whether he scans the rows from left to right, as you tried to help him learn at the beginning, or looks at the cards at random.

If he fails, try the various approaches outlined for direct matching under (a), such as *reducing the number* of choices, *using lower numbers alone,* then *higher numbers alone,* then *recombining the whole set.*

Since he has succeeded in perceiving the configurations when only direct matching was demanded, this item gives an opportunity to *explore his ability to recall the image from memory.* This may give a clue to his future ability to learn to read as well as to learn arithmetic.

If he has *unusual difficulties and fails* after you have tried the different approaches for finding from memory that were described for finding by direct matching under (a), see *modifications in chapter 9. For deaf children and those who do not understand language, also see modifications in chapter 9.*

The ability to find configurations up to seven from memory can be expected of children whose level of development is under that of six years of age. The material is used here only for children of six and over for the purpose of confirming intactness of functioning, where it exists, and of revealing specific difficulties, if they happen to exist, before the child is exposed to academic instruction.

VI-6 — and up.

c) finding matching amount when configuration and color are different.
Level: 6-9 to 7-0 and up.

Main areas:	Other areas:
ability to abstract above the level of identity;	probably, spatial reconstruction of configuration done mentally;
ability to arrive at a solution by a process of elimination.	ability to count;
	ability to shift from previous mind-set.

MATERIALS: same as 37a. (Part of material appears in Fig. 7.)

PROCEDURE : *with the cards in the stand* as they remained after the conclusion of item 37b, say : *"Now we will play one last game with these cards. This time I am going to show you one like that."* Hold up the *yellow card with the five dots* and say : *"Which one does it go with?"* Allow as much time as the child needs. If he wishes, hold it over each of the seven cards in the stand in turn while he tries to figure it out. If he succeeds, ask : *"How did you know?"* Find out by this inquiry whether he succeeded by chance, by approximation, by counting or by mentally reconstructing the dots. His replies will be :

a) "Because I think so," or, "It just goes," or, "It looks like it, a little," or, "Doesn't it ?"
b) "Because this is a square and here is a square (see Fig. 7), "Because it has more than that one" (indicating the configuration of four).
c) "Five here and five there," or, "They are both five."
d) "Because the dot should be inside," or, "You could put this dot in the middle."

Present in turn the *yellow card with the configuration of six* and of *seven* in the same way. If he *succeeds, no further inquiry is needed. If he fails* to arrive at the solution for a while *but does succeed finally, inquire.* He may have been able to discard a less suitable way to arrive at the solution for a more advanced one.

If he fails, it may be worthwhile to *reduce the number of cards* inserted to just the three highest numbers. Give *another trial with each card.* DO NOT TELL HIM TO COUNT THE DOTS. You are trying to find out how he learns and, if he finally succeeds, are observing the pattern by which he did so.

Describe in the Inventory of Development all the pertinent observations about his way of attacking a task of some degree of complexity.

IV-0 — VI-0 and up.

38.   TACTILE SENSITIVITY.

Level: 4-0 to 6-0 and up.

Main areas:	*Other areas:*
ability to perceive slight differences in texture by touch alone;	ability to cooperate on a task requiring this degree of awareness;
ability to recognize familiar objects by touching their form and texture without seeing them.	ability to give information about this type of personal exploration.

MATERIALS : one zwieback and a wooden block, similar in shape, size and weight, covered with sandpaper. Also : ball, scissors, penny, crayon. (Fig. 19, left corner of table.)

PROCEDURE: prepare for this item by having the four familiar objects *handy but not in sight*, (ball, scissors, penny, crayon) since they are to be recognized by touch without having been seen beforehand. Present the other two pieces of material: *zwieback and sandpaper block. Place them* before the child and *ask him* if he knows what they are. Then *let him feel* each of these two objects and *call his attention to their rough* texture. *Name* them for him: "toast" and "sandpaper block." Then say: *"I want to find out if you can tell WHICH one I put in your hand while you are NOT looking."* While arranging his chair so that he faces away from you, or stepping in back of him, or asking him to stand up and turn around, challenge him on his level to try his best. Some children become apprehensive, perhaps expecting an injection when they are told to look the other way. They can be helped if they are told that they will get one of these two objects in their hand and *"if they are good detectives* (use a television hero if the child is receptive to this), *they cannot be fooled."*

Use the *leading hand first,* hold it in back of the child or under the table out of sight, standing ready to cut off his involuntary attempt to look, and place in his hand the *zwieback,* closing his fingers around it but retaining your hold on his hand to prevent a sudden withdrawal for an instinctive look. Ask: *"What did I put in your hand? Is it the sandpaper block or the toast?"* After he answers, permit him to look at it if he so wishes. Return his hand out of sight and place the *ball* in it. If he does not spontaneously name it or throw it to show that he recognizes it, ask: *"What did I put in this time?"* Next give the *scissors* and repeat as before. Last give him the *sandpaper block* and repeat as before.

If he has succeeded with all objects, *repeat* the same presentation on the *nonleading hand,* starting with the *sandpaper block,* then the *penny,* next *zwieback,* last the *crayon.*

If he has succeeded on every object without error and without looking, it can be assumed that his tactile sensitivity *is probably grossly intact. This observation is described in the Inventory* for the information of the teacher and the therapist.

Intactness of tactile sensitivity should always be determined before a child, especially one with a known or postulated brain defect, is started on such self-care learning as buttoning, lacing and other dressing activities. It is of equal importance to determine his functioning in this area before he is taught to use crayon and pencil.

If he has failed, either in tactile sensitivity or in the recognition of familiar objects by touch alone, use the modifications in chapter 9 (see Fig. 19). *Impairment of* tactile sensitivity in a child *without visible motor handicap* must be called to the attention of the medical specialist.

III-6 — VI-0 and up.

39. RECOGNITION OF SYMBOL AND FORM: BLACK OUTLINE HALF-INCH
     SYMBOLS.

  a) matching.

Level: 4-0 to 6-0 and up.

Main areas:

ability to perceive likeness and difference in outline drawings ½ inch in
diameter;

attention to detail;

vision;

eye-motion.

Other area:

conditioning for the ability to perceive
word-pictures.

MATERIALS: two sets of five cards each, 2 x 2 inches, white cardboard, with
½ inch black outline drawings of circle, square, triangle, cross, and diamond.
(Material visible in Fig. 18.)

PROCEDURE: screen the stand and *insert one set of five cards* at positions
most suitable for the individual child. Place at random, the only consideration is to *avoid placing diamond and triangle next to each other.* Keep the
second set of cards in back of the stand for your use. Expose the stand and
allow a moment for the child to look at the cards. *Observe* his eyes. If he
strains to see or remarks that they are hard to see, adjust the position of
the stand or the placement of the cards. After he indicates that he is ready,
present for his inspection the card of the reserve set with the *cross.* Say:
"Which of yours looks exactly like that?" If he succeeds, present in turn
the *circle, triangle, square, diamond.*

  *If he succeeds with each card without difficulty, present the next Item,
39b. If he succeeds with a few of the symbols but fails* with the triangle,
diamond, and perhaps the square, remove the ones he was able to match and
give a *second trial,* with the *choices reduced to the two or three cards he
failed. Try again,* if he succeeds with at least one of the ones failed earlier,
until it is demonstrated whether or not he can perceive, or understand the
significance of, the difference between the ones he has consistently failed.

  If he again has failed, perhaps with the diamond versus either one of the
other two cards, indicating them interchangeably, *place the cards on the
table before him* and *help him to trace the outline with the index finger* of
his leading hand. Ask him what they look like and help him *to name them,*
either "triangle, square and diamond," or "clown's hat, box, kite." Then
give another trial and *observe* whether he can now succeed or not. If possible,
try to *watch* by what means he attempts to solve the task, whether spontaneously or by tracing the outline in the air or on the table, or by closing
his eyes for a second, probably in an attempt to recall either the name or

the motor-memory of tracing it. If he verbalizes, *observe* his comment closely. If he seems to *count the lines or the corners, give a trial with only the square and the diamond* in the stand and watch his way of solving the task. If he can recall them by using the names you gave them or by any of the devices you are able to *observe* him use, make a note of it for later recording.

If he fails on all five cards, give trials with a reduced number of cards until you can demonstrate to your own satisfaction *that he either can or cannot learn* to match the symbols. *If he begins to succeed when the choices are reduced in number, increase the number slowly* one by one and try to help him hurdle his difficulty by gradual increase of difficulty rather than by an overwhelming demand. (To a child, a choice of five cards with abstract little symbols on them may be overwhelming.)

If he is unable to match any of these cards, try to find out by verbal inquiry what he sees on the cards. If he says or indicates that they are all the same little cards, *show him the circle and tell him that you can see a little ball.* If he still indicates that they are all the same cards with little things on them, *terminate the task.*

IV-6 — VI and up.

b) finding from memory after short exposure.

Level: 4-6 to 6-0 and up.

Main areas:	*Other areas:*
same as in(a) ; also:	eye-motion ;
ability to form a mental image of a perceived symbol and hold it in mind for immediate recall.	pattern of learning ; role of forgetting and of incomplete recall ; role of distractions.

MATERIALS: same as 39a. (Material visible in Fig. 18.)

PROCEDURE: keeping the stand exposed, ask the child to watch what you are doing. *Slowly place each of the five cards* in the stand, at the best angle for his vision but preferably in one row. Encourage him to talk about them and ask a few times: *"What does this one look like?"* and similar things to help him occupy himself with the cards intensively. Then say: *"Now we are going to play one last game with them. We are going to play Hide and Seek. Ready?"* Screen the stand from view, hold up the card with the *circle,* say: *"Take a good look at it. Try to remember what it looks like."* Bring the card as close to his eyes as he wishes and if he wants to hold it, let him or help him until he indicates that he is ready. *Remove the card, count silently to five* and then take away the screen *and expose the stand.* Say: *"Which one was it?"*

If he succeeds in indicating the circle, present in turn the *cross, diamond, square, circle,* and *triangle.* Hold each card you present at the spot he may have indicated as his best way to see it on the first trial, but expose it only for as long as it takes you to say in a normal way of speaking: "Take a good look at it. Remember what it looks like." If he is physically handicapped and takes his time to get ready to watch each time, wait until he indicates that he is ready and expose the cards to him for the same period as for other children.

If he succeeds with every card, go on to the next item.

If he fails with some cards and succeeds with others, check which cards he failed on direct matching. If he failed the same cards there, do not give any more trials with (b) to him. *Go on to item 40a* and give *only the matching* of item 40. OMIT the recall item 40b.

If he succeeded without error on direct matching of item 39a, *but begins to make errors on this item,* 39b, *experiment with reducing the number of choices* and then *slowly increasing the choices one by one,* until it becomes clear whether *his difficulty is an inability to recall the after-image* or whether *he becomes distracted and "thrown off the track"* when he tries to select his choice and *has to examine four DIFFERENT symbols until he comes to the one he is trying to hold in mind.*

Note the working pattern of the child who succeeds either immediately or eventually for *later utilization in the Inventory of Development.*

Give the next item, 40a, only if the child has been able to succeed on 39a, or on both (a) and (b), but do NOT present item 40 to any child who has already had difficulty with 39a.

V-9 — VI and up.

40. NUMBER SYMBOLS AND WORD PICTURES.
   a) matching.

Level: 5-9 to 6 and up.

Main areas:
ability to perceive likeness and difference in unnamed number symbols and word pictures;
reversal tendency;
left-to-right eye sweep.

Other areas:
endurance and stamina;
recall of familiar objects or shapes resembling unfamiliar ones, as a learning device utilized spontaneously;
use of other spontaneous aids for learning.

MATERIALS: two sets of six cards each, 2 x 3 inches, white cardboard, with black manuscript printed words: home—cat—tac—sat—and the number symbols: 2—4. (See Fig. 18; cards shown inserted in stand, with one sample card inserted also.)

PROCEDURE: say: *"This is our last game. This one is a regular school game. Watch what I do."* While the child watches, place in the stand *one set of the cards,* starting on the child's left: *2—sat—home—tac—4—cat.* Allow a few moments for him to look at the cards. Then say: *"Ready?"* If he indicates that he is ready, present the card with *"cat"* on it, *hold it slowly over each card* in the stand, going from his left to his right, until you come to the last card. While still letting your hand remain over the card on the child's right in the stand (which is the card with "cat" on it), say: *"Which one looks exactly the same as this one?"* Then hold *the card over the center of the stand* and wait for his reply. It may be necessary to say: *"Look at all of them until you find one just like the one I am holding. There is no hurry."* If he wants to hold it himself or have a closer look, *oblige* him. Move the stand into the best position for his needs if, for material of this size and difficulty, he must strain to see.

Whether he succeeds or not with this first card, go on and present in this order: *2—home—4—sat—tac—2—cat,* in the same manner. *Remind him* that he need only look at or point to the card; he need not lift it out of the stand.

If he succeeds with all six cards, go on to Item 40b.

If he succeeds with all but "cat," "tac," "sat," *give a trial using only these three cards.* If he eventually can match all of these three correctly, add the card with *"home"* on it and *give one more trial,* now using a *choice of four cards.* Then go on to Item 40b.

If he consistently confuses "tac" and "cat," but does succeed in finding *"sat"* correctly, *ask him to tell you what he sees.* He may only be able to make comparisons between "c" and "s," the initial letters and may not yet have the ability to understand or to appreciate any significance in the sequence in which the letters are arranged. *His responses may show how he sees the word pictures.* He may tell you that two have "airplanes" (the letter *t*) in them and a sort of "moon" (the letter *c*), while the other one only has an airplane and a little "snake" (the letter *s*). Such a response would indicate that while he can see and perceive the details correctly, he sees no need to be particularly accurate about either the sequence of the letters or the direction of his eyesweep. *To explore his way of functioning further,* tell him that you can see that this card has the airplane right at the front while the other one has it at the end (tac—cat). *If he agrees, give another trial* and observe whether he can now succeed with all of the three cards.

If he can succeed after this sort of explanation, his earlier failure can be *evaluated as immaturity rather than a tendency to reversals. If he consistently fails,* especially with these two cards, even after you have discussed it with him as directed, *this should be evaluated and described in the*

Inventory as a possible tendency to reverse. Check his performance with your findings on handedness, preferred eye, turning the handle on the music box, performance in the pellet and bottle item and findings on the item testing tactile sensitivity, eye-motion, left-to-right progression in scanning a row of material and on the items to test orientation in space.

If he succeeds eventually, go on to item 40b. If he persistently confuses these two or three words but *succeeds with the other ones, go on to item 40b. If he has failed* with all cards or all but two of them, *OMIT item 40b.*

VI-6 — and up.

b) finding from memory after short exposure.

Level: 6-6 and up.

Main areas:
intactness of visual perception for letter-like symbols on a very simple level;
intactness of immediate recall of a mental image;
awareness of space and sequence in simple letter-like patterns.

Other areas:
eye-motion and left-to-right progression;
learning pattern.

MATERIALS: same as item 40a.

PROCEDURE: with the cards still in the stand from the preceding task, say: *"And NOW we play it as Hide and Seek once more and that is ALL."* Encourage the child to *look at the cards,* then *screen* the stand from view but *do not turn it away* from the child. Present the card with *4* on it, hold it up for the child's inspection, say: *"Take a good look at it. Try to remember it."* Make the necessary initial adjustments as directed earlier, until the child indicates that he is ready. Then *remove the card, silently count to five,* and expose the stand. Present in this order: *home—sat—4—tac—2—cat.*

Give three trials with any word picture the child fails, alternating it with a number symbol. *It is not necessary to reduce the number of choices* since, at this level, *you are trying to find out* the child's ability to function without consideration of any difficulty he may encounter. *Repeat the reminder* that he need not pick up the cards and have him indicate his choices by pointing or regarding the card fixedly.

Observe his pattern of functioning in the areas significant for this item and *note* any difficulties which may be revealed during his performance.

Only for *children who are, or who function on the level of, above six years and who fail,* use the modifications in chapter 9.

9. Modifications of items and indications for their use

Use the modifications of the standard item when a child fails to respond appropriately to the standard presentation of an item. In chapter 8, which describes the items and gives directions for their presentation, there is a notation at the end of the directions for those items which can be presented in a modified form.

The modifications are marked with letters of the alphabet, starting with a. Each successive letter marks a lowering of the demand; thus, e signifies a modification four steps lower than the demand inherent in the modification of the same item marked a.

Use the modifications to help motivate the child to respond by more closely approaching the level on which he can function; the modifications serve also to enable children who have difficulty in auditory reception, language reception or in comprehending English to understand the request. Modifications which will serve to present the item in question also to deaf, aphasic and non-English speaking children are marked with an asterisk: (*).

At each step, directions are given as to what to do next if the child has succeeded. If he still has failed, use the next lower modification and continue to retreat gradually, step by step, to lower levels of demand until the child begins to function. The level on which he is finally able to succeed or to function must be evaluated as the developmental level which he has achieved in this area.

In some instances where it appears both feasible and desirable to explore deviations in functioning more minutely, the modifications for the area being examined by the standard item will be found to afford the possibility of lateral exploration as well. Uneven functioning and specific obstacles to learning by conventional methods of instruction can thus sometimes be detected. Approaches that may circumvent or accommodate the defect may become obvious by the child's reaction to the various modifications; a description in the report of the performance and the underlying cause will inform and possibly aid the child's teacher.

You need not use the modifications mechanically. Be guided by your observation of the child and by your recognition of the specific kind of motivation he may require. Utilize his spontaneous reactions and responses. If they demonstrate that he can reliably comprehend or recognize whatever is to be recognized or comprehended by the use of the particular item, it may not be necessary to use the described modification to evaluate his level. Should an apparently successful performance require a more conclusive demonstration to confirm the validity of the response, check by using a suitable modification.

Always make a note of when it was necessary to use a modification. Note the level on which the child responded. If it appears indicated, add a pertinent comment about the deviations or apparent deviations in an area if his responses indicate that such may be present.

1. RECOGNITION OF CONCRETE FAMILIAR LIFESIZE OBJECTS, WHEN NAMED.

MATERIALS: same as in standard item (Fig. 3).

OTHERS: doll (Fig. 15).

(a) Reduce the material to two choices and ask for each in turn by name. If the child succeeds, enlarge to three, then to four choices, and ask for each in turn by name. If the child now succeeds, go on to item 2.

(b) Restore four choices, introduce doll and ask for each object in turn in relation to the doll (i.e., "Give me the doll's shoe. The dolly wants her shoe.") If he succeeds, go on to item 2.

(c) Reduce choices to two; ask for each object in turn by name in relation to the doll. If he succeeds, enlarge to three, then to four choices, and repeat. If he succds, go on to item 2.

(*) (d) Restore four choices, retain doll, and use pantomime to request each object in turn in relation to the doll (i.e., indicate the doll's foot by lifting it up, gesture toward all four choices and expect child to help out by giving you the shoe).

(*) If he succeeds, cross-check by using the pictures (Fig. 9) of item 4; in pantomime, ask for each picture in relation to the doll.

(*) If he succeeds, use sound blocks and other sound items (item 14) now.

(e) Reduce to two choices, retain doll and in pantomime request each object in turn in relation to the doll. If he succeeds, enlarge to three, then four choices, and repeat. If he succeeds, try item 2.

(f) Move objects aside and place doll in front of child or on his lap. Place in his hand one of the objects and encourage him to use it in relation to the doll. Use each object in turn in this way. (Assist manually those who need help). If he succeeds, try item 3. Omit item 2.

(g) Leave objects moved aside or remove them from view altogether if they are in the way (as when child flings them to floor or when he has involuntary motions or when he wants to chew them.) Remove doll. Place spoon or comb in child's hand and encourage him to use it, either on himself, the mother or the examiner. If he succeeds, place two objects before him, one that he has just succeeded with and another one. Encourage him to help himself, by pantomime and verbal suggestion. If he succeeds, go on to item 9, using the modifications rather than the standard item. Omit items 2 to 8.

(h) Using only the spoon, approach the child's mouth, using verbal and gestured encouragement. If he succeeds (opens his mouth), check by approaching his foot with the shoe.

If he succeeds, approach his mouth with the cup.

If he succeeds, bring the comb and brush near his head.

If he succeeds (inclines his head expectantly), check by approaching his mouth with the shoe.

If he succeeds (refuses to open his mouth, turns his head away, smiles, pushes the shoe away), double-check with the cup by offering it to his foot, as if to put it on.

If he succeeds (refuses to lift the foot, turns away, looks puzzled, brings his mouth or head nearer to the cup), it may be assumed that he recognizes these familiar objects in direct relationship to himself. Go directly to item 9; use modification. Evaluate his reactions with a consideration of his handicap. Children raised in institutions may not know shoes. Children hampered by braces or physical limitations may not ever have seen the shoe on their foot. Very concrete children will not be able to translate their personal recognition of their own glass or cup to an unfamiliar cup. Bottle-fed children similarly may not recognize a cup.

(i) Remove the child's own shoe while he watches. Make him aware of the fact that he is now stocking-footed by letting him stand on the foot or tickling it. Offer his own or the test shoe to him while he is seated, as if to put it on for him.

If he succeeds (lifts foot, tries to push foot in shoe, even the one with a shoe on), double-check by removing other shoe. (You must first put the first shoe actually back on his foot to make the whole situation completely concrete to him; if you fail to do so, a subsequent failure to comply on his part might be because you have confused him; he cannot comprehend that you are looking for answers and not for his foot. You must put yourself on his level, since he cannot put himself on yours). To the other foot, after that shoe is removed, offer the hair brush or the cup.

If he succeeds (refuses to offer his foot, smiles, turns away, pushes the object away), it is assumed that he recognizes at least one article of personal clothing in very concrete use directly related to his own person. Go on to item 9, using the modifications immediately. Omit items 2 to 8.

(j) If he has failed, go on to item 9, use one of the lower modifications. Omit items 2 to 8 and the standard presentation of item 9.

His response is evaluated as indicating that he is unable to recognize or is unaware of familiar objects and possibly is only vaguely aware of himself.

2. RECOGNITION OF CONCRETE LIFESIZE FAMILIAR OBJECTS,
 WHEN DESCRIBED IN TERMS OF USE.

MATERIALS: same as in standard item (Fig. 3.)

OTHERS: doll.

(a) Reduce the choice to two choices, ask for each in turn by describing it as in the standard presentation. If he succeeds, increase the number of choices and repeat. Indicating each object in turn, ask each time the same question (e.g., "Is this the thing we eat with?") and continue until each object has been asked for by a description of its use, while pointing out each object in turn.

If he succeeds, go on to item 3.

(b) Restore four choices, introduce the doll. Ask for each object in turn by a description of its use but in relation to the doll (e.g., "What do we use to fix the dolly's hair?") until all four choices have been requested. Avoid gestures. If he succeeds, go on to item 3. His performance must be evaluated with the qualification that he can recognize objects when verbally described in terms of use, if the situation is concrete.

(c) Reduce to two choices; retain doll. Ask for each of the two objects in turn by a description of its use in relation to the doll. Avoid gestures. If he succeeds, add a third object and repeat. If he succeeds, add the fourth object and repeat. Exchange the unused objects for the used ones if he has difficulty when the choices are increased, until he has unmistakably selected each one when described verbally in terms of use in relation to the doll. His difficulty may be intellectual limitation or may be related to some difficulty in hearing or in the reception of language symbols. Observe these areas for further clues. If he succeeds, go on to item 3. If he succeeds only partially or with difficulty, try d, the next lower step.

(*) (d) Restore four choices, retain doll. Ask for each choice in turn, in relation to the doll, but combine pantomime or gesturing with the verbal description of the use of the object.

If he succeeds, repeat, but omit any verbalization, using nothing but pantomime.

If he succeeds, cross-check by using the pictures of item 4, relating them to the doll using only pantomime (e.g., gesture to the three pictures in general, then hold up the doll's foot and point to it and indicate that you need one of the pictures to go with her foot). Ask for each in turn by using appropriate pantomime. If he succeeds, use sound blocks and other sound items now (item 14).

(e) Reduce choices to two, retain doll, and using only pantomime, ask in turn for each object, relating it to the doll (same as modification (e) of item 1). If he succeeds, go on to item 3.

No further downward modification is used. Ability to recognize the function of objects nonverbally is tested with the modifications of item 1 and need not be repeated. Item 2 tries to test language comprehension. A further nonverbal modification would be noncontributory. Modification d serves to elucidate whether there is disproportionally higher functioning in nonverbal situations. A successful performance would definitely point to some interference with the reception of language. Continue to keep the whole area of language reception under specific scrutiny as the interview progresses.

4. RECOGNITION OF LIFESIZE FAMILIAR OBJECTS IN IMAGE, WHEN NAMED.

MATERIALS: same as in standard item (Fig. 9).

OTHERS: doll, mirror, objects of item 1, red ring, cookie.

(a) Reduce choices to two and ask verbally for each in turn. Repeat by exchanging used picture for unused one, confining the choice to two each time, until each choice has been asked for. If he succeeds, go on to item 5.

(b) Restore choices to three; introduce doll. Ask for each picture in turn by relating it to the doll (e.g., "Find the comb and hair brush for the dolly.")

If he succeeds, try item 5.

(c) Reduce choices to two, retain doll, and ask for each picture in turn verbally by relating it to the doll. Exchange used picture for unused one and repeat. If he succeeds, you might try item 5. (He will probably demonstrate that he needs modifications for item 5 as well.)

(*) (d) Restore choices to three, retain doll. Using pantomime ask for each in turn by relating them to the doll (e.g., mimic feeding the doll with your fingers, gesture questioningly to the three pictures and expect the child to help you). If he succeeds, repeat once more in verbal presentation related to doll. He may only gradually have realized that this is make-believe and may now be ready to perform.

If he succeeds, go on to item 5.

(*)(e) Reduce choices to two (shoe and hairbrush and comb): remove doll. Using pantomime, ask for comb and brush by pointing to your own hair or the child's hair and gesturing to the two pictures, expecting him to help. It may be useful to place both pictures in his hands and to bring your head close to the child, between the two pictures. (Surprisingly frequently, the immediacy of the situation helps the child to catch on and his performance will demonstrate whether he can differentiate and recognize the pictures.) Ask for the shoe by holding both pictures near the child's foot as if trying to put the shoe on his foot. Say: "Put your foot in the shoe." He should try to bring his foot over the picture of the shoe.

If he succeeds, add the spoon, reverse the former position of the pictures; using pantomime, ask for the spoon by gesturing to your or his mouth, making lip-motions as if eating.

If he succeeds, go on to item 5, but do not insist if he fails with the first two pictures presented in the standard mode of presentation. Instead, go on to item 7. Omit item 6.

(*) (f) Remove the pictures. Place the mirror before the child. If he demonstrates that he sees a face in the mirror, bring the actual shoe or the cup (of item 1) behind him and let the image of the object appear in the mirror next to his face. Hold it somewhere in back of his peripheral visual field so that he is not forewarned by the motion of your hand. If he fails to spot the image of the object, move it slowly up and down and sideways to attract his attention. If he shifts his eyes toward the mirror image of it, move it slowly to determine whether he conclusively sees it in the mirror. If he turns around and looks for the actual object, he demonstrates that he can reliably recognize the mirror image of an object. If the performance was not conclusive, check with another object, until it is possible to observe the validity or invalidity of the response.

If he succeeds, go on to item 9, omit items 5 to 8.

(*) (g) Remove the mirror; dangle the red ring on a string before the child's eyes, 6 to 10 inches distant; move it sideways and up and down to make him follow it with his eyes. If he is disinterested in the ring, show him a cookie (round), and make him follow it with his eyes. Then place the mirror in front of the child and after he has focused upon the image of his own face, hold that one of the two objects (red ring or cookie) which aroused the most interest in him so that the mirror image of it appears near his face in the mirror, as described in f. If he does not spot it immediately, move it around until he does. Observe whether he follows it with his eyes in the mirror or turns to the actual object in your hand or looks in back of the mirror. If he succeeds, his performance is evaluated as being on a level where he can recognize the mirror image of an object when highly motivated but does not yet habitually seem to recognize or see the mirror image of familiar objects. Go on to the modifications for item 9 to explore his form perception next. Omit items 5 to 8 and item 9 in the standard form.

(*)(h) With the child facing the mirror, whether he seems to perceive the mirror image or not, ask his mother to step silently in back of him so that her face appears in the mirror near his own; warn her not to call to him or wave her hand in the mirror for the time being. (If the mother or father are not present, the examiner must use his own face.) Observe whether the child focuses upon the face of the adult, smiles at it, or turns around to see the real face, or fails to do any of these actions which would indicate that he can perceive the mirror image of a familiar face. If he does not seem to spot it, wave your hand, move your head up and down, and smile, but silently, or have the parent perform all these motions intended to arouse the child's attention and help him spot the image.

If he succeeds, his performance is evaluated as being able to perceive (and perhaps recognize) a familiar face in the mirror image, but not yet the mirror image of a familiar object, even when motivated. Go on to the modifications for item 9 and start at one of the lower levels. Omit items 5 to 8 and item 9 in the standard form.

(i) Read the modifications of item 30 and decide whether the mask should be used now or later. If later, try modifications of item 9 next. Start on the lowest level. Omit items 5 to 8.

5. RECOGNITION OF LIFESIZE FAMILIAR OBJECTS IN IMAGE, WHEN DESCRIBED IN TERMS OF USE.

MATERIALS: same as in standard item (Fig. 9).

OTHERS: doll.

(a) Reduce choices to two. Ask verbally for each in turn, but avoid naming the object pictured. Instead, ask: "What do we put on the baby's foot?" or: "I see something that goes on your foot. Is it that one or this one?", pointing to each of the two choices in turn; or: "I can see a picture of something that goes on your foot." (The difficulty for concretely thinking children is that, while they may be able to recognize the picture, they cannot easily make the transition from the representation of a shoe in a picture to the real and concrete article which "can be put on." They see the paper on which the picture is printed and cannot see how *it* could be put on their foot. Conversely, some children will be found to hesitate or fail altogether when the picture is only named but will immediately select each picture correctly when it is described in terms of use. This performance may point to a possibility of difficulty or delay in the recall of nouns or of the meaning of nouns, while no similar difficulty may be present in the reception, recall and comprehension of verbs.) If the child has needed modifications for item 4, down to (d) where the use of the object depicted was indicated by gesturing and relating it to the doll, or even lower, to (e) and still has difficulty now, go on to item 7, omitting item 6, and if he fails item 7, go on to item 9 without using the modifications for item 7. He probably is not ready for pictures of any degree of complexity.

If he succeeds in a choice of two, exchange one picture for another that was not used, and repeat until each choice has been asked for. Proceed to item 7.

(b) Restore choices to three; introduce doll. Ask for each picture in turn verbally, relating the request to the doll. (E.g., "I want to fix the dolly's hair. What do I need? Show me.", at the same time indicating the row of pictures and waiting for the child to show you which one you must use. Avoid naming the depicted objects.) If the child says "comb" or "hair-brush," accept the word silently but indicate that you want him to show you which of the three pictures he means. If he succeeds with all three in this mode of presentation, go on to item 7.

(c) Reduce choices to two, retain doll. Ask for each picture in the same way as described in (b). Exchange used picture for unused one and repeat. If he succeeds, try item 7.

(*) (d) Reduce choice to presentation of one single picture, either shoe or brush and comb, retain doll. This time gesture toward the doll and then back to the picture, or you might place the picture in the child's hand. Let him see that you expect him to show you what one does to the doll with the object in the picture, or where, on the doll, one would use the depicted object. He may point to or look at the correct part of the doll (for shoe: foot; for comb and brush: head or hair). Success even with this modification would indicate that he can make the necessary transition described under (a) although not in response to a request using language. His correct performance is evaluated as the ability to use this level of imagery but without having achieved a corresponding level of language comprehension and usage. This ability is expected at two and one-half to three years. A correct performance with one picture should be checked with another picture, also presented singly. (If picture of comb and brush was used on first trial, use picture of shoe now.)

If he succeeds, try item 7.

No further modifications are used. Pantomime and mimicry were used in modification 4 (d) and a repetition here would be noncontributory.

For the child who succeeded on item 4 in the standard presentation but failed item 5 in the standard presentation and in the modifications down to (c), the examiner may wish to try cross-checking item 5 (d) with that of item 4 (d). By this method, it may become clear whether the child was able to get the idea gradually, whether his initial difficulty was in language comprehension or in imagery. The finding is noteworthy and should be recorded; the presentation of succeeding items should be adapted if the level of comprehension of language is lower than the level of imagery. Nonverbal presentation of the higher items (as for deaf children) may reveal the child's true level more accurately.

If he has failed, go on to the modifications for item 9; omit items 6 to 8.

7. Recognition of Action in Image.

MATERIALS: same as in standard item (Fig. 10).

OTHERS: piece of brown or red cloth, 2 or 3 inches square, teaspoon (use spoon of item 1) (see Fig. 16).

(a) Offer both pictures to the child and say playfully: "Kiss the children goodnight." Use any special word the mother might suggest ("beddie-bye," "nightie-night," etc.). Correct response is to direct kiss toward picture of children in bed. Check with second request, if child has succeeded, by pointing to, or helping him to hold, the spoon, and saying: "You feed the children." Correct response is to approach with the spoon the picture of the children seated at table.

The need for concreteness and for an emotional appeal indicates a degree of immaturity, but correct responses indicate conclusively the ability to perceive and comprehend a picture of this level of complexity.

If he succeeded, go on to item 9 or 10, depending on his age and level. Omit item 8.

(b) Present one picture only. Use that of the children in beds first. Say: "What are they doing?" If he succeeds (mimics going to sleep, snores, closes eyes), check with other picture and repeat the question. If he succeeds (mimics eating or feeding), he demonstrates that he can perceive a portrayed scene. He may have difficulty in keeping the request in mind or in making a selection among two choices, or both, on the standard level.

If he succeeded, go on to item 9, omit item 8.

(c) Present one picture only. Ask: "What do you see?" Observe whether he enumerates a few of the details without conceiving the scene as a whole, meaningful, portrayed action. The nonspeakers may point to or indicate some of the details adequately. Coming after failing modification (b), this would also show that details are seen and recognized correctly but there is no concept of the meaning of the scene. A response of this type is sometimes indicative of visual impairment. Keep that area under observation if the child has shown some hesitation or failure on other items which might point to difficulties in vision.

Whether child has succeeded or not on (c), go on to (d) next.

(*) (d) Present both pictures, in stand or flat on the table depending on the child. Place the teaspoon and the piece of cloth between the pictures, as if undecided. Pantomime the action of covering a bed with the cloth, then the action of feeding, moving questioningly from picture to picture and expect the child to show you where to apply each material, or let him hold the materials and push the pictures conveniently close. If he succeeds (covers sleeping children with cloth, feeds children seated at table with spoon), his actions may indicate that he fails to comprehend, hear or hear well enough to respond to the verbal request but that he has no difficulty in perceiving and comprehending the pictures adequately.

A review of his performance on the earlier items to check them against this performance is then indicated. If he has apparently had difficulty in responding to verbal requests on earlier items and has frequently performed more adequately in response to pantomime, check with the use of the sound blocks (item 14) to rule out or confirm a hearing deficit. (Apply sound blocks in pantomime also.) Explore further by use of the modifications for item 14, if necessary. If hearing appears significantly impaired, present the rest of the items for his level, as given for deaf children. Keep in mind that lack of hearing will have proportionally restricted language acquisition.

Consider also the possibility of difficulty in the reception of language symbols in spite of adequate auditory functioning. If child has succeeded, go on to item 9 or 10, depending on his age or level. Omit item 8. Accommodate his difficulty and the result of his difficulty (poor language acquisition), if you suspect such a difficulty, in the presentation of items from here on.

(*)(e) Present one picture only. Offer teaspoon and cloth, pantomime a request to use the materials to help the children in the picture. If child succeeds (applies either spoon to eating children or cloth to sleeping children), check by using the unused picture, also presenting it alone, with both materials. Correct response would show that he is able, or has learned during his exposure to the pictures, to comprehend them adequately when presented singly and with a concrete and nonverbal suggestion.

This would mean that he uses imagery on a two and one-half to three year level, but can do so only in direct relationship to one picture at a time and only in response to a nonverbal suggestion. The areas of language development and of intellectual adequacy must then be observed as the interview progresses. Hearing and receptive language difficulties would likewise warrant close attention.

If he succeeded, go on to item 9 or 10, depending on age and level. Omit item 8.

If he has failed, try item 9, using modifications.

RECOGNITION OF FORM, SHAPE AND SYMBOL (Items 9, 10, 11) (Fig. 18).

Note: The area of the function to perceive, recognize, differentiate and recall forms is given extensive consideration in the Educational Evaluation. In addition to the standard items (items 9, 10, 11, 17, 28, 29, 36, 37a and b, 39a and b, and 40a and b), the test kit contains a hundred-hole peg board and pegs for modified approaches. The user of this manual who has an opportunity to test great numbers of children who may or may not have difficulty in the area of form perception will want to add to his test kit some of the experimentally used materials illustrated in Fig. 18 on the right side of the picture. Children for whom they are useful are those with brain defects, with and without motor involvement, and some retarded children, with or without brain defects. Figure 18 shows most of the items of the standard sequence used in this area and a collection of experimentally used materials as well. Figure 14 shows a formboard which is adapted for use with physically handicapped children with manual involvement. These illustrations may serve as suggestions; and may perhaps motivate other workers to think of further everyday materials which can be utilized to obtain clues to a child's ability to recognize and differentiate form and shape on a concrete level of functioning.

9.   RECOGNITION OF FORM AND SYMBOL IN CUT-OUTS.

MATERIALS: same as in standard item (visible in Fig. 18).

OTHERS: two boxes of the same height and color, preferably white, three to four inches in diameter, one square and one round; doll; several cookies, round and square, of approximately equal size; small toy, such as red ring with string, short string of colored wooden beads, or similar object; penny or pellet will do, if child is old enough.

(a)   Present three cards of the standard item, placed with the circle in the middle. Introduce doll; as you ask for each card in turn, relate each to the doll. Place circle on her lap as suggested in standard item, call it "ball;" hold triangle against her hair, call it "hat;" place square between her hands, call it "book." Return each choice to the former position on the table. Place the sample circle on doll's lap and ask child to give her the other ball, indicating the row in general. Then repeat in similarly playful style with triangle by "putting a hat on the dolly," the child, or the mother, and ask for another hat for that person or doll who is hatless. Repeat with square in similar mode of presentation.

Correct performance is evaluated as the ability to differentiate and match the forms but only when the task is made concrete and related to a doll or person. The difficulty may be in concept formation rather than in perception. The child may be unable to abstract, even on this simple level, the quality of form from the cards unless they can be made meaningful and the form is related to a familiar object within his experience.

If the child has not gotten the idea after this mode of presentation, there is little advantage in trying to repeat the task with a reduction of choices to two. The examiner is free to retreat to that step, however, if he feels that the child might be able to function there. It may be more profitable to conserve the child's energy and present to him, if he fails on (a) the lower step, (b) next. If the child has succeeded, go on to item 12. Omit item 11.

(*) (b) Remove cards and doll; present the two boxes; open each box and show the child the empty inside of each. Making certain that the child watches, place one round cookie (if the mother informs you that he does not like cookies, use a small toy, pellet or penny, depending on child's preference) in the round box, again holding the box so that child can see the inside. Close box. Show child empty square box and close it while he watches. Hide both boxes from view for one minute (under table), during which time you can tell the child that he may eat the cookie if he can find it in the right box when you bring back the boxes. (Motivate the others with a promise that they can play with the surprise in the box.) Use pantomime combined with verbal request in all phases of this task. Bring back the two boxes, place them in reversed positions on the table before the child. Invite him with gestures and words: "Where is the cookie?" Assist him in opening the box he indicates. Prevent him from shaking any of the boxes. If he succeeds (finds correct box at first attempt), give him the cookie and repeat the test, using another round cookie but hiding it in the square box. Proceed exactly as the first time. Be sure child watches, show empty round box, and hide both boxes for one minute. Return them to table, reversing former positions, and ask with gestures and words as before: "Where is the cookie?" If he indicates correct box at first attempt, he shows conclusively that in a concrete situation he can perceive and differentiate between these two shapes. Now indicate with gestures and verbally: "It's your turn. You hide something for me." Place the two boxes, open, next to each other, about five to six inches apart and place the covers in a vertical row between child and the center of the open boxes. Help the child to drop a toy or cookie (his preference) into the round box and wait for him to select the matching cover to close it. If necessary, remind him to hide it so that you won't see it any more. If he succeeds (selects the correct cover for each box), he demonstrates that he can match these two shapes in a concrete task. (It may be necessary to go through the motion of placing the boxes under the table and for the examiner to "find" the one in question; this depends on the child and can be decided by the examiner.)

If he has succeeded, go on to item 12.

(*) (c) Present both boxes, introduce doll. Invite child's attention as before, place toy or cookie in round box, close it, show empty square box, close it, hide both boxes for a few seconds only, return them to the table in reversed position. Use gestures and verbal request simultaneously, but make the appeal more convincing by relating it to the doll: "Find the toy (cookie) for the dolly." Prevent the child from shaking the boxes. Help him to open the box he indicates. If he succeeds (finds correct box at first attempt), repeat in similar fashion with other box. (If a child wants to open the second box when he finds the first one empty, he indicates that he remembers that something was hidden, that he can deduce that if it is not in one box, it must be in the other, but he does not demonstrate an ability to perceive the two forms.) A successful performance on this level would be evaluated as the ability to recognize two shapes in a concrete situation under high motivation.

If he has succeeded, go on to item 12.

(*) (d) Remove boxes and doll. Line up a row of cookies, alternate round and square ones. With gestures and words, invite the child to take a cookie. Note which shape he selects. Unless used to being given square cookies, children usually select round cookies. (If they prefer square ones, the repeated selection of square ones demonstrates ability to perceive and differentiate shapes on this level.)

Either after he eats one cookie or "for his mother" and to "take home with you," let him select a few, always restoring the row to one of alternating forms. Even with the child who does not, or does not yet, comprehend language, this invitation seldom needs any repetition. (If he is the rare child who refuses to accept a cookie, you might place the two contrasting box covers before him. If he spontaneously reaches repeatedly for one of them (usually the round one) exclusively, no matter where you replace it each time in relation to the other cover, he demonstrates on this level the ability of preference on the basis of visual functioning.)

Observation of the child's spontaneous reaction to cookies or boxes of these two shapes affords an opportunity to detect whether form can be perceived by the child on this level. The performance is not on the level of awareness of perceiving differences in form, but rather on that of a preference for the more appealing simple round form. The other form may be ignored rather than rejected.

There is on this level neither success nor failure since the situation is a motivation to react, not a directed task, but the examiner will gain insight into the ability of the child to function, if he shows a form preference. More than half of the children ever presented with this situation showed such a preference. The examiner must remember that other than perceptual functioning may play a role in the child's reaction. He may simply reach for the cookie nearest him at each trial, or for the one nearest his empty hand. This does not necessarily indicate a lower level of intellectual functioning.

Make a note of the child's reactions. Go on to item 12 or a modification of item 12.

10. RECOGNITION OF SYMBOLS AND FORMS. MATCHING.

MATERIALS: same as in standard item (visible in Fig. 18).

OTHERS: materials of item 9; materials of modification of item 9.

(a) Remove cards from stand; place before the child two cards of item 10, circle and triangle, about four inches apart. Give child the second card with a circle and say: "Put this ball with the other ball," indicating simultaneously the two cards placed on table. If he succeeds, remove the top card again, offer child the second triangle and say: "Now put the funny clown's hat (use any name child may have previously used for triangle) with the other clown's hat," and again indicate the two choices on the table. If he succeeds, exchange circle for square. Repeat verbal instruction, avoiding gestures except to point in a general way to the available two choices. Ask for square, calling it anything the child may have named it earlier or just call it a "box," a "block" or even a "square." If the child has been able to perform correctly so far, increase the choices to three. Place the circle in the middle of row and repeat the task once more with each card, verbally, using concrete designations for the cards. A correct performance indicates that the child is able to perceive visually the three forms and to comprehend verbally the directions given when the task is reduced in demand and verbally reformulated to concretize it.

If he succeeds, go on to item 12. Omit item 11.

(b) The presentation of modification (a) when given up to the point before choices are increased to three, serves as modification (b). If a child succeeded on (a) when the choices were two in number but failed when they were increased to three, his performance is evaluated as an ability to perceive the likeness and difference of the symbols printed on the cards and to demonstrate this, acting upon verbal instruction alone. The fact that he can function with such adequacy, but only in a very simplified situation, points to a more generalized lower level of achievement in all spheres; neither a specific difficulty in perception nor a specific difficulty in auditory functioning or language reception should be assumed to be responsible for his performance.

Go on to item 12 or a modification of item 12. Omit item 11.

(*) (c) Increase choices to three cards, placed on the table before the child, with four inches between the cards and the circle in the middle of the row. If child has difficulty in looking down at the table top, adapt the presentation by using a tray with rim or place cards on board or cardboard and tilt to desired angle. Without verbalization, pantomime the sorting of the second set of cards, demonstrate comparing each sample card to the three choices on the table and place sample card on top of matching choice; make sure the child watches. After all three choices have been displayed, with the sample card placed on the corresponding matching one, indicate the finished task to child. Remove sample cards; hand circle to child and invite him nonverbally with gestures to imitate your earlier demonstration. Assist manually those who need it, but leave initiation and decision up to the child. Continue until all choices are placed. Correct sorting is evaluated as an ability to perceive similarity and differences of the symbols visually and to match them in a choice of three. Previous failure to succeed on (a) and (b) would point to some interference in hearing or comprehension of language. If he succeeds, go on to item 11. The child may need a nonverbal demonstration to comprehend item 11. Watch the areas of hearing and language reception.

(*) (d) Reduce choice to two (circle and triangle); place before the child as directed above. Without using verbal instruction, demonstrate matching of the two cards as directed above. Invite child to imitate. If he succeeds, replace the circle with the square and repeat demonstrated task with triangle and square; if he succeeds, add third card and repeat. A correct performance is evaluated as the child having some difficulty initially but being able to sort the three symbols after practice and in a nonverbal presentation with demonstration. The area of auditory functioning should be observed further, but the perfomance may simply indicate that at this time the child does not yet understand language adequately enough to follow verbal directions without demonstrated example.

Go on to item 12. Omit item 11.

(*) (e) Present two cards only; if the circle has been causing no difficulty but the triangle and square have, use the latter two. Help the child to trace with the index finger of his leading hand the outline of each of the symbols printed on the cards. Offer him a sample card (triangle) and help him to trace outline also. If he does not spontaneously want to place it on top of the triangle, demonstrate. Then remove top card, reverse the position of the two cards on table, and invite child to place triangle where it goes. Use verbal instruction combined with gestures. If he succeeds, repeat with square.

A correct performance is evaluated as the ability to learn with practice by combining motor experience with visual perception, while remembering the aspect of each, to match these cards in a choice of two.

If he succeeds, go on to item 12. Omit item 11.

(*) (f) Remove cards; introduce paper and crayon or pencil. Make one vertical line on the side of the paper farthest from the child's leading hand. (If he is right-handed, your line is placed on left side of paper as seen from his point of view. Offer him choice of crayon or pencil. (Most young and most manually involved children prefer, or work better with, crayon. Very concretely thinking children will reach for the examiner's crayon; they may think that the line has to be made, or can only be made, with the same tool; oblige.) Encourage him verbally and by gesture to imitate your line. If he makes a horizontal line, turn paper to blank side and demonstrate again. It might be best to draw the line toward the child (away from examiner) since this is the way it will look more natural to him. Request that he imitate or copy. If he fails, take another paper, move over to child's side of table, draw vertical line from top of paper to bottom and tell him to do the same. Help the manually involved child to close his fingers around the crayon but be guided by his own decision as to where to place and where to start the line.

If he still is unable to do this and draws either horizontal lines or circular ones, hold his hand (even if he is not motor-handicapped) and draw several distinct vertical lines with him. Then encourage him verbally and by gesture to imitate. If he still fails, give him a new paper and let him use his crayon spontaneously. Observe whether he dots the paper, marks it, makes lines in any one direction repeatedly. Save his papers, thank him and go on to the modifications of item 9. If he seems willing, try standard form of item 9 first.

The child who succeeded in imitating a vertical line should be given the horizontal line next. Demonstrate as directed above. Invite child verbally and by gestures to imitate. (Note the one who seems to perseverate and is unable to shift.) If the child succeeds with a horizontal line, give circle next, using demonstration as directed. Use always that side of paper opposite his leading hand. Give as many demonstrations as necessary, and if the child has difficulty, demonstrate a final circle holding his hand in yours.

If the child succeeds with the circle, either immediately or finally, and if he is three years of age or older, or functions on a three year level or above, try a cross next. Make certain that he watches your performance and not only the finished product. You might call the cross an airplane to concretize the task.

Save the child's productions for later perusal. Go on to item 12. Omit item 11.

(g) *An attempt can be made toward the end of the interview to present item 9 to any child who has failed item 10 and the modifications of item 10. If he is found to have difficulties with item 9 in the standard form, retreat to modifications of the item.*

11. RECOGNITION OF SYMBOLS AND FORMS. FINDING FROM MEMORY.

MATERIALS: materials of item 9.

OTHERS: boxes as in modifications of item 9.

(*) (a) Remove the cards of items 10 and 11. Place on the table in a row one set of three cut-out card symbols, with the circle in the center of the row. If the table is a light color, the cards must be placed on a dark board or paper. Make certain the child looks at each card. Tell him and show by pantomime that you will hide the cards and then will let him find one. Cover row with cardboard; make sure the order is not disturbed. Place on the cardboard for the child's inspection the second circle of the set (cut-out card), instruct him verbally and by gesture to look at and remember it. Then remove it, lift the cover to expose the three originally placed cards. Ask verbally and nonverbally which one you just showed him. If he succeeds repeat the procedure until each card has been found from memory in this way. A correct performance would indicate that the child is able to re-visualize or has an after-image reliable enough to find these three symbols among a choice of three when the symbols are represented as distinctly as they are in cut-out forms but not when they all appear on similar square cards.

Review child's earlier performance on item 10. If he was able to succeed on item 10, his difficulty would not be one of possible figure-background confusion. If he has succeeded, go on to item 12.

(*) (b) Reduce the number of choices to two. Repeat the request to find from memory exactly as directed in (a), but keep the choices to two always, exchanging an unused form for a used one until each has been presented.

If the child succeeds, go on to item 12. His difficulty might be on the basis of intellectual inability to cope with three elements of a task simultaneously, while the perceiving of forms may not present any unusual problem to him.

(*) (c) Remove cards. Present the two contrasting boxes. Open both boxes; let the child see that they are empty; place cookie or small toy or object (depending on child's level and preference) in square box, call the child's attention to it, show him once more that one box is empty while the other one is not, then close both boxes while the child watches. Tell him verbally and also in pantomime that if he can remember later which box has the surprise in it, he will "win the game" (or "get the cookie," if he needs this motivation). Place both boxes out of sight but remember their original position on the table. Keep boxes hidden for three minutes.

You might gainfully occupy the intervening time either by giving the child paper and pencil tasks as described in modification (f) of item 10. Or you might present item 17 to him (two halves of a circle) in the meantime. Then return the two boxes to the table, reverse their former positions, and tell the child to find the surprise. Do not permit him to shake the boxes. *(You should make a mental note of his attempt to do this because it demonstrates insight and resourcefulness.)* If he succeeds (indicates correct box at first attempt), go on to item 12.

If his performance did not satisfy you conclusively and might have been a lucky guess, repeat the task, using the round box this time to hide the toy. If this second trial is considered necessary, the intervening time might be used to present item 22 (pellets and bottle). After three minutes, return boxes, reverse their former position, and repeat exactly as directed above. A correct performance would be evaluated as the ability to keep in mind one shape reliably enough to recognize it after time has elapsed, in a concrete and meaningful situation.

If he has succeeded, go on to item 12.

(*) (d) Present two contrasting boxes, open, and let the child hide a toy or cookie in the one he selects for the purpose. Help him to close both boxes. Remember their present positions on the table. Remind him verbally and in pantomine to be sure to remember which one he has used. Hide them for one minute and return them to the table in reversed position. Invite child to find the hidden treasure. A correct performance would be evaluated as the ability to keep in mind one of two contrasting shapes under high motivation and for a limited time only. If he succeeds, go on to item 12 or a modification of item 12.

(*) (e) Remove covers from both boxes and place them out of sight. Elicit child's attention. Turn both boxes bottom up. Place pellet or cookie *under* the square box on the table and hide it while the child watches. Now push both boxes rapidly into several different positions, sliding them to the far end of the table and back, keeping the hidden toy always safely under the square box bottom. Leave the two boxes finally in a vertical line in the center of the table with the square box the farthest away from the child. Invite the child to remember under which box the surprise was hidden and let him indicate his choice. Since it is unlikely that the child has succeeded in following the box in question during all these maneuvers, a correct performance (indicating the correct box at first attempt) would be evaluated as being able, in this playful and highly motivating situation, to keep in mind the shape of one of two contrasting shapes in boxes.

If he has succeeded, go on to item 12 or a modification of item 12.

Auxiliary materials, which have been experimentally used and which the interested examiner will find illustrated in Fig. 18 on the right side of the picture, and which have not figured in the modifications described here, are:

1. *Three small pill boxes, round, square and rectangular.* These can be used in choice of two and then of three. A penny or pellet can be hidden. Or the child can be asked to put the cover on the one in which the examiner places a pellet. Placing the boxes in a horizontal row before the child and the covers in a vertical row between the child and the boxes, he is requested (verbally or nonverbally) to put the cover on the box. This can be repeated with every one of the three boxes. The child's choice of a correct or incorrect cover for any box will demonstrate his ability, or lack of it, to match shapes in this concrete situation. The motor-handicapped child can point out his selection for the examiner, who will follow his directions.

2. *Rectangular boxes (here gray in color) one marked with a square* cut from gold paper and pasted in center of cover, *the other marked similarly with a diamond.* This material can be used for a six or seven year old, especially if he

has failed on other testing instruments to copy a diamond. Hide something in one of the boxes. Hide the boxes for times varying from one to seven minutes, during which time the child may go ahead with other tasks, return the boxes and ask child to find the one containing the surprise. His performance will provide some insight into his ability to perceive the difference between a square and a diamond and into his ability, or lack of it, to keep one of these two contrasting forms in mind.

While the drawing of a diamond requires a sensory-motor development which is on a higher level than that needed to perceive the shape and to be able to differentiate it from a square, even the ability to perceive this difference and to keep in mind a mental image of the shapes gives us some insight into the child's ability to function in the area of perception.

3. *Solid wooden blocks, cubes and triangles, all painted the same color.* These blocks can be used with very immature children or with those in whom an examiner suspects the existence of a real disturbance in perception. Start a tower of two cubes; leave cubes and triangles in front of the child and encourage him to make the tower higher. The child who places a triangular block on top and then persists in placing next either a square or another triangular block shows lack of insight into the property of the block which comes to a point by his persistent effort to force another block on top of it or to balance one somehow on top. The child who develops insight after a while into the fact that somehow the triangular block can rest on the very top but is not useful otherwise in making the tower higher (this is how it is figured by a child) will show by his ability to discard all but one triangular block for his tower his developing ability to perceive the difference in these two shapes. The child who really begins to appreciate the differences between the two differently shaped blocks and the properties of each will eventually make several small towers and top each one with a triangular block.

With some children who function very concretely, these blocks can be used to test their ability to perceive differences in shapes by substituting the blocks for the yellow cut-outs of item 9. The triangular block can be called "hat" and can playfully be placed on the doll's head. The cube can be called chair, and she can be placed upon it to sit down. The child can be asked for another hat or another chair for a second doll or for the doll who has "lost" hers. Asking him to give another while he still can see the one used by the examiner would constitute matching. Requesting him to find another when the first one is out of sight ("lost") constitutes finding from memory.

4. *Cookie cutters.* These concrete objects may be known to a child and he may even have developed a preference for one of the shapes, so that the use of cookie cutters may permit recognition by the child on his own level. They can be used in choices of two, three and four. A cookie can be hidden under one and the task presented as was described with the bottoms of boxes in the modifications for item 11, level (e). If you use this material, insure validity of the child's response by covering the open slits near the handle of the cutters with adhesive tape so the hidden surprise cannot be spied.

5. *Doll cooking pots with lids.* These and others which an examiner will collect eventually are very suitable "warm-up" toys. In addition, the child's ability to select the fitting lid at first attempt will demonstrate his ability to see the matching shapes, while his ability to succeed eventually by trial and error will give insight into his resourcefulness and persistence. A pellet or cookie placed in the pots will make the game more realistic and childlike. Placing the small lid in the oval baking tin and covering it with the oval lid without a further attempt to retrieve the small lid for the round pot and other random utilization of the material is observed in very young, immature, and sometimes in very disturbed children. The latter may simply give up in frustration or indifference, without further attempts to figure out the correct placement of lids.

It is possible to use the cooking pots to test the ability to recall on this very concrete level. Hide something which the child has obviously preferred and which is small enough to fit in either pot while he watches. Push both pots out of reach. Let him retrieve his toy after a brief pause and so demonstrate his ability, or lack of it, to recall in which of two containers you have placed his toy.

6. *Four forms of adapted formboards* (for illustration, see Fig. 14), two round and two square forms, one of each form white and one orange-colored. These forms are made especially suitable by the peg placed on the surface which serves as a handle. By resting the forms on the point of the handle, the round forms can be made to roll, while the square ones will not respond to attempts to roll them. The author has been taught by very low functioning children how to utilize even these qualities of the formboard material. Children who were unable to fit formboards sometimes began to play with the forms. By offering square and round forms simultaneously, with the squareness and roundness presented face-on, not on the table where the rolling motion would give clues to the child, it was sometimes possible to demonstrate that, after practice (such as using square forms in a futile attempt to play rolling them on the table), children might begin to reach selectively for the round forms only and play their game with them. The selection is made purely on an empirical level by the child and he may need practice, if one attempts the same test ten minutes later, in order to "re-learn" his feeble ability to perceive differences in forms. (In free-field observation, such a child may demonstrate something of the same incipient ability to use form perception, when it serves his egocentric purpose, by turning toy cars upside down and turning their wheels.)

12. Discrimination of Colors. Matching.

MATERIALS: three pairs of small socks, red, yellow, blue (Fig. 15) and doll.

(*)(a) Remove color blocks; place before child, about five to six inches apart, one red and one yellow sock. Introduce doll. Proceed with a combination of verbal and pantomimed approach, which will be suitable for either hearing or non-hearing children, as well as for those who do not comprehend verbal directions. On that foot of the doll which is nearest to the displayed red sock, put the second red sock of the pair, with the doll's feet extended in the direction of the child. (Her bare foot should now be directly opposite the yellow sock.) Ask verbally and gesturing toward the two choices in a general way: "Give me the dolly's other sock." Lift up her bare foot and show that she needs one more, then lift up the foot in the red sock to show (but do not name the color) what kind of sock she needs. Expect child to help you dress the doll and to provide you with the correct sock. A correct performance would indicate that in a choice of two and in a concrete situation, the child can discriminate between these two primary colors.

A further exploration in this area utilizes the concrete approach to determine whether *the three primary colors* can be discriminated in a similar way.

(*) (aa) Check the validity of the child's correct response to the request for the red sock by presenting the same two socks (red and yellow) in reversed positions. Saying that the dolly wants her other socks today, put the extra yellow sock on the foot nearest the yellow sock on the table, and proceed as directed above to request yellow. The fact that the child needs to secure the sock farthest away from the bare foot gives the assurance that his reaction is based upon a considered decision and choice. If responses appear too inconclusive to an examiner, perhaps due to the child's involuntary motions or due to other factors, repeated checking is possible. Since, however, to the child the task looks different than to the examiner, the child being intent on helping to dress the doll while the examiner is preoccupied with finding out whether the child can differentiate colors, the examiner should proceed with the child's point of view in mind. This means following through with slipping the second sock on the doll's foot after the child has found it, since an omission of this would look to the child as a rejection of his sincere desire to help dress the doll. Similarly, the use of another color sock has to be put in a reasonable light, since the child may wonder why the adult cannot make up his mind. Devices are: the dolly cries because she does not like the socks that were put on; a second doll, if available, who also needs socks; using one pair as "gloves" because the dolly is cold today.

After red and yellow have been found correctly, add one blue sock to the row on the table. Use the other blue sock on the doll's foot or arm as directed, reverse the position of the three choices, and request verbally and in pantomime the sock that the dolly needs to go with the one she is wearing. If the child succeeds, he demonstrates that in a concrete situation he can match the three primary colors and discriminate the colors in a choice of three. Go on to item 14.

(*) (b) Reduce the choices to two, red and blue only. Repeat task as described above, requesting in two trials the blue and then the red sock in a choice of two. Exchange the red sock for a yellow sock on the table and repeat, until each color has been found from a choice of two. Success is evaluated as the ability to match and differentiate between primary colors but only as long as the choice is limited to two each time and only in a concrete situation. Failure on (aa) is credited to an intellectual inability to cope with three choices at once, rather than to an inability to see colors.

If he has succeeded, go on to item 14.

(*)(c) Remove doll. Take off the child's own shoes and socks on both feet. Show him the red and yellow socks, both of the pairs. If he reaches selectively for one of the colors, use one sock of that pair and put it over his toes. If he did not reach selectively, use the red sock to put on him. Hold up his own foot with this sock on it and admire it, ask his mother to admire it and then point out (or tickle) his other (bare) foot and request verbally and in pantomime the second sock that he needs for his other foot. Make certain that the correct choice is not the one accidently nearest his hand, so that he has to demonstrate his ability to decide among two choices. Correct performance would indicate that he is able to see the difference between these two primary colors in a concrete situation related to himself. (Girls may be a little more capable of success on this task. Underprivileged children of both sexes have been found to be more indifferent to the colors of a pair of socks than children who are usually dressed in matching pairs.) Go on to item 14.

(*)(d) Inquiry into the ability to see and differentiate colors can be carried further by using balls or lollipops of contrasting colors, red and yellow for lollipops, red and blue for balls. A repeated selective choice of one color would provide some information about the child's ability to see and differentiate colors. The mother may be able to volunteer some information about preferences for a color in clothing, hair ribbons, neckties, socks, or balloons. Notation should be made in the recording form of such information if the item did not elicit direct demonstration from the child.

Go on to item 14.

14. Sound Blocks and Related Sound Items. Hearing.

materials: comb, spoon and cup, wooden cubes (from item 12), box of crackers or a similar wrapped box with crackly wrapper. (All material must be kept out of sight before and during initial use.)

(*)(a) Stepping in back of the child, keep his attention focused toward the front. This can be accomplished by verbal instruction to the older child and by more indirect means with the younger or more immature child. The dangling red ring may be used with a younger child since it is a noiseless toy and will probably keep him looking as long as it is moved. Paper and crayon may serve to keep the child occupied without looking back. Produce a noise by stirring the spoon in the tin cup in back of the child's head. Observe his reaction. If he reacts, it may be the familiarity and meaningfulness of the sound which motivated him to listen and react. Make a mental note of his reaction, whether negative or positive.

(*) (b) Still in back of the child, produce a noise by opening the box of crackers directly in back of his head. If he reacts, observe whether his subsequent actions indicate that he not only heard the noise but identified it and therefore must have recognized its similarity to previously heard, familiar sounds. Make a note of the reaction in either case.

(*) (c) Drop a wooden cube to the floor in back of the child. Observe his reaction. If the reaction was slight, place yourself opposite the child so that you can observe his eyes. Without his knowledge, under the table, fling another cube to the floor. See whether his pupils dilate. Make a note of his reaction.

(*) (d) Show him the comb. Let him watch you produce a sound by sliding your finger over the teeth of the comb. Offer the comb to him and observe whether he wants to imitate and whether he shows by any sign that he knows why he is doing this trick. Show by holding your hand to your ear that you are listening.

(*) (e) Remove all materials. Remove the table so that the child is seated opposite you without any separating furniture. Make certain that he watches your face and say soundlessly: "Come to me." If he comes to you or if the motor-handicapped child tries to get up to come to you, say: "Good boy (girl)" in the same inaudible manner but making certain that the child watches your face. If he smiles or tries to repeat (with or without sound) the words you used, let him know that you are pleased with him. Then step in back of him or hold your hand over your mouth and repeat the same words in a loud voice. Watch his reaction. If he reacts when he can see you speak, even if you speak without sound, he may spontaneously have begun to catch some words by lip-reading. This may be because he cannot hear, or cannot hear well, or because spoken word symbols, even though he hears them, are not comprehensible to him. By cross-checking by speaking in a loud voice but in such a way that the lips and mouth cannot be observed, it may become clear whether he is aware that you speak, whether he fails to realize that you are speaking, or whether he responds minimally to spoken language which he either sees or hears with incompleteness and difficulty.

In chapter 7, difficulties in the area of the function of hearing were discussed in greater detail. If a child reveals puzzling behavior on the item using sound blocks, the examiner is referred to the description of the various underlying factors given there.

Observations on hearing made during the interview and especially *during the use of the sound blocks* are an integral part of the report on the child.

Any pertinent, and especially any unexplained and puzzling, findings must be called to the attention of the medical specialist.

A finding of adequate response to familiar meaningful sounds in the absence of adequate response to the sound blocks and other sound items may have several explanations. It is sometimes found in the extremely retarded child, who almost seems to exhibit a conditioned-reflex reaction to a few sounds and noises directly related to his bodily comfort. It is sometimes found in the autistic child, who seems to be selectively inattentive or selectively attentive to sounds and who may be attentive only intermittently even to sounds he sometimes reacts to. Findings of this type should be called to the attention of the neurologist and psychiatrist in charge of the child's care.

19. RECOGNITION OF SIZES IN SMALL OUTLINE CIRCLES.
    GRADING.

MATERIALS: same as in standard item. (Material illustrated in Fig. 8.)
OTHERS: nest of cubes.

(*)(a) Observe whether the reason for the child's failure to grade the circles might possibly be due to his tendency for right-to-left progression rather than the more traditional left-to-right progression in which the circles are demonstrated in the standard presentation. This can be recognized as a possible base for apparent failure if the child *persistently* tries to grade *the correct next larger circle* on the wrong side, to the left of the line-up. If you suspect this reason or have good cause to think that he is trying to solve the task with comprehension but is confused by some obscure difficulty, remove all cards from the stand. Either in the stand or on the table, wherever the material has been presented to him on previous trials, demonstrate the graded row but this time start on the right side with the smallest circle and continue toward the left side so that the largest circle is placed at the extreme left side. In gesturing to the child, go from right to left in order to indicate the graded sizes. Leave the first three cards in place and scramble the others on the table or place them at random in the stand (depending on the child's needs). Now invite the child to try once more. If he succeeds (places the remaining cards in correct order in the row, going from right to left), his performance is evaluated as adequate, with the comment that he has only succeeded when the direction was reversed.

If the child is old enough and appears mature enough to profit from an immediate discussion of his difficulty, an attempt can be made to point out to him why he had trouble at first and to remind him during the remainder of the interview to practice looking at things from left to right. If he is self-conscious, young, immature or otherwise seems not ready to profit from such a discussion, the report must contain a description of his difficulty and performance on this item for the benefit of his teacher or future teacher, who in turn will aid him with retraining methods.

If he has succeeded, go on to item 20. Allow for the same difficulty when you present item 20.

(*)(b) Remove cards; present the nest of cubes; remove the smaller cubes and scatter them upon the table; demonstrate fitting of the nest of cubes, making certain the child watches. Offer him the nest of cubes and conveniently scatter them so that they are not in exact order of sizes. Do *not* explain verbally the principle of fitting the next smaller cube in a larger one, but give a second demonstration if necessary, making it quite clear by your actions that you are comparing sizes in order to learn which one you need to place in the nest of cubes next. The principle of this material is roughly the same encompassed by the graded sizes of circles, but the cube material provides a self-teaching or self-correcting quality by presenting a physical obstacle which alerts the child to his error. If he succeeds with the cubes after failing on item 19 with the circles on cards, it may be worthwhile to call his attention to the fact that with the cards, too, it is a question of looking for the very small difference in size between those which are to follow each other. If he then expresses a wish to try the circles again, he should be given the chance. A successful performance with the card material now would probably mean that he was a little slow in catching on and needed either practice or a concrete example to get the idea, and it would conclusively eliminate the possibility that his earlier failure might have been due to an inability to perceive small differences in sizes.

Go on to item 20.

(*)(c) Consider next the possibility that the visual functioning of the child made it difficult for him to see the material with sufficient accuracy in the position in which it was first presented. Some children may be able to see the pictures and larger symbols clearly enough, but may be less able to judge the small differences in size of the outline circles. Be guided by the child's own readiness to go on with a renewed presentation, either now or toward the end of the interview. Experiment, or let the child experiment, with holding the cards upright, at a slant, flat on the table, or wherever either he believes he can spot the differences or where his performance demonstrates that he can tell the difference better. If such a difficulty exists and the placement of the cards can accommodate it, the child should be permitted another chance. If he succeeds, the performance and adaptation needed should be described in the report. If he has succeeded, go on to item 20. You should consider the consequence of an apparent visual difficulty in the presentation of item 20 and other items of similar demand on visual functioning, and accommodate his needs suitably.

21. RECOGNITION OF SIZES IN SMALL OUTLINE CIRCLES. INSIGHT.

MATERIALS: same as in standard item (Fig. 8).

OTHERS: nest of cubes as in modification of item 19.

(*) (a) The child who fails the standard presentation of item 21 may have the same difficulty with a tendency to right-to-left progression described under modification (a) of item 19. If his performance during his initial attempts to solve the task or his manual tendencies during other observed activities make you suspect such a possibility, remove the inserted cards and present the item once more, but now going from right to left, as directed in modification of item 19, level (a). Gesture now in the right-to-left direction as you indicate to the child what you have inserted and where he is to continue.

If he can now succeed without needing any further repetition of the request, he should be evaluated as having performed adequately. The need to reverse the direction must be described in the report.

Go on to item 22. Review his performance on item 20 and possibly on item 16, both tasks requiring grading and both presented in the conventional left-to-right progression in the standard presentation. If indicated, repeat the items in a way adapted to his needs. Keep in mind his tendency and accommodate it where needed.

(b) Use as the next lower level item 19 in the standard mode of presentation. If the child still has difficulty, retreat further to the various suitable modifications of item 19. This may be postponed to the end of the interview if the child is uncomfortable about having failed. In that case, go on now to item 22.

24. AMOUNT CONCEPT: "ONE ONLY" AND "MORE THAN ONE."

MATERIALS: same as in standard item (Fig. 11).

OTHERS: doll, cup and cubes, drumstick or similar object (pencil), cake tin (desirable but not essential), cookies in box.

(*) (a) By using a verbal request combined with gestures, the modifications try to detour existing or possible difficulties in verbal comprehension. Retain milk bottles, introduce doll. Point to doll, hold up one finger, say: "Give the doll a bottle of milk." Gesture from doll to bottles and back. If necessary, repeat: "Give her a bottle." Sometimes this verbal formulation, which avoids emphasis on the number one, is comprehended, while the request for "one" seems to confuse the child. If he succeeds (gives one bottle only), return the bottle after suitable motions of using it for the doll; hold the doll near you, gesture to both the doll and yourself, hold up two fingers, point back to doll and yourself, gesture toward the bottles and back to the two "people" wanting milk. Say: "Let us have our milk, we need two bottles, for her and for me." Point once more with emphasis to doll and self. Correct performance (giving one bottle each to doll and examiner) would indicate that in a concrete situation, by matching object to person, he can supply up to two people appropriately with one object each ("one only"). The ability to comprehend the verbal symbol "one" for a number may or may not be present.

If he has succeeded, go on to item 28 or 30, depending on the child's age and level.

(b) Remove milk bottle set; present cup and cubes. Demonstrate dropping one cube in the cup, while child watches. Say: "You put one in." If he succeeds, (stops after one cube), praise him, empty the cup, say: "Can you put two blocks in the cup?" If he succeeds (places two or more in the cup), he demonstrates that he has a beginning concept of amounts. The object of this item is to probe the ability to respond in a differentiated way to the request for "one" and for "more than one." If he has succeeded, go on to item 28 or to item 30, depending on the child's age or level.

(*)(c) Remove cup and cubes; bring back doll; present cake tin and drumstick or use a long pencil. Pretend that the doll is holding the drumstick and let her hit the cake tin (or table surface) just once. Say: "Boom" or "Bang" while hitting the cake tin. Offer the cake tin and drumstick to child and invite him to imitate. Say: "You make bang." Aid the manually involved child to grasp the stick but leave the initiative up to him. If he succeeds (hits with stick just once, even if he does not aim at the cake tin), praise him. Take back the drumstick, or use a second one, and let the doll hit the cake tin two times, very distinctly. Say: "GOOD GIRL," emphasizing one beat for each of the words. Invite the child to imitate. Say: "You do it. GOOD BOY (girl)." It may be necessary to demonstrate a few times, repeating each time the two words as well. If he succeeds (hits distinctly more than once, not involuntarily but intentionally) he demonstrates that he is aware of the difference between "just one" and "more than one."

If he has succeeded, go on to item 28 or item 30, depending on child's age and level.

(d) Remove cake tin and drumstick. Present open box of cookies, offer them to the child and say: "Have a cookie." If he succeeds (takes just one), present the box again, hold out your other hand and say: "Give me two cookies." If he succeeds (gives you more than one, even if he does not stop at two), he indicates in this concrete and familiar situation an ability to adapt to a verbal request using number words. If he fails, repeat the request, but this time place the box before him and hold out your two hands to receive the two cookies. This level is parallel to the matching of an object to one person at a time. The two hands provide him with a visible reminder. The material is more familiar than that used in level (a) and the situation is more meaningful to the child. Correct performance demonstrates that he can adapt to a non-numerical mathematical task in an extremely concrete situation to the extent of differentiating between "one only" and "more than one."

If he has succeeded, go on to item 30. Omit items 28 and 29.

The performance of the young and immature child on this item will show his level of awareness of "one" as against "more than one" and his incipient conceptualizing in this area. But it is *the older retarded child* whose performance on this item and the next can provide us with an insight into his potential for useful tasks around the house. The ability to supply in a concrete situation a given number of persons with one object per person, even if no further growth of amount recognition can be anticipated in an older, severely retarded youngster, can be utilized to teach him table setting, meaningful fetching and carrying and other simple routine tasks.

(*)(e) Further inquiry into the ability to be aware of amounts can be made by encouraging the child to play with two objects, such as two spoons, two balls or two drumsticks, then hiding both under a tissue or a towel while he watches, securing the towel with the hand in such a way that only one object at a time is visible to the child as he tries to retrieve them to resume his former game. If he is content with finding just one of them and does not bother to look further, his performance would suggest that he probably has forgotten that he had more than one. His awarness of more than one is probably limited to the brief attention he is able to give to visible, tactily felt, present objects.

A review of his earlier performances and reactions during the interview will result in an accumulation of other pertinent data about his incipient ability to be aware of two and of the twoness of concrete things, such as pot and lid, box and cover, two socks for two feet, father and mother, mother and examiner. If he has inserted pegs in the peg board, he may have revealed an absence or presence of awareness of more than one. The very severely retarded child can insert only one peg unless another peg is placed in his hand to remind him to go on with the task; this difficulty exists in the nonphysically handicapped child as well, even though he has no problem in using his hands except that based upon his intellectual limitation. This helps to explain the lack of self-direction sometimes found in such activities as self-feeding, where a severely retarded youngster in spite of good manual equipment fails to learn a continued activity.

25.   AMOUNT CONCEPT. SEPARATING A STATED NUMBER OF OBJECTS FROM A LARGER GROUP.

MATERIALS: same as in standard item (Fig. 11).

OTHERS: doll, pennies (use some of item 26), drumstick and cake tin, pegboard and pegs, paper and crayon or pencil.

(a) Retain the milk bottle set, table bell and the cardboard on which deliveries are to be made. Go back and order in the manner described in the standard formulation ONE bottle. As child hands you the bottle, pay him with the pennies, placing ONE penny directly in front of the bottle and impressing him with the fact that for ONE bottle you pay him ONE penny. Give back the bottle and order TWO. Whatever amount of bottles he gives you, accept them, but then again emphasize: "I give you TWO pennies because I want TWO bottles of milk." Match pennies to two bottles by placing them directly in front of two of the bottles he gave you and explain that TWO are all you want to buy. If he wants to collect the money or put it in his pocket, help him to do so. Return the bottles, introduce the doll and let her order in the former manner just ONE bottle of milk. After he gives one bottle, let the doll match it as above with one penny. Return the bottle. Let the doll order TWO bottles. Let two pennies be seen and say: "She can only buy two bottles because she has only two pennies." If he succeeds (gives two and terminates the giving conclusively after that), repeat with examiner ordering THREE bottles and paying THREE pennies. Carry it up to four, in the same manner, if the child succeeds with three. Correct performance (giving correct number asked, for at least up to TWO) can be evaluated as the ability to learn in a concrete situation and with visible clues and to correct his own performance in response to such clues.

If he has succeeded, go on to item 28.

(*)(b) Place one bottle before the child, one bottle before the examiner, remove both. Place two bottles before the child and two before the examiner. Remove them. Then place one before the examiner and with gestures and words invite the child to: "Take one. Just like I have." If he succeeds, remove both bottles, let him know that he is doing fine, and place two bottles before yourself. In pantomime and verbally, invite him to imitate. If he succeeds (takes just two), try to repeat the task with three, but do not insist if he refuses or wants to terminate the task. A correct performance (matching up to two bottles) is evaluated as the ability to adapt to a non-numerical mathematical task in a concrete situation up to an amount of two or three, whichever limit the child achieved. Comprehension of the words for numbers may or may not be present.

If he has succeeded, go on to item 28.

(*)(c) Remove pennies, retain bottles, introduce doll. Placing one tissue each before the child and doll as a napkin or similar symbol of table setting, indicate that he is to bring enough bottles to the party or meal for himself and doll. Use pantomime and verbal request combined. If he can stop after giving just two, whether he places them near self and doll or just takes them out of the stand, praise him and try to repeat the task but ask for three, using one more tissue to indicate examiner's place. Correct performance up to at least giving two reliably is evaluated as the ability to supply at least two people conclusively with one object each. Comprehension of the number word may or may not be present. If he has succeeded with at least two, go on to item 28.

(*) (d) Remove bottles, introduce pegs and peg board. Place two pegs in the board, one each at the extreme upper corners, while he watches; call his attention to the pegs, take his hand and touch each of the two pegs with it. Remove the pegs, push the board near him and hand him both pegs. Assist the manually involved child but let the initiative come from him. With pantomime and words request that he imitate the demonstrated placement of pegs. Correct performance (placing the two pegs in the upper corners of the board or in any two extreme corners, such as both lower corners or upper and lower corners of either left or right side of the board, but not random placement even if one peg should happen to be inserted in a corner) would indicate a beginning ability to conceive of a related linking of two, which probably is a forerunner of the ability to have a concept of two.

If he has succeeded, go on to item 30. You might attempt item 28, but he will probably be unable to understand it.

(*) (e) Remove peg board and pegs. Introduce drumsticks and cake tin (table surface will do). Demonstrate one tap with the drumstick, saying "Bang" as you hit the cake tin, then demonstrate two taps, using the child's name if it is a two-syllabic one or *"Good boy* (girl)" if it is not. Give the drumstick to the child and indicate by pantomime and verbally that it is his turn. Observe whether he can spontaneously make a creditable attempt to produce a rhythm. Whether he does or not, demonstrate (using a second drumstick) one single tap, pulling back your hand in an emphatic manner to show the termination of the beat. Encourage him to do the same. After he does, demonstrate two beats, using the above suggested words to indicate the rhythm. Encourage him to imitate. If he succeeds (stops after just two beats), repeat with three and four beats in subsequent trials. Assist the manually involved child but let him direct. It is helpful to use words to go with the rhythm, such as: "Good   big   boy   (girl)" for three beats, "I like mommie" for four beats. Successful performance of either two conclusively terminated beats or three or four, indicates an ability to keep in mind a stated amount of beats, or a rhythm. This means that the child performs in response to a request perceived either auditorially or visually and comprehended as to a limited unit of beats; the size of the unit depends probably not only on his auditory or visual memory but may also reflect musical responsiveness. Observe closely the child who seems unable to stop after two, although his expression or an attempt to nod his head in time with the rhythm indicates clearly that he followed the demonstration. Some children cannot inhibit a repetitive motion, once it is initiated, but must follow the intentional beats with a few unintentional, fainter ones.

If he has succeeded, go on to item 30.

(*) (f) Repeat the task described under (e) but let the nonhandicapped as well as the handicapped child use his hand or foot for hitting the table or tapping the floor. Using his own body sometimes seems to motivate a child who cannot perform as well when using "tools," such as a drumstick.

Further inquiry in this area should include a review of the child's performance on earlier items. When using the table bell of item 23, did he try to hit the bell button with each finger of each hand without needing a reminder? Was he able to select among choices of three and four, which would show some ability to deal with several elements of a situation? If he did any pencil and paper tasks, was he able to imitate a cross, which requires an awareness not only of two related strokes but of two differentiated directions?

If feasible, you might let him use paper and crayon or pencil now. Demonstrate two vertical lines parallel to each other and placed on that side of the paper farthest from his leading hand. Ask him to imitate what you did. Observe whether he makes two lines or less or more. If he made two, demonstrate a cross, let him imitate. Observe whether he succeeds, whether he just makes two lines, or whether he attempts to approach the first line with a second line in a way which shows an awareness that it is in some way to be related to the first line. If he is willing, give a second demonstration by holding his leading hand with yours and drawing the two crossing lines very slowly and emphatically. Observe whether this motor experience serves to improve his own production. Save the papers for later perusal and go on to item 30. A disproportionally adequate performance on imitating a cross in a child who has difficulty with amount concepts as low as two might point to a specific weakness in one or another of the factors which together go to make up the ability to form concepts of amounts.

30. Recognition of Wedgie Doll and Miniature Toys.

MATERIALS: same as in standard item (see Fig. 12).

OTHERS: small three-dimensional doll, doll nursing bottle, two beds (of item 31), mask, mirror, cup, spoon, doll.

(a) Retain the wedgie man, remove horse and car; place the larger of the two beds on table. Say: "Put daddy in his bed." If the response is conclusively correct (man is placed in or across bed), the child is evaluated as being able to recognize the wedgie man in isolation and in a familiar activity. The fact that he accepts the wooden bed is an additional evidence of his ability to accept miniature toys as replicas of real things and people.

His difficulty might have been an inability to cope with three choices and unfamiliar objects all at once.

If he succeeded, go on to item 33.

(*) (b) Remove bed; stand man upright before the child and place spoon and cup near child or hold it conveniently for the manually involved child. Indicate the man and by pantomime, using the spoon, demonstrate how you can feed him; then, returning the spoon to the cup, offer one spoonful to the child and another one to the man. Invite the child to take over. Help with the holding of the spoon but wait for the child to use spoon as he wishes. Gesture to the man as if indicating that he wants to be fed. If the child meaningfully brings the spoon near the man, even if he does not point accurately toward the mouth, nod encouragingly and expect him to repeat it. By his expression it should become clear whether he engages with some degree of conviction in make-believe play or whether he simply apes mechanically a demonstrated, incomprehensible motion. A correct performance would show that with a familiar life-size implement, he is able to learn to engage in a directed imaginary activity. Review in your mind his response to the imaginary telephone in item 24 and evaluate whether or not he can make believe at this time when the adult provides the motivation to do so.

If he has succeeded, go on to item 33.

Incorrect responses include: placing the man in the cup, chewing the man, ignoring the man and occupying himself with the spoon and cup.

(c) Remove man, bring back the bed, and introduce three-dimensional doll and doll nursing bottle. Place the doll in the bed and give the bottle to the child; say: "Give the dolly her bottle." Observe whether he approaches the doll approximately between head and middle with the nipple of the bottle. If he does, thank him, pick up the doll and hold it near his face; say: "Kiss the dolly." If he does, hand him the doll and say: "You put her back to bed." If he succeeds, his responses would indicate that with a three-dimensional doll he can accept the figure as a replica of a real baby (i.e., he can accept a miniature toy appropriately) but cannot accept a more abstract representation, such as a wedgie doll. The additional acceptance of the bed, after it has been demonstrated before, would indicate that he can translate from the real object to a make-believe representation.

If he has succeeded, go on to item 33.

(*d) Present the same material nonverbally by demonstration and pantomime to children who are deaf or who can hear but do not comprehend language or English. Use the same criterion.

(e) Remove doll and man, remove bed and bring back the horse. Observe whether the horse alone will elicit a conclusive response from the child. If not, introduce the three-dimensional doll, say: "The dolly wants to ride on the horsie." If he succeeds (uses the doll to place it on the horse), it might indicate that the familiarity of the one toy helped him to get the idea of the less familiar one (horse). He may be just at the beginning of being able to imagine a little. If he has succeeded, go on to item 33.

(*) (f) Remove toys, bring back car. If the child has not used the car meaningfully during the standard presentation of the item, an attempt should now be made to make the car meaningful and recognizable to him by pushing it and making appropriate sounds for motor and horn. If he now imitates meaningfully, he may have begun to see it as a car (replica in miniature of a real object); only from observation will it be possible to judge whether he can accept a miniature or whether he has obediently but noncomprehendingly aped the examiner's demonstration. If you are not sure, the car can be given back to him after item 33. His subsequent use of it may enable his first response to be judged conclusively. (This is a fairly important observation when testing older retarded children who reportedly have never played with toys, although they recognize concrete cars, horses and people and imitate real activities with real tools. The ability to translate the aspect of concrete things into make-believe and miniature representations of them may be lacking. An explanation of the level and the consequences of the level to the parents sometimes works miracles. A child mistakenly judged to be destructive with his toys and as always wanting to "hang around the mother and get underfoot in her work" may actually only comprehend real things, like the objects his mother handles, while his toys are entirely meaningless to him.)

Go on to item 33.

(g) If the child has only started to exhibit difficulties now and no modifications using the 10 inch doll have been needed on earlier items, an attempt should be made to observe how he reacts to the larger doll. Present the doll and nursing bottle, or if the child is long past his own infancy, give him the spoon and cup instead. Suggest that he feed the doll. If necessary, demonstrate. If he succeeds, go on to item 33.

(h) For the sake of completeness, a suggestion as to how to demonstrate conclusively the ability to recognize the human face will be given; although this inquiry chronologically belongs to a lower level, it is placed here since this item concerns itself with awareness of the body image.

Place the mask ready but keep it out of sight. Either ask the mother or attempt yourself to engage the child in as lively a face-to-face contact of smiling and talking as it is possible to establish. Warn the mother quietly beforehand. Then ask her to hold the mask over her face, while continuing the attempt to hold the child's attention. Observe the child's reaction. A startle reaction or a cessation of the former smiling response should be forthcoming at about four months of age or in a child functioning at this level. The more mature child may simply remove the mask or even play hide and seek with the mother by holding the mask alternately before her face and his own.

Although the author has many misgivings about establishing the child's awareness of the human countenance by such an unchildlike approach, and has substituted a towel to blot out the mother's face in the case of very vulnerable children, the mask has its established value. When children are to be evaluated who give almost no evidence of intellectual or emotional response, the reaction to the mask has the advantage of showing whether there is awareness of the mother or of persons in general. When blindness is suspected but not yet conclusively demonstrated, a reaction to the mask may help to repudiate the suspicion. With schizophrenic and autistic children who appear to live in a world of their own, the use of the mask helps to illustrate the remoteness of the child. He may wander around the room, use materials here and there, glance at his mother's knees or lap once in a while, and never once appear to be aware of a mask placed over her face. When he is placed on her lap, he may stare at the mask and then become inattentive again.

Children who have been raised in institutions or who have been hospitalized for extended periods at younger ages may not react appropriately with a startle reaction unless the mask is used over the face of a favorite attendant or nurse. This may be because they see, and are looked at by, such a multitude of faces that one strange face more or less does not register.

Even if the child has failed and has not reacted to the mask, he should now be presented with item 33.

32. UNDERSTANDING OF RELATIONSHIPS OF PARTS OF A WHOLE.

MATERIALS: same as in standard item (Fig. 1).

OTHERS: small cake of soap, cup.

(a) With the material still in place as in the standard presentation, hold piece of soap visibly between your hands, motion to the three main objects (doorknob, faucet handle, electric plug), and say: "Turn on the water, please. I am trying to wash my hands." If he successfully indicates or pretends to use the faucet handle, thank him and remove the soap. Return to the standard presentation, since this little piece of immediacy may be all he needed to help him get the idea.

(b) Remove the three auxiliary objects (key, electric bulb, sink stopper). Hold the cup toward him and say: "Turn on the water, please. I want a drink." If he succeeds now (indicates or turns the faucet handle), he may have needed a reduction in choices and was confused by six items in the earlier presentation. Replace the faucet handle if it has been moved, remove the cup, and present *individually* each of the other auxiliary objects until he indicates which object is used with which. (To illustrate: hold up the door key and motion toward the three objects on the table; say: "Do you know what this is?" If he says correctly: "Key," nod and say: "Which one of these (indicating the three objects) do we use it with? Which one does it go with?") Continue until each pair has been correctly identified and matched. If he succeeds, his performance is evaluated as the ability to associate related objects even out of a concrete context. He must be able to revisualize the concrete situation of which the parts constitute vital elements in order to be able to perform on this level.

If he has succeeded with all three or at least two out of three, go on to item 33.

(c) Remove all objects. Offer him the key and help him to walk around the room. Say: "What do we do with this?" If he pulls you toward the door, or if the walking child goes to the door and tries to insert the key, use the electric plug next. Offer it to him and say: "You know where this must go, don't you?" If he tries to find a wall socket, or even if he carries it to the electric light switch or desk lamp, use next the faucet handle. Ask him what we use it for. He may mimic washing his hands or make a sound indicating water running in a tub. If he does not respond, place the sink stopper, key and the electric bulb on the table, motion to them in general and, holding up the faucet handle, say: "Which of these do we need when we use that one (faucet handle)?" If he succeeds with two out of three, his performance indicates that he can associate in the visible and concrete environment the related objects of a few very familiar situations. If he has succeeded, go on to item 33. There are no further downward modifications.

(*d) The material can be presented by pantomime to children who do not hear or who hear but do not comprehend language or English. If the child is slow in getting the idea, it may be necessary to demonstrate, using the soap and selecting deliberately and slowly, while the child is certain to see it, the faucet handle; then use both objects in pantomime and again invite the child to go ahead. Lower the choices gradually, as described above, if the child fails in the standard presentation. Use same criteria. Go on to item 33.

35. ORIENTATION IN TIME: SEASONS.

MATERIALS: same as in standard item (Fig. 13 and Fig. 17).

OTHERS: small three-dimensional toy Santa Claus (or picture).

(*a) For children who do not hear or comprehend language or English place both pictures wherever the child can see them best (in the stand or on the table); show the child the toy Santa Claus and indicate that he belongs to one of the pictures. Motion to both pictures, in general, and place the figure between the pictures, as if undecided. Look to the child to help decide where it might best be placed, indicating that you expect him to show you.

Allow a reasonable amount of time for him to peruse both pictures. Help the manually involved child when he gets ready to place the figure. At age four, or when functioning is at a four year level, children are expected to point out the winter scene.

36. SPATIAL RELATIONSHIPS. (b) two halves of a square.

MATERIALS: same as in standard item.

OTHERS: paper, pencil, scissors, crayon.

(*) (a) While child watches, cut two square pieces of paper, approximately 4 or 5 inches square, and mark the borders of each with a fairly strong black crayon line. Pretend to spread butter on the "inside" (the unmarked sides) of each, place them on top of each other, sandwich fashion, and offer the make-believe sandwich to the child with a pantomimed suggestion that he pretend to eat it. Before he can pick it up, pretend that you remembered only now that you did not cut it, place it very visibly on the table (the black border will emphasize the impression of a square), and cut it diagonally in two (from corner to corner), using the scissors. Now place one of the resulting two-layer triangles before the child in the same position in which the standard cardboard triangles were presented originally, pretend a moment's hesitation and then, as if deciding to let him have the whole sandwich, place the other two-layer triangle next to it, also in the standard starting presentation. Motion to him that he can put his sandwich together since he is to have it all for himself anyhow. Assist manually so that the two layers do not confuse him by slipping out of alignment. If he succeeds, his performance would be evaluated as the ability to fit two halves of a square when the task is made meaningful and concrete; the black border (representing the crust of the sandwich) provides a clue to the original shape. Repeat with one more trial of the standard material now, again placing the two cardboard triangles in the same starting position, as directed in the standard presentation. If he can perform correctly now (fitting two halves of a square), it would indicate that practice and insight gained with the help of more concrete material have served to improve his visual recognition and spatial orientation sufficiently for him to succeed. His earlier poor performance has probably been on the basis of inability to perform because the abstractness of the task and material is above his present functional achievement level. Visual perception would be evaluated as adequate, since he can perform adequately when he can relate the task to a meaningful familiar experience. Immaturity or intellectual factors rather than perceptual factors have thus been responsible for his failure on the expected level.

If he has succeeded, go on to item 37.

(*) (b) Move around to the child's side of the table. Present the cardboard triangles of the standard item in the directed starting position. Guide the child's hands through the actual task until the square is fitted. Observe his reaction to learn whether or not he recognizes that this is the completed task. If he expresses or acknowledges his awareness of the correctness of the performance, suggest that he should try it once more. Return the two triangles to their original starting positions and this time let child manipulate the material alone. The child who appears unaware of the completion of the task obviously is not on the level on which he can be expected to perform it adequately. The child who succeeds after these learning approaches can be evaluated as being able to comprehend and perform the task after maximum stimulation; he may require the same favorable conditions for successful performance when presented with the task again at another time. The explanation for a poor performance would lie in the intellectual area and probably not in some perceptual difficulty.

After he has succeeded, go on to item 37.

(*) (c) If the child fails to fit the two triangles even after having been guided through the motions but expresses his recognition of the correctness of the finished performance when the square is fitted by assisted motion, he may have some difficulty in orientation in space. Present the standard material, a piece of paper and a pencil. While the child watches, fit the square on the piece of paper and trace its outline. Make room between the two halves and mark the diagonal line on the paper. Lift off the two triangles and point out the tracing on the paper. Present the two triangles once more, but this time suggest that the child use the outline on the paper. Hold the paper while he tries to place the cardboard shapes. If he succeeds, his performance seems to indicate a real problem in space perception, of which he appears aware and which may require special approaches in his educational program. This must be described in the report so that his teacher will benefit from the evaluation and in turn will be able to help train him. If the child succeeds, go on to item 37.

(*) (d) Only to a child who expresses an awareness of having difficulty and a willingness to find out how he might learn to perform should you present the next modification. Give the child a square piece of paper and take one yourself. Demonstrate folding it once diagnoally. Let him fold his, but if he starts to fold it horizontally, assist him to fold it "like a paper napkin for a party." Then demonstrate several times how to open it up into a square and fold it back into a triangle. Present the cardboard triangles of the standard item, and after fitting them into a square, "fold" one triangle over the other along the diagonal line while the child watches and "unfold" them by placing them next to each other in a square again; repeat several times. Let him try. Then present the two pieces once more in the standard starting position and let the child try once more. If he has difficulty, ask him to figure out which sides must be placed next to each other (longer sides). If he succeeds only now, his difficulty points to a real perceptual difficulty.

After he has completed the task to his satisfaction, go on to item 37. Omit item 36(b).

(*His ability to utilize other faculties* to supply the information by association and reasoning which his perceptual functioning does not give him *may point the way to retraining methods.* The *report on the child* should contain a description of his performance and the means which led to an improvement in it. Memory of details (three corners, length of sides: two the same, one longer), association by relating abstract shapes to familiar objects (triangle and folded napkin), mathematical insight (longer sides from diagonal corners) may play a role in re-enforcing his weak area. Since the child, having had such difficulties from the beginning of his life, may not really be aware of the need for, or possibility of, better functioning, he will need guidance in learning resourceful utilization of other faculties. He may have developed a pattern of taking his difficulties for granted, or he may assume that all people function in the same way. Additionally, the implications of his particular difficulty for his adequacy in other areas, such as self-dressing, tying a bow, learning to write, reading, must be considered.)

36(c). FITTING FOUR QUARTERS OF A CIRCLE.

MATERIALS: same as in standard item.

OTHERS: paper, pencil, crayon, scissors.

Before using any modifications with a child who has been unable to fit the four quarters of the circle correctly after the various approaches suggested in the standard presentation have been tried, you should mentally review his earlier performances on such items as form and symbol recognition (items 10 and 11). Did he have difficulty in finding the correct symbols from memory? Did he need to be given modified approaches? Can he be expected to remember the round form which he is to piece together from the four quarter pieces? If he has a poor memory for forms or for forms of such an abstract character, his failure may be based on this latter factor. If you have found that recall from memory is one of his poorer areas, check back to his performance on the recall of a missing picture (item 6); was he slow in his responses? Did he succeed at all? If his memory is poor for recall of a meaningful picture, it will be poorer for recall of an abstract form.

If you have found that he is unable to follow through on an assignment alone, a quality needed for successfully completing the grading of circles and color shades (items 19 and 20), he may be equally unable to persist with his efforts in fitting the four parts of the circle.

Check particularly his performance on the items testing his concept of amounts (items 25 and 26); at what number did he begin to be unreliable in his responses? If his amount concept is solid only up to three, with spotty successes above three, he may fail the fitting of the circle simply because he cannot intellectually master a task which requires that four parts are to be placed in a prescribed relationship to each other. Did he perform better on the penny matching than when required to count out a given number of milk bottles? Perhaps this means that he depends in his performance more on visual cues than on his verbal or visual memory, abstract reasoning or comprehension. Once the demonstrated circle of the standard item is broken up again, he may be unable to proceed in any organized manner.

From this review you should arrive at a considered opinion of his capacity for successful performance on a task requiring him to place four unfamiliarly shaped pieces together to form a previously demonstrated but no longer present and visible circle, and you must decide whether it is justified to expect him to learn to perform when the task is presented in a modified form.

(*)(a) Using pantomime and verbal communication, help the child to trace with his finger the outline of each quarter circle. They should be placed roughly in a circle, with sufficient space allowed at the radii to show the separation. As you hold his index finger and trace the shapes with him, impress upon him the roundness of the outer side and the squareness of the corners where they meet in the center. Let him experience the straightness of the radii and show him how the pieces meet at the straight line. Then permit him to scramble the circle into four parts himself, without insisting on the original position used in the standard presentation. Encourage him to try again. If he succeeds, his initial difficulty should be evaluated as due to immaturity and inexperience or possibly to a mild intellectual slowness, but probably not as due to a specific perceptual deficit. His performance has to be evaluated in the light of his over-all functioning during the interview.

If he has succeeded, go on to item 37.

(*)(b) Place the four quarters of the circle together while he watches. With the completed round form between you and the child, smile at him and begin to sing or hum: "Happy Birthday to you," encouraging him to join you. At the end of the song, pretend to "blow out the candles on the birthday cake" and invite him to help. (Avoid having the pieces blown out of the circle alignment.) Make an elaborate pretended effort to "cut the cake" along both center lines, leave three-quarters of the circle in place and "offer the child a piece of birthday cake" by pretending to serve him with the fourth quarter. Pretend to take two pieces for yourself and give the child another piece, until the four quarters have been removed from the circle. By pantomime and with words, suggest that the game should be played once more and ask the child to "bake the cake," giving him the four quarters in any kind of position, not insisting on the standard starting placement of the material. If he can succeed when he has been helped to associate the abstract material with a familiar and pleasant concept, his initial difficulty can be evaluated as one of difficulty in abstracting, and he would be described as not fully ready to use constructively learning materials of this simple degree of abstractness.

If he has succeeded, go on to item 37.

(His *need to be guided slowly from the concrete and tangible to the more abstract* should be *described in the report.* This will provide information for his teacher, or future teacher, and permit her to *meet his educational needs* on the level on which he is ready to function adequately.)

(*)(c) While the child watches, trace the round outline of the fitted circle on a piece of paper, move the sections slightly apart and trace the separation lines. Remove the four cardboard quarters of the circle and point out the traced outline of the circle on the paper to the child (as in the similar approach with the triangle). Let him place the four pieces together on this outline. If he should not succeed, it may be worthwhile to use a black crayon to emphasize the tracing on the paper so that it will stand out and provide him with guidelines, and let him try again. If he succeeds now, it may be an indication that his space perception is immature or disturbed, as demonstrated by his particular performance.

If he has succeeded, go on to item 37.

(His *difficulty or suspected difficulty* and the *approaches used* to guide him to a more adequate performance should be described *in the report* for the benefit of his teacher or future teacher.)

(*)(d) If the child is willing to go on with experimental approaches to help him find a way to function in this area and if he is mature enough to cooperate with comprehension, it may be worthwhile to suggest that he should feel the outer round edges of each piece with his hand, tracing them slowly first while the four quarters are fitted into a circle, and with his eyes open, then with his eyes closed; next, that he trace them again when the pieces are separated, first with his eyes open, then with them closed. Suggest, but do not insist, that he might want to try, with his eyes closed, fitting the four quarters into a circle after having learned about the pieces with his fingers. Or, and if he is willing, simply darken the room while he makes the attempt. If he should succeed, let him scramble the pieces himself and try a second time while using his eyes in combination with his hands. Compare the two results. Observe the child's own reaction to a successful performance.

If he can succeed now, or if he can succeed better without seeing how his hands perform the task, it will be necessary to evaluate his performance and his way of functioning very cautiously. Tentatively, he might be thought to have a sensory-motor difficulty. Further study of his functioning in this and other areas related to it would be required to arrive at a clearer picture of his difficulty and his need for retraining or for accommodation in a school program. Some insight may be gained by observing his way of performing on the next items, which probe visual perception but not in combination with a visual-motor act. Continued inadequacy with such material would point more toward a difficulty in perceiving, while adequate performance would suggest that perception might be intact but that visual-motor co-ordination might not be.

37. AMOUNT RECOGNITION IN CONFIGURATIONS. (a) matching.

MATERIALS: same as in standard item (Fig. 7).

(*) (a) Only those children whose difficulties on this item appear disproportionate to their general level of functioning should be presented with modifications of this material. In order to rule out inadequate performance due to a misunderstood or incompletely comprehended concept of the purpose of the task, the cards should be presented once more and the task demonstrated nonverbally. Place only the three pairs of one, two and three dot configurations on the table. Whether the child is motor-handicapped or not, guide his index finger in tapping the dots on each card. If he counts them, let him, but counting should not be suggested as a device to differentiate the cards since it is not only amount concepts but the perception of designs which is under scrutiny. Demonstrate sorting of the six cards in this way: place three cards so that from left to right in one row, separated by about four inches, you display the one dot, then the three dot, then the two dot card. Spread out the three reserve cards and demonstrate how you compare by holding them next to those in the row until you find the one that looks exactly the same. Continue until you have sorted the three cards. Motion toward the three piles and remove the top card of each; spread them out before the child and gesture to him to place each card with the one in the row that is the same. If a child who previously seemed unable to succeed when confronted with making a choice only among three now does begin to function adequately, he may really have failed to comprehend the nature of the task earlier.

If he succeeds now, he should be given a second chance to perform in the standard presentation, or an alternating presentation in the stand and on the table may be experimented with to discover whether some unexplained factor has prevented success before.

If the child fails to comprehend the nature of the task or is unable to succeed because he fails to appreciate the significance of the differences in the dot configurations appearing on the cards, he obviously is not ready for this task and it should be terminated.

(b) Continue modified approaches only with the child who has been found to have an amount concept adequate to his age level (items 25 and 26) but who has experienced difficulties when the cards were presented in the standard form. Present the first six cards at random in the stand. Without attempting to have him match them, discuss with him what he sees; if he has difficult speech, try to find out what he sees by pointing to one eye for the one dot card, indicating a diagonal line in the air for the three dot card, outlining roughly the shape of a square for the four dot card, and similar pantomimed devices. Observe whether he agrees. With both the speaking and the nonspeaking child, now ask for the cards on the basis of the verbal designation agreed upon. To illustrate, you might trace a diagonal line in the air to ask for the three dot card or use the word "house" to ask for the four dot card. If he can succeed with such a device, his initial difficulty is more likely to have been due to the vague and abstract aspect of the cards and their essential similiarity. As they assume more meaning by being associated with known things, he can perceive their different aspects more readily.

If the child has responded in this way, go on to item 38.

(c) Deliberately teach the child to count the dots so that he will be able to select the cards which you want him to match. Increase the number of cards from which to select the one to match each time. If he succeeds, you might try to present item 37(b), but the item will now serve only to probe his amount concept and will no longer be a device to probe visual perception, if such an inquiry should still be desirable.

(d) The child who continues to experience difficulty with the configuration cards after having been given the various opportunities for learning provided by the earlier modifications deserves cautious and concentrated study. It must be demonstrated that his amount concept is adequate and reliable up to at least seven. His vision should be observed, and his performance on earlier pictorial material should be reviewed. If the colored pictures of the earlier items (items 4 and 7) and the black and white pictures (item 35) have been perceived adequately, and if his performance on symbol recognition (items 10 and 11) and his ability to see colors adequately (items 12, 13 and 20) have given no reason to question visual functioning, it may be tentatively considered possible that he has a figure-background disturbance. When the child, in spite of real effort and great willingness, continues to perform unreliably, or, rather, inconsistently, on the configuration cards, whether the request is to match the cards by calling out the number of dots, or by sorting, or by giving their suggested names (e.g., "house" for the four dot card, "peppermint stick" for the three dot card), it must be assumed that he does not reliably see or perceive what we think he should see or perceive. In the evaluating of preschool children the inquiry in this area is extremely difficult. The child may always have had the difficulty and may not know that he perceives differently than everybody else. Visual materials presented to preschool children are usually of a nature and size that allow him to see, and see with comprehension, those materials he is given, and the environment may be unaware of his problem.

If possible, an attempt should be made to learn from the child himself what he thinks is on the cards. He may be able to report that they sometimes look like one thing and then change and look different. Or he may not think that he is looking at the same cards. The seven dot card may look like seven dots at one time and like two windows or a ladder another time; the five dot card may look like five dots now and like a white circle moving around the next time.

When you suspect a difficulty of such subtle nature in a preschool child, the finding should be confirmed by repeated observations, and it should be checked by special tests when the child is mature enough to perform appropriately. His eyes should be checked and the difficulty discussed with a neurologist. In the performance of preschool children, factors like fatigue, uneven effort, and inattention play a greater role than in that of school age children. Therefore, the *report on the finding* should either be postponed or given with due reservations as a tentative suspicion *until later work serves to confirm or eliminate this possibility.* In 17 years of using the material, the author has found only three genuine cases of this type; two were children, one an adult.

37 (b.) finding from memory.

MATERIALS: same as in standard item.

(*) (a) Demonstrate the task after moving over to the child's side of the table and sitting down next to him. Reduce the number of choices to three, placed in the stand at random at the best level for him to see them. Use the cards with one dot, three dots, and four dots only. Screen the stand from your and the child's view. With your other hand, hold up the one dot card and emphasize looking at it. Make certain the child sees what you are doing and invite him in pantomime to look also. Then remove the card and the screen. Pretend to look the choices over carefully until you "spot" the one dot card. Pick up the discarded sample card, hold it next to the other one dot card and indicate to the child that they are the same. Repeat with the four dot card; as you remove the screen to look for it, observe whether the child is beginning to join in the game; draw him into it by tacitly looking for his approval as you pretend to remember which card you are trying to find. When it is found, repeat bringing back the discarded sample card and comparing the two similar cards, for the child's benefit. Suggest that he have a turn, and after screening the stand, hold up the one dot card again, remove it, expose the stand, and look to the child for his response. If he performs correctly, praise him; if he indicates that he, too, wants to compare his choice, oblige once. Repeat with the three dot card, to make sure that the child has understood the purpose of the task, then move back to your side of the table, from where you can observe him better, or remain by his side if he wants you to. Add the other cards one by one; as you insert them, call his attention to the new card and make sure that he studies it before you screen the stand again. After all cards have been found from memory, or after you have satisfied yourself that he has performed to the limit of his ability, go on to item 38.

(b) Insert just the three cards (one dot, three dot, four dot cards) in the stand. If the child fails to find from memory one of these three cards but has been able to match them all adequately when only matching was involved, present the card to be matched next and let him trace with his finger the form of the configuration (a line for three dot card, a square for four dot card) or help him to trace it. Then remove it and expose the stand. If he succeeds, try a few of the cards, six dots, five dots, added to the ones in the stand. Always let him trace the one which he is to find from memory, briefly, before removing it, while the stand is screened from view. If this tactile or motor experience helps him to remember the aspect of a card after it is removed and until he sees a similar one in the stand, he gives a clue to the way in which he can re-enforce his visual perception. If he has found from memory all cards or all the ones he appears ready for, go on to item 38.

(c) Practice with the number of choices the child can cope with at any one time, if he, even with the device of tracing the configurations, begins to fail at finding cards from memory as soon as the number of choices is increased. Exchange unused cards for used ones until all have been tried. His disability must be evaluated as probably being due to a difficulty in visual recall and mild intellectual slowness. These two bases may be related or may exist independently of each other.

(d) Observe the child for any sign that he is aware that the cards have given amounts of dots on them. Give a tacit clue by removing all cards and inserting, while he watches, the one dot card; screen the stand, show him the other one dot card, remove it, expose the stand, and let him "find" it. Add the two dot card next to the one dot one. Call his attention to it. Screen the stand, show the reserve two dot card to be found, remove it, expose the stand, wait for him to find it. Continue in this silent teaching process, placing each higher card next to the lower one, until you have in the stand a row from one to five, each of them having been "found" as they were added. Show the four dot card and observe whether he now can perform correctly. If he succeeds, it is possible that the essential similarity of the cards, all bearing black dots, makes it difficult for him to differentiate one from another unless he can see both of the cards to be matched simultaneously (since he has succeeded in direct matching). When he is forced to remember the particular aspect of the one to be found, rather than having it before him, he may simply lose the image of it. It may be worthwhile to present to him modification (b) of 37(a), where it is suggested that each configuration be supplied with a name, such as "house" for the four dot card. He may have a verbal memory better than his visual one, and may manage to remember more reliably when he can use verbal and visual recall together. Go on to that modification.

(e) The approach described in the modification of item 37(a), level (d) is used to probe a possible figure-background disturbance. Since the child has been able to match the cards in direct matching, this possibility is slight. But it can be argued that a perceptually distorted image may look exactly alike on two matching cards presented at the same moment, while the mental image of one card and the physical presence and aspect of a similar card at different moments of perceiving might look unlike each other to the child. (Go on to modification 37(a), level (d) for further exploration.)

38. TACTILE SENSITIVITY.

MATERIALS: same as in standard item (Fig. 19).

OTHERS: hair brush (item 1), pellets (item 22), music box and table bell (item 23), pegs and peg board, chalk, Scotch tape, ice (if available, for extreme cases), crayon and paper. Auxiliary: child's own shoe and clothing.

Modified material and approaches in the area of tactile sensitivity are used to serve three main purposes: testing the tactile sensitivity of the very young handicapped child, especially if he has, or appears to have, impairment of vision; testing the tactile sensitivity of the child who appears to reveal impairment in this area; and probing laterally for the implications of suspected impairment for other activities.

(*) (a) *To explore tactile sensitivity in the very young child who cannot cooperate consciously,* use the *hairbrush.* Bring the child's palm and fingertips in touch with the bristles of the brush and move the brush back and forth to continue the sensation. Observe the child for his reactions. Reactions that indicate that he perceives the sensation include cessation of other activities for the time his hand is exposed to the bristles; beginning to move his own hand spontaneously over the bristles, returning to this game when the brush is withdrawn for a few seconds and then made to touch his palm and fingertips again; loss of interest and attention when brush is turned around so that wooden back of brush touches his fingertips and a contented grunt or smile when bristles once more contact his fingertips; startle withdrawal of hand each time it is touched with brush, pursing of mouth or getting ready to cry; recall of this "game" after three to five minutes. Somewhat older children will search with their hand if the brush is turned around so that the wooden back touches their hand, and will resume rubbing their fingertips against the bristles after they find them.

Use a piece of *ice* to touch the child's fingertips, cheeks, and chin. The most frequent reaction is a violent withdrawal, sometimes a brief outcry or whining. Less frequent reactions are bringing the mouth to the piece of ice and licking or sucking it, and the child taking the ice in his own hand and waving it around with a frightened half-laugh, half-sigh. Using *Scotch tape,* paste an inch (too big to be swallowed before it can be retrieved by examiner) on the tip of the index finger and observe the child's reactions. He may feel it accidentally when the fingers meet, may try to withdraw from it by pulling his hand back toward his body or may pull it off with the other hand.

These reactions, when present, indicate that a child's ability to receive impressions from and through his fingertips appears to be grossly intact. An absence of such reactions to the stimuli listed points to the possibility of impaired tactile sensitivity, or possibly to extreme immaturity; it is sometimes but not always found in children with extremely severe retardation.

(*)(b) *To explore the tactile sensitivity of a child who appears to have revealed impairment in this area* let the child write or scribble with *chalk* on a blackboard, if available and if he is old enough, or on a piece of dark paper, then observe how he reacts to the feel of chalk dust on his fingertips. Observed reactions that indicate the child feels the chalk dust on his fingertips include wiping his fingers against his clothing, asking for a tissue to wipe his fingers, or commenting on it even though there is no attempt to do something about it. Observed reactions that appear to confirm a lack of tactile sensitivity include a return to other tasks without any attempt to at least rub the fingertips against the palm of hand or against each other; when offered a tissue, holds it uncomprehendingly because he does not feel any need for it; observes with polite interest examiner's own use of tissue to wipe fingertips without becoming aware of a similar sensation that could cause this need.

Review the child's earlier use of the *pellets and bottle* or present them again. Observe whether both hands can pick up the pellets equally well or whether perhaps with one hand the child drops the pellets accidentally, if only one hand has revealed a lack of tactile sensitivity. Does he have trouble picking them up and needs repeated attempts to get hold of them? Does he instinctively look very carefully with his eyes when he tries to pick them up? Does he use the second joint of the finger and thumb rather than the tips? These observations would tend to confirm a possible lack of tactile sensitivity.

Review the child's previous performance with the *music box* or present it once again and observe whether he can grasp the small knob on the winding crank without difficulty. Does he tend to lose his grip on it? Does he alternate his hands? Does he hold the knob with his thumb in opposition to his bent index finger, with the four fingers closed into a fist? Such performances would tend to confirm a possible lack of tactile sensitivity.

The performance with the *table bell,* in which he had to hit the push button, may have revealed that the same difficulty of accurately feeling the button was present. This must not be confused, however, with inaccuracy of directing the finger to the button. This is one of the observations which an examiner learns to judge after seeing the performances of many children with and without cerebral palsy.

If the child has not previously used the peg board and *pegs,* his performance when trying to pick up the match-size pegs will gives clues to any subtle difficulty in this area. Always manage to offer a few pegs to the non-leading hand also, in order to establish whether both hands function in an intact way.

Observe, if you have not observed during the interview so far, his grip on a *crayon or pencil.* Lack of tactile sensitivity may reveal itself in this activity by the child's inability or marked difficulty in controlling the slant on which the crayon meets the paper. Observe his use of crayon for unexpected (and possibly unnoticed), sudden changes in this slant when the child draws or makes lines. His sensation may be comparable to yours if you attempted to write while wearing heavy gloves or when your hands were numb from cold.

Observations which help to confirm lack of tactile sensitivity as apparently revealed during the standard item (38) or, in the case of children too young or immature to be presented with the standard material, as observed in their use of the above listed materials, must be described in the report. As explained in chapter 7, such findings are of value to the teacher and the therapist. In the case of children who are not obviously motor-handicapped and in whom a diagnosis of cerebral defects may or may not have been made, findings in this area must be brought to the attention of the medical specialist who is responsible for their care.

(*) (c) *The implications of suspected impairment in this area for routine self-help and for classroom activities* can be probed by making such observations as those described above in relation to the use of a *crayon or pencil.* The child and his teacher will need to be alerted to the child's problem. The teacher can train him to substitute with his eyes for the missing clues other children receive from their fingertips, until he develops a conscious pattern of making sure that his writing utensils remain under the combined control of his hand and eyes.

During the interview the examiner should further observe whether the child can unbutton *larger and smaller buttons;* lace a *shoelace* through eyelets while holding the lace by the tip; *make a bow* if he is functioning on or above a seven year level; use a *key* in an actual keyhole; pick up *pennies.*

These observations and the child's ways of functioning are described in the report. If the child is sensible enough to profit from it, the difficulty can be discussed with him by the examiner, who can suggest the above-mentioned aid of using visual clues to supplement his sense of touch. Frequently, a child's unhappy and self-debasing attitude about what he feels is his stupidity and clumsiness can be relieved by an appropriate explanation.

Adaptations in the child's clothing can be suggested to the mother if the difficulty is severe. Zippers can replace small buttons; large coat buttons can replace rows of tiny ones; shoes with buckles can replace shoes with laces; ready-made neckties can replace those tied by hand. If he learns to use Scotch tape to avoid having to cope with string (as in wrapping packages) and other sensible adaptations, the difficulty which he experiences can be reduced to a necessary minimum.

(d) The child who has been discovered to have *difficulty in naming objects placed unseen in his hands* must be studied further. Here, two possibilities must be considered, that of impaired recognition by touch alone and that of an inability or difficulty in recalling the correct name for the object, which may have been correctly recognized.

Systematic inquiry will frequently serve to rule out one or the other underlying cause. Try first to probe the area of language as it might have affected his performance. When he tried to feel the scissors with his hand, did he fumble for the correct word? Repeat the test by inserting in his hand, unseen, a series of other objects taken from the various test items, such as spoon, comb, key, faucet handle, shoe. Observe whether he continues to have difficulty or whether the apparent difficulty may have been due to his unfamiliarity with this kind of request.

If there is no or very little delay in naming a new series of familiar objects at a second trial, the child may demonstrate that both his ability to recognize by touch and to connect name and object adequately are intact, but that he may be a little delayed in adapting readily and alertly to unfamiliar demands. A different problem is revealed if he can immediately mimic the function of the object when he feels it in his hand (mimics eating when given the spoon to feel; mimics fixing his hair when given the comb) but brings out the wrong word or delays in naming the object verbally. At first glance, this suggests that he is unsure of the object placed in his hand, but on closer inspection, the difficulty is found to be in the language area. The kind of response may vary; some objects may be named readily, while others are given nearly correct names, such as "door" instead of "key," or "foot" instead of "shoe ;" at other times, the name of the last object may be repeated without the child noticing the error. The correct use of appropriate mimicry, even in the presence of delay in finding the word, rules out tactile inability to recognize objects. This response would have to be compared to other language behavior observed during the interview. It points in the direction of mild aphasic difficulty. Only by ruling out possibility after possibility can the real disability become known.

A child who is unable to indicate which object he has been given but is able to name it the moment he is shown the same object probably demonstrates a delay, difficulty or disability in the recognition of objects by touch alone. Children who demonstrate this kind of impairment may feel even the round rubber ball with a tormented expression and finally guess "tomato, apple, roll," only to shout "a ball" the moment they are allowed to look. The scissor may be called "key, knife, cold thing, fork," and again be named completely correctly immediately after it has been seen. Difficulty in recognizing objects by touch appears to be related to impairment of tactile sensitivity, but not every child who has impairment of tactile sensitivity has difficulty in the manual recognition of objects. This is why you must inquire in every individual child for every one of these faculties. The opportunity to gain further insight into the language and speech area is an added advantage of such an exploration.

40. NUMBER SYMBOLS AND WORD PICTURES. (b) finding from memory.
MATERIALS: same as in standard item.

OTHERS: pegs and peg board; materials of item 9: cut-outs of circle, square and triangle; materials of item 28: similar cut-outs in three colors.

Modifications at this level are used mainly to explore laterally the *specific nature of a difficulty which appears disproportionate to the over-all level of functioning.* The modifications need not be presented to young children who have performed without marked difficulty on the earlier items testing form perception, spatial orientation, amount concepts and language comprehension but begin to demonstrate mild difficulties of a maturational nature on item 40. The children whose specific weak areas may possibly be pinpointed by the following modifications are primarily school-age children who have been referred for an Evaluation because they appear to perform with a marked disability in some phase of their schoolwork. Finding from memory is an essential ingredient of learning to read. Words which the child has learned to recognize in one connection must be spotted and recognized again in another connection. Such an ability is composed of several factors. No claim is made that the Educational Evaluation investigates reading disabilities. What is investigated is intactness of functioning in significant areas related to learning.

A preliminary review of the child's performance on the earlier items may show that you have already picked up a persistent delay or weakness in one or another area. Using the modifications will then serve to confirm or rule out such a hunch.

(a) Screen peg board from view and insert three rows of pegs in the upper part of the board horizontally. Going from left to right, insert only yellow pegs except for one red peg in the fourth hole of the first row, one red peg in the ninth hole of the second row and one red peg each in the second and sixth holes of the third row. Remove the screen and present the board, with the three filled rows now in the upper part of the board as seen by the child. If necessary, the board can be raised slightly on a slant if the child indicates the need for such an adjustment. Secure the child's attention and guiding your hand from his left to his right (Caution: this means from the right side as seen by you to the left) along the first, then second, then third row try to guide his eyes along in the conventional left-to-right progression of eye-sweep. Then direct him to look over the three rows in that way very carefully and try to find any pegs that look different than the others. If he hesitates, tell him to find any that do not look the same as most of the pegs look. The manually impaired child can eyepoint his responses. Observe, as you sit opposite the child, how his eyes function. Note whether both eyes seem to fuse. Note whether he scans the rows in the way you have indicated, returning to the beginning of the second and third rows when he has come to the end of a row, or whether his eyes begin to stray and he scans the next row from right to left. Give a second and third trial, increasing the difficulty by filling more rows and by inserting more red pegs in some and none in others, to keep him on the alert. His performance will give insight into the level of his ability to carry through under supervision, following verbally given instructions with added demonstration, a simple task of directed and controlled eye-sweep. Inability or inconsistency here would simultaneously influence the same activity when he is to follow reading material on the blackboard, an experience chart or in a primer.

(b) Remove peg board and pegs; screen table from view. Use the cut-out cards of item 9. Place on table a pattern of *five* cards: from left to right: square, circle, triangle, circle, square. Remove screen. Secure the child's attention. Tell him to look at the cards carefully because he will have to copy the pattern exactly as you have them now. Screen them again, remove them, and then give the child the *six* cards and ask him to make the same pattern you made. Even manually involved children can push these cards into position, or they may indicate which card comes next as you place them. (If the table top is light in color, you may need to use the dark fiber board or a dark paper to make the yellow cards stand out sufficiently.) Observe the child's performance. Note whether he starts at the left side of the row (seen from him) or whether he places two similar cards at each end and works toward the middle; whether he remembers the pattern well enough to ignore the extra triangle of the set or seems to wonder where it is to be placed because he has not been able to keep the number of cards in the original pattern in mind; note especially whether he appears to remind himself verbally of the order of the line-up, perhaps having memorized the names of the cards better than their visually perceived forms. Although these symbols have an element of greater abstractness than have letters of the alphabet, which to some children assume meaning and character very rapidly, failure on copying a five-part pattern of cut-outs two inches in diameter would point to a real difficulty in the recall of a simple pattern from memory.

(c) Screen the table from view; remove cards of item 9. Use cards of item 28. Place in one row from the child's left to his right: blue square, red circle, blue circle, red square. Remove screen and secure the child's attention. Direct him to look at the pattern very carefully and ask him to name each card for you (from left to right), so that he can remember what he saw. Screen the row from view again, but do not remove it. Ask the child to tell you from memory the order in which the cards are lined up from left to right. Observe whether or not he has difficulty in correctly recalling the three elements of this task: sequence, form, color. If he drops one of these elements, which one does he lose? He may recall the order and forms correctly but not the colors, or the colors and forms but not the order in which they were arranged, or the order and colors but not the forms. If he had difficulty, let him see the orignal pattern again and observe whether he recognizes his error or not. Repeat the same presentation, exchanging the two red cards for two yellow cards. Observe whether practice has helped to improved his recall or not. Then remove the cards of item 28 and use those of item 9 once more. Present in similar fashion only the four yellow cards, using the same pattern of square, circle, circle, square. Remind the child to remember their places, their names and the number of cards he sees. Screen them from view without removing them. Ask him to tell you how the cards were placed by naming them in order from his left to his right. Observe whether his recall of sequence and form improves when the third element, that of color, is eliminated; observe closely any hesitation in naming the cards (he can use any appropriate designation, such as circle and square, or ball and block, etc.) or a complete disability to name them from memory but an instant recognition when asked to copy the pattern from memory. Some children may trace the forms in the air or on the table in an effort to recall their names. Vary the demand of the task, by using either copying from memory or naming from memory if his difficulty points to one of these areas, until you feel you are coming closer to pinpointing the weak area. Since recall usually occurs through a combination of recall of a visual image and a verbally made mental note, his trouble may become clearer.

(d) Remove the cards of item 9; use the cards of item 40. Either put them in the stand or place them on the table before the child, depending on his preference; use five cards, arranged in this order: *cat—4—home—2—sat*. Secure the child's attention and encourage him to look at all of them closely, telling him that you will take one away and he must remember which one it was. After he indicates that he has seen it sufficiently, screen the stand from view, remove the card with 2 on it, push the other cards closer together to camouflage the empty space, and expose the stand and ask child to tell you which card is gone. If he can remember the location where one is missing but not what is on the missing card, screen the stand from view once more, leaving the cards in place, and line up before the child the six cards of the complete reserve set, not in the order in which the cards are in the stand, but at random, or even in a stack. Let him look over these cards and try to find the one that looks like the one you took away from the stand. If you observe that when he can see the possible choices, he has no difficulty in finding and recognizing the missing one, give a few more trials, asking for a different card each trial. Reduce the numbers of cards in the stand to four, then increase them to five, and reduce them again to four, or even three if his disability seems severe. Permit him to name each card of the displayed row and to trace each figure on it with his finger before screening it from view. Always ask first for recall of the verbal designation, then of the remembered form, and finally, if he still fails, give him the stack of reserve cards to look through for the one he is trying to recall. Real disabilities in immediate and delayed recall, in either the verbal area or the visual area or even in a combination of both, will be revealed by these modifications. Such disabilities may range from mild delay to a complete inability to recall the card, as if the missing card had been obliterated from his memory, until he can actually see it again. The problem must be described in the report for the teacher's benefit. It must also be brought to the attention of the neurologist who cares for the child.

(e) Exploring a different aspect, remove all cards, returning them to their correct envelopes, and present the pegs and peg board again. Move to the child's side of the table and seat yourself next to him so that he can see you perform exactly as he is to copy later. Insert one red peg in each corner of the board, starting at the upper left hand corner and going clockwise. Next insert one yellow peg in the second and ninth holes of the second row, in that order, and in the ninth and second holes of the ninth (one before last) row in that order (Fig. 4B). You now have two pegs at each one of the four corners, placed as though at the beginning of a diagonal line from each corner going toward the center, with the red pegs on the outer end. Encourage the child to look at the pegs, feel them, name them, and in every way possible to make a mental note of the exact placement of the pegs. Screen the peg board from view; remove the pegs and give him only these eight pegs. Do not confuse him by making him select the pegs from a number of mixed colors. Ask him to make the same pattern you had made. Help the manually involved child by placing the pegs he indicates in the holes he indicates by eye-pointing or gross motions or signs of assent and negation as you try to follow his instructions. Observe the child for his plan of attack; does he follow a consistent order of inserting the pegs? Does he succeed? Does he have to work hard or can he perform with ease? Does he change the position of the colors, such as placing the yellow pegs on the outside, the red ones on the inside? Or does he change the order of colors from corner to corner? Does his placing become less assured as he comes to the third and fourth corner? Are the first two or four pegs placed correctly, as if at the beginning of a diagonal direction, but the later ones next to each other in a vertical or horizontal direction? Is he aware of difficulties or not? At age seven and above, children are expected to be able to place the eight pegs, in this form of presentation, correctly from memory. In a nonretarded child of that age, difficulties would make one suspect some interference with space perception. If he has failed, therefore, reduce the number of elements necessary for success by one, i.e., use only red pegs (eight), give another demonstration, and observe his response. Can he succeed in correct placement when he does not have to think simultaneously of the two colors? If this is the case, perhaps the difficulty is not as much in spatial orientation as in adequacy of recall of details, such as colors, or in inattention to colors as an essential detail of the pattern. If he has failed again, reduce the number of elements by one more and insert four pegs only in the two upper corners in the same formation. If he can succeed in placing the two pegs in each corner in the correct alignment, perhaps his difficulty is in remembering the various aspects but not the correct direction of pegs in the corner placements. Observe once more, if you have missed it previously, the child's handedness, his preferred eye, his tendency of progression of eye-sweep, if any. Check his number concept. His basic weakness will frequently then become more clear.

(f) In order to pin down a possible difficulty based on a reversal of direction when called upon to copy from memory, place two red pegs in the left lower corner of the board, again in the beginning of a diagonal direction, and two yellow pegs in the same formation in the right upper corner of the board. Ask him to be sure and remember where the pegs are placed because he is to copy the pattern exactly. Screen the board from view, give him just the four pegs needed, and ask him to place them as you had them placed. The child who automatically inserts the pegs in the left upper and right lower corners, or use the yellow pegs on the left side of the board and the red pegs on the right side, reveals an interference in his functioning when called to copy a simple, related, juxtaposed pattern which seems to point to some difficulty in space perception.

These *subtle but real difficulties* found in some children with or without motor handicaps and with or without a diagnosis of brain lesion, although more frequently with such a diagnosis, *present learning difficulties in reading and writing. Frequently affected as well* is the child's ability in learning *mathematical concepts* with the ease with which they are acquired by non-handicapped children. As discussed in chapter 7, it will be more helpful to the teacher who has to plan the child's educational program if the examiner describes the performance of the particular child and substantiates the report with illustrations which the teacher can translate into the child's classroom performance and needs, rather than stating that the child has difficulty in visual perception and letting it go at that. Although much has to be learned about methods of retraining children with such an impairment, a first step is to pinpoint the nature of the difficulty and to rule out those difficulties which do not figure in the particular child's performance. By narrowing down the weak area or areas, it will sometimes be possible to train the child to utilize his stronger areas to complement his deficiencies to a degree.

MATERIALS NEEDED TO MODIFY STANDARD ITEMS
*(Those included in the Test kit are marked **.)*

**Doll with rooted hair, 10 to 12 inches. (Items 1, 2, 3, 4, 5, 9, 12, 24, 25.)
**Framed mirror, 10x12 inches. (Items 1 and 30.)
Red ring on string, 2 to 3 inches in diameter. (Items 1 and 14.)
Boxes, round and square, 3 to 4 inches in diameter. (Items 9, 10, 11.)
**Three pairs of small socks, red, yellow, blue. (Item 12.)
Nest of cubes. (Items 19 and 21.)
Drumsticks (2). (Items 24 and 25.)
Cake tin or drum or small tambourine (Items 24 and 25.)
**Mask. (Item 30.)
Small doll, 2½ to 3 inches, three-dimensional. (Item 30.)
Doll nursing bottle. (Item 30.)
Cardboard tube (as found inside of rolls of paper towels or wax paper). (Item 34.)
**Peg board and pegs. (Items 24, 25, 38, 40b.)
**Toy Santa Claus, 3 to 4 inches, unbreakable. (Item 35.)

RECOMMENDED AUXILIARY MATERIALS

Two boxes of cookies, round and square. (Items 9, 10, 11.)
Doll cooking pots, small, larger, round, oval. (Items 9, 10, 11.)
Adapted formboard (see Fig. 14). (Items 9, 10, 11.)
Small string of colored wooden beads (Items 9, 10, 11.)
Soap (Item 32); Chalk (Item 38); Pencils and paper.

RECOMMENDED "WARM-UP TOYS"

Spinning top.
Jack-in-the-Box music box.
Pull toy.

10. Recording the interview

The record of the interview should contain the specific responses to the items and a full report of observations in the areas outlined in chapter 6, which describes the nature of the structured interview. A sample record form is reproduced at the end of this chapter which illustrates the systematic survey the examiner is expected to have made during the conduct of the interview. It will serve to help the examiner recall his own mental notes on the child's performance and those aspects of the child's physical and sensory functioning which impressed him for one reason or another during the conduct of the interview.

Except for brief check notes, the recording of the interview should be done at leisure after the child has been dismissed. This method permits the examiner's full attention and energy to be devoted to conducting the interview. Recording of the results must not be postponed, however, and time should be scheduled for this purpose immediately after the interview while the picture of the child's behavior pattern is still fresh in the examiner's mind.

The specific responses to the items can be marked directly under the Arabic numerals which are on the right hand side of each item. A plus sign when the item has been responded to adequately, a minus sign when failed, an abbreviated "n.g." when an item was not given, and, finally, in the space to the right of the item, a comment on the level and nature of the response to any modification used will preserve the essentials of the child's performance. Such a record is necessary to any later re-evaluation by the same or another examiner. It further serves as a vivid picture of the level the child has been able to achieve in the various areas. On the basis of the child's levels in the different areas, the examiner will arrive at his estimate of the functional level; evenness or unevenness of development; and comparative adequacy, inadequacy or acceleration of the functional level when measured against the chronologic age level. Disproportionate levels of functioning will become obvious, and may lead the examiner to analyze carefully the many observations of behavior patterns which he recalls from the interview.

On the first pages of the record form, under the specific headings provided for the purpose, observations about the child's physical and sensory development and functioning, as they gradually take shape in the examiner's mind during the child's responses to the items and to the other opportunities created by the examiner, are entered in cable style. The child's behavior pattern is sketched briefly under the heading provided for these notes. The language behavior is described systematically in the space reserved for this area on the final page of the record form. The two main aspects, compre-

261

hension of language and the child's way of communicating with the environment, the examiner and perhaps the doll, are evaluated as they are described. The level of comprehension, as revealed by the child's responses to those items testing language comprehension, such as the first eight items and the story item and those items presupposing a four year level of comprehension for the understanding of verbal directions (items 15, 16, 32 and 38), is evaluated in retrospect. The level of communication is considered carefully, both of a speaking child and of a nonspeaking one. This area was described in full in chapter 7 in the fictional interview with a child with cerebral palsy, and the examiner is referred to that description if a child's way of communicating leaves him puzzled.

The examiner will discover that the interviews, since they always follow the same sequence with every child, will eventually unwind themselves before his inner eye like the reels of a film. The particular characteristics of a child will stand out against the background of the sequence. Recording the results of the interview then becomes a crystallized and deeper evaluation of the whole sum of accumulated findings, contradictions, and meaningfully related manifestations. The examiner will find himself flipping the pages of the record-form backwards and forwards in order to enter not only the result of his educated observations but also the considered recognition of the meaning of those observations, as they become illuminated in this leisurely recreation of the child's performance. Interpretation of the findings will be discussed in the next chapter.

EDUCATIONAL EVALUATION OF PRESCHOOL CHILDREN.
RECORDING FORM

Name: Date seen:

Birthdate:

Chronologic age: Examiner:

Presenting Problem:

I. GENERAL STATEMENT ABOUT TESTABILITY AND NECESSARY MODIFICATIONS

II. PHYSICAL DEVELOPMENT:

1. GENERAL:

a. Balance and Locomotion:

b. Upper Extremities:

c. Self-help Functions:

Feeding:

Dressing:

Toilet Care:

2. BODY CONCEPT:

a. General Orientation:

b. Graphic Expression:

3. SENSORY INTACTNESS:

a. Vision

Eye Motion:

Visual Functioning:

b. Hearing Behavior:

c. Tactile Sensitivity:

III. OBSERVATION OF BEHAVIOR PATTERN DURING THE INTERVIEW:

IV. SPECIFIC RESPONSES TO ITEMS:

Present to ages:	No. of Item:	Description of Item:	Age level expected:
II-0 to VI	1.	Recognition of objects, when named	2-0 to 2-6
II-0 to VI	2.	Recognition of objects, described in terms of use	2-6 to 3-0
II-0 to VI	3.	Recognition of sizes, concrete	2-6 to 3-0
II-0 to VI	4.	Recognition of objects in image, when named	2-0 to 3-0
II-6 to VI	5.	Recognition of objects in image, described in terms of use	2-6 to 3-0
III-6 to VI	6.	Recall of missing picture from memory	4-0 to 5-0
II-6 to III only	7.	Recognition of action in image	2-6 to 3-0
III-0 to VI	8.	Recognition of (action in image and) time of day	3-0 to 3-6
II-0 to III only	9.	Recognition of form and symbol, cut-outs, matching	2-0 to 2-6
II-6 to VI	10.	Recognition of form and symbol on square cards a) matching	2-6 to 3-6
III-6 to VI	11.	b) finding from memory	4-0 to 4-3

Present to ages:	No. of Item:	Description of Item:	Age level expected:
II-6 to VI	12.	Discrimination of colors a) matching	3-0 and up
III-6 to VI	13.	b) when named	4-0 and up
II-0 to VI Not to be omitted	14.	Sound blocks and other sound items a) hearing	2-0 and up
III-6 to VI	15.	b) matching	4-0 and up
IV-0 to VI	16.	c) grading	4-6 and up
II-0 to VI (see 36)	17.	Spatial relationship a) two halves of circle	2-6 and up
II-6 to IV only	18.	Recognition of sizes in outline circles a) big and little	3-0 to 4-0
IV-0 to V-6 only (see 21)	19.	b) grading	5-0 to 6-0
IV-6 to VI	20.	Discrimination of colors c) grading shades within a color	5-6 and up
V-6 and up	21.	Sizes in circles: c) insight into principle of ascending serial grading	6-0 and up
II-0 to VI Not to be omitted	22.	Pellets and bottle a) dropping in bottle	2-0 and up
II-0 to VI Not to be omitted		b) finding pellet on floor	2-6 and up

Present to ages:	No. of Item:	Description of Item:	Age level expected:
II-0 to VI Not to be omitted	23.	Push button table bell and music box	2-0 and up
II-6 to IV only	24.	Amount concept (milk bottles) a) "one only" and "more than one"	3-0 to 3-9
III-6 to VI	25.	Amount concept (milk bottles) b) separating a stated number of objects from a larger group	4-0 to 6-0
V-6 to VI	26.	Amount recognition (pennies) c) matching	6-0 and up
V-6 and up	27.	Familiarity with non-numerical mathematical terms (more-less few-many pair across morning-afternoon)	6-0 and up
III-0 to VI	28.	Multiple choice color—form a) sorting	3-6 and up
IV-6 to VI	29.	b) shifting	5-0 and up
II-0 to III-6 only	30.	Recognition of wedgies and miniature toys	2-6 to 2-9
IV-0 to VI	31.	Story comprehension	4-6 and up

Present to ages:	No. of Item:	Description of Item:	Age level expected:
IV-0 to VI	32.	Understanding of relationship of incomplete parts of a whole to each other	4-0 and up
II-0 to VI Not to be omitted	33.	Flashlight and sparkler toy	2-0 and up
II-0 to VI Not to be omitted	34.	Preferred eye (tube)	2-6 and up
III-0 and up	35.	Orientation in time: seasons	4-0 and up
III-6 and up (see 17)	36.	Spatial relationships b) two halves of square	4-0 and up
IV-6 and up		c) four quarters of circle	5-0 and up
IV-6 and up	37.	Amount recognition in dot configurations a) matching	5-0 and up
VI-0 and up		b) finding from memory	6-0 and up
VI-6 and up		c) finding matching cards in dissimilar configurations	6-9 and up
IV-0 and up	38.	Tactile sensitivity	4-0 and up
III-6 and up	39.	Recognition of symbols, black outline a) matching	4-0 and up
IV-6 and up		b) finding from memory	4-6 and up
V-9 and up	40.	Number symbols and word-pictures a) matching	5-9 and up
VI-6 and up		b) finding from memory	6-6 and up

V. LANGUAGE BEHAVIOR:

    1. COMMUNICATION PATTERN AT HOME:

    2. COMPREHENSION OF LANGUAGE:

    3. COMMUNICATION:

VI. CONCLUSIONS:

VII. RECOMMENDATIONS:

11. *Interpretation of the findings*

The interpretation of the findings is an ongoing process in an Educational Evaluation. The examiner learns to become and remain cognizant of the areas probed by any particular item, the lists offered under the heading of each item being a reminder of those areas needed for adequate response to the item. Thus, as he conducts the interview, the examiner is engaged in a constant process of evaluation and re-evaluation, cross-checking, and confirming and ruling out tentative leads and trends. At the conclusion of a structured interview of such a flexible character, the pattern of the child's functioning in pertinent areas has become revealed. Intactness or impairment of functioning in these areas has manifested itself in response to items eliciting such functioning.

What remains to be done is to summarize the findings and explain their meaning. The levels achieved in specific responses to items, or to modifications, as recorded in the recording form, are examined. They show the level of functioning. The adequacy, acceleration, or inadequacy and degree of inadequacy of this functional level in relation to the chronologic age of the child gives the examiner information about the comparative status of the child as measured against the expected level for his age-group.

What is more important than such a comparison is an understanding of the quality of functioning and an answer to the question of whether functioning is intact or not. The Evaluation gives insight into the levels of functioning in each of the areas tested, and if functioning is found to be impaired, further inquiry attempts and frequently succeeds in sounding out the area. It is then demonstrated whether or not the child can function at all in an impaired area, and, if he can function, in which way he functions. Thus, the cause of a poor performance often becomes clarified. Similarly, abilities, assets and probable potential are demonstrated. The opportunity to observe not only the result of a performance in response to an item but the how of the performance, the way the child mobilizes assets and abilities to perform, even in a weak area, gives the examiner data on which to base his conclusions about potential functioning. Specific teaching techniques can then sometimes be suggested which may serve to accommodate, circumvent or retrain a weak area.

The relationship of sensory functioning to intellectual performance, of physical impairment to classroom functioning, of emotional handicaps to adequacy of adjustment can become known by the nature of the responses. Conclusions summarizing the findings and pointing out demonstrated or suspected difficulties and their nature and implication for development must be conveyed to those in charge of the educational planning for the child.

An inventory of the developmental levels in the areas investigated, whether there is evenness of development or not, will give the child's teacher a true picture of his pattern and a basis for her educational approach to the child.

A description of the language and communication behavior of the child with poor or almost no speech, based upon intensive contact with the child during the interview, frequently serves to facilitate communication by and with him in his home environment.

While an Educational Evaluation produces a wealth of information, and while it aims to and succeeds in serving to insure more appropriate educational and training programming for the individual child, it must remain an individual evaluation. It would be a misconstruction of the aim of this procedure and be entirely meaningless to attempt to average the findings in the various areas or to compute a numerical quotient. Its value consists in the thoroughness of the inquiry into functional intactness and in the descriptive report based upon such an inquiry.

12. Reporting the findings

The reporting blank at the end of this chapter provides space for the inventory of developmental levels, for a condensed description of the physical functioning, and the levels achieved in the areas of self-help functions, and for a brief description of the sensory equipment as observed in functional use. A description of the language behavior is included. Another heading provides for the description of poor performance and causes of such performance, as well as for a statement of abilities, assets and probable potential. Based upon the findings the conclusions are summarized and recommendations are suggested.

Constant reference has been made throughout the text to the obligation to make the findings available in a form which will render them directly helpful to those who can utilize them for the benefit of the child, in school, in rehabilitation programs, and in the family setting. Fndings which will be useful to the medical specialists concerned with the child's care or which suggest a need for medical checking have been pointed out in the text, with the recommendation that such findings be brought to the attention of the responsible physician.

An Educational Evaluation is not an end in itself. The most searching and productive Evaluation of any child is only as useful as skilled reporting can make it.

EDUCATIONAL EVALUATION REPORT FORM.

Inventory of Developmental Levels.

Name:

Birth date: Date:

Chronological Age: Examiner:

Presenting Problem:

    I. PHYSICAL DEVELOPMENT:

        1. GENERAL:

           a. *Balance and Locomotion:*

           b. *Upper Extremities:*

           c. *Self-Help Functions:*
             Feeding:

             Dressing:

             Toilet Care:

2. SENSORY INTACTNESS:

a. *Vision:*

Eye Motion:

Visual Acuity Observable in Functional Use:

b. *Hearing:*

c. *Tactile Sensitivity:*

3. BODY IMAGE:

GENERAL ORIENTATION, GRAPHIC EXPRESSION, REACTION TO DOLLS.

II. INTELLECTUAL DEVELOPMENT:

1. LANGUAGE BEHAVIOR:

REPORTED DEVELOPMENT AND COMMUNICATION PATTERN AT HOME:

a. *Comprehension:*

b. *Communication:*

2. LEVELS OF FUNCTIONING:

Possible Causes and Implications of Poor Performance:

Assets and Possible Potentials:

III.   OBSERVATION OF BEHAVIOR DURING THE INTERVIEW:

IV. Conclusions:

V. Recommendations:

Bibliography

BENDA, C. E.: Developmental Disorders of Mentation and Cerebral Palsies. New York, Grune & Stratton, 1952.

——: Mongolism and Cretinism. New York, Grune & Stratton, 1949.

BIBER, B.: Children's drawings from lines to pictures. New York, The Cooperating School Pamphlets, No. 6. No date given.

BIRCH, H. G. and LEE, J.: Cortical inhibition in expressive aphasia. Arch. Neurol. & Psychiat. 74:514, 1955.

BLUM, L. H., BURGEMEISTER, B. and LORGE, I.: Columbia Mental Maturity Scale, New York, World Book Co., 1953.

BUEHLER, C.: The First Year of Life. New York, John Day Co., 1930.

—— and HETZER, H.: Kleinkinder Tests. Leipzig, Barth, 1932.

——: Testing Children's Development from Birth to School Age. New York, Farrar & Rinehart, 1935.

BURT, C.: The Backward Child. London, London University Press, 1937.

CARLSON, E. R.: Born That Way. New York, John Day Co., 1941.

CASS, M. T.: Speech Habilitation in Cerebral Palsy. New York, Columbia University Press, 1951.

CATTELL, P.: The Measurement of Intelligence of Infants and Young Children. New York, Psychological Corporation, 1940.

CLARK, J. P.: Testing hearing of children with noise makers—a myth. J. Except. Children. 22:326, 1956.

COOPER, W.: Problem of social and emotional adjustment in cerebral palsy. Am. Acad. Orthop. Surgeons, Lect. 11:283, 1954.

CRUICKSHANK, W. and RAUS, G.: Cerebral Palsy, Its Individual and Community Problems. New York, Syracuse University Press, 1955.

DOLL, E. A., PHELPS, W. M. and MELCHER, R. T.: Mental Deficiency Due To Birth Injuries. New York, Macmillan, 1932.

——: Mental evaluation of children with expressive handicaps. Reprinted from Am. J. Orthopsychiat. No date given.

——: Neurophrenia. Am. J. Psychiat. 108:50, 1951.

——: The Vineland Social Maturity Scale. Vineland, N. J., Publication of the Training School, 1941.

DRISCOLL, G.: How to Study the Behavior of Children. New York, Columbia University, Teachers College. Bureau of Publications, 1941.

DUNSDON, M. I.: The Educability of Cerebral Palsied Children. London, Newnes, 1952.

EISENSON, J.: Examining for Aphasia, A Manual. New York, The Psychological Corporation, 1954.

FEATHERSTONE, W. B.: Teaching the Slow Learner. New York, Columbia University, Teachers College. Bureau of Publications, 1941.

FOURACRE, M. H.: Realistic educational planning for children with cerebral palsy. Pamphlets 1–7, New York, United Cerebral Palsy Associations, Inc., 1952.

FRAMPTON, M. E. and GALL, E. D.: Special Education for the Exceptional. Boston, Porter Sargent, 1955.

GANS, R.: Guiding Children's Reading through Experiences. New York, Columbia University, Teachers College. Bureau of Publications, 1941.

GESELL, A.: Infancy and Human Growth. New York, Macmillan, 1928.

—— et al.: The First Five Years of Life, New York, Harper, 1940.

—— et al.: An Atlas of Infant Behavior. Vols. I & II. New Haven, Yale University Press, 1934.

—— and ILG, F. L.: The Child From Five to Ten. New York, Harper, 1946.

GOLDBERG, I. I.: Current status of education and training for trainable mentally retarded children. J. Except. Children. 24:146, 1957.

GOLDSTEIN, K.: Language and Language Disturbances. New York, Grune & Stratton, 1948.

GOODENOUGH, F. L.: Measurement of Intelligence by Drawings. Yonkers, N. Y., World Book Co., 1926.

GRIFFITHS, R.: The Abilities of Babies, New York, McGraw-Hill, 1954.

HAEUSSERMANN, E.: Fundamental problems in the formulation of the reading program for children with cerebral palsy. Cerebral Palsy Review 17:92, 1956.

HEILMANN, E.: Appraisal of the abilities of the cerebral palsy child. Am. J. Ment. Deficiency. 53:606, 1949.

Helping the Physically Limited Child. New York, Board of Education, Curriculum Bulletin Series No. 7, 1952/1953.

HILL, A. S.: Cerebral palsy, mental deficiency and terminology. Am. J. Ment. Deficiency. 59:587, 1955.

HOPKINS, T. W., COLTON, V. C. and BICE, H. V.: Evaluation and Education of the Cerebral Palsied Child. Washington, D. C., I.C.E.C., 1956.

HUGHES, J. G.: Early detection of cerebral injury. J. Pediat. 40:606, 1952.

ISAACS, S.: Intellectual Growth in Young Children. London, Routledge & Kegan Paul, Ltd., 1950.

ITARD, J.: The Wild Boy of Aveyron. New York, Century, 1932.

JERSILD, A. T.: Child Psychology. New York, Prentice-Hall, 1941.

JOHNSON, G. O., NEELY, J. H. and ALLING, R. C.: A comparison of the 1937 revision of the Stanford-Binet (Form L) and the Columbia Scale of Mental Maturity. J. Except. Children. 22:155, 1956.

KATZ, E.: The "pointing modification" of the Revised Stanford-Binet. Am. J. Ment. Deficiency. 62:698, 1958.

KIRK, S. A. and JOHNSON, G. O.: Educating the Retarded Child. Boston, Houghton Mifflin Co., 1951.

LAMM, S. and FISCH, M. L.: Intellectual development of the cerebral palsied child as a factor in the therapeutic progress. Am. J. Ment. Deficiency. 59:452, 1955.

LORD, E. E.: A Study of the Mental Development of Children with Lesions in the Central Nervous System. New Haven, Psycho-Clinic, 1929.

——: Children Handicapped by Cerebral Palsy. New York, Milford, 1937.

McCARTHY, D. A.: The Language Development of the Preschool Child. Minnesota, University of Minneapolis Press, 1930.

The Mentally Subnormal Child. Geneva, W.H.O. Technical Report Series, 1954.

MEYER, E. and CROTHERS, B.: Psychological and physical evaluation of patients with cerebral palsy studied for periods of ten years or more. Am. J. Phys. Med. *32*:153, 1953.

MICHAL-SMITH, H.: The Mentally Retarded Patient. New York, Grune & Stratton, 1956.

MYKLEBUST, H. R.: Auditory Disorders in Children. New York, Grune & Stratton, 1954.

O'BRIEN, V.: Treatment of children with cerebral palsy. New York J. Med. *45*:1546, 1945.

ORTON, S. T.: Reading, Writing and Speech Problems in Children, New York, Norton, 1937.

PEIPER, A.: Die Eigenart der kindlichen Hirntätigkeit. Leipzig, VEB. Georg Thieme, 1956.

PHELPS, W. M.: The management of cerebral palsies. J.A.M.A. *117*:1621, 1941.

PIAGET, J.: The Language and Thought of the Child. New York, Meridan Books, 1955.

———: The Origin of Intelligence in Children. New York, Internat. Univ. Press, 1952.

PREYER, W.: Mental Development of the Child (Brown, H. W., Transl.) New York, Appleton, 1893.

ROGER, G. and THOMAS, L.: New Pathways for Children with Cerebral Palsy. New York, Macmillan Co., 1935.

ROSENZWEIG, L. E.: Report of a school program for trainable mentally retarded children. A. J. Ment. Deficiency. *59*:181, 1954.

SCHROEDER, P. L.: Behavior difficulties in children associated with the results of birth-trauma. J.A.M.A. *92*:100, 1929.

STRAUSS, and KEPHART, N. C.: Psychopathology and Education of the Brain-Injured Child. New York, Grune & Stratton, 1955.

——— and LEHTINEN, L.: Psychopathology and Education of the Brain-Injured Child. New York, Grune & Stratton, 1947.

——— and WERNER, H.: Comparative psychopathology of the brain-injured child and the traumatic brain-injured adult. Am. J. Psychiat. *99*:835, 1943.

——— and WERNER, H.: The mental organization of the brain-injured mentally defective child. Am. J. of Psychiat. *97*:1194, 1941.

STROTHERS, C. R.: Evaluating intelligence of children handicapped by cerebral palsy. The Crippled Child. *23*:82, 1945.

TERMAN, L. M. and MERRILL, M. A.: Measuring Intelligence, Revised Stanford-Binet Tests. Boston, Houghton Mifflin Co., 1937.

WERNER, H.: Perception of spatial relationship in mentally deficient children. J. Gen. Psychol. *57*:93, 1940.

WERNER, H. and STRAUSS, A. A.: Causal Factors in low performance. Am. J. Ment. Deficiency. *45*:213, 1940.

———: Development of visuo-motor performance on the Marble-Board Test in mentally retarded children. J. Gen. Psychol. *64*:269, 1944.

——— and STRAUSS, A. A.: Disorders of conceptual thinking in the brain-injured child. J. Nerv. & Ment. Dis. *96*: 1942.

——— and STRAUSS, A. A.: Pathology of figure background relation in the child. J. Abnorm. & Social. Psychol. *36*: 1941.

—— and STRAUSS, A. A.: Types of Visuo-motor activity in their relation to low and high performance ages. Proc. Am. Assoc. Ment. Deficiency. *44:* 1939.

WEST, R.: The Rehabilitation of Speech. New York, Harper, 1937.

WISHIK, S. M. and MACKIE, R. P.: Adjustment of the school program for the physically handicapped child. Am. J. of Public Health. *39:*8, 1949.

WORTIS, H. and COOPER, W.: The life experience of persons with cerebral palsy. Am. J. Phys. Med. *36:*4, 1957.

WORTIS, J.: A note on the concept of the brain-injured child. Am. J. Ment. Deficiency. *61:*204, 1956.

Index

281